SECOND EDITION

Language and Literacy Development in Children Who Are Deaf

Barbara R. Schirmer

Kent State University

Allyn and Bacon

Boston ▪ London ▪ Toronto ▪ Sydney ▪ Tokyo ▪ Singapore

Executive Editor: *Stephen D. Dragin*
Marketing Manager: *Richard Muhr*
Editorial-Production Service: *Omegatype Typography, Inc.*
Composition and Prepress Buyer: *Linda Cox*
Manufacturing Buyer: *David Repetto*
Cover Administrator: *Jenny Hart*
Electronic Composition: *Omegatype Typography, Inc.*

Library of Congress Cataloging-in-Publication Data

Schirmer, Barbara R.
    Language and literacy development in children who are deaf / Barbara R. Schirmer.—
2nd ed.
        p.   cm.
    Includes bibliographical references and index.
    ISBN 0-205-31493-7
    1. Deaf—Means of communication—Study and teaching (Elementary).   2. Deaf
children—Language.   3. Deaf—Education.   I. Title.
    HV2443.S33   2000
    305.9'08162—dc21   99-049357

Printed in the United States of America

10   9   8   7   6   5   4   3   2   1   04   03   02   01   00   99

Photo Credits: Will Faller, pp. 2, 98, 218; Will Hart, pp. 46, 132, 180, 200

To my children—
Alison, who read the complete first edition
Todd, who updated the references for the second edition

CONTENTS

PREFACE

Like the first edition, the purpose of this text is to provide teachers with comprehensive information regarding how children who are deaf learn to use language in face-to-face communication, reading, and writing. The audience is preservice and inservice teachers who want to know how to create classroom environments that foster the development of language and literacy in children who are deaf.

Throughout the text, I have tried to maintain a balance between theory and practice because I believe that outstanding teachers of deaf children understand the theoretical foundations on which their teaching strategies are built. Trends in education come and go. The best teachers examine a trend in light of what they know about the processes involved in learning language for deaf children, using what is valuable and ignoring what is unproductive.

The theories, models, and strategies discussed in this text are those that are currently relevant to teachers of children who are deaf. To this end, I have drawn on the literature in deafness, special education, early childhood, linguistics, bilingual education, psychology, child language, reading, cognition, research in education, educational technology, communication disorders, child development, children's literature, curriculum, and language arts.

Chapter 1 focuses on the acquisition of linguistic knowledge in the child who is deaf, the application of this information to language goals for classroom instruction, the role of language assessment, methods and techniques for using informal approaches and formal tests to assess the language of children who are deaf, and the classroom teacher's use of assessment information to develop individualized language goals for each child.

Chapter 2 presents language as a curricular base on which the full school day is organized. It explains how to embed each deaf child's language goals into an array of daily learning experiences. The central role of conversation, teaching models and strategies, interdisciplinary curriculums, and the use of technology are all described and used to illustrate how the teacher can encourage language growth in children who are deaf. A final feature of this chapter is a discussion of bilingual ASL–English programs for deaf children.

In Chapter 3, balanced literacy is defined, and the rationale for using balanced literacy principles to teach children who are deaf is discussed. This chapter also includes a thorough description of current views of reading and writing development, the kinds of reading materials that can enhance the development of literacy in youngsters who are deaf, and the instructional implications of the relationship between language, literacy, and cognitive development.

Chapter 4 builds on the theoretical framework of literacy development that was presented in Chapter 3. In this chapter, theory is linked with practice through descriptions of teaching models and strategies that form the core of a literacy program for children who are deaf. Included are activities that foster emergent literacy, that promote growth in reading and writing, and that enable children who are deaf to become autonomous readers and writers.

Chapter 5 presents strategies for helping deaf children to read and write in the content areas. This chapter includes descriptions of reading models and strategies that enable deaf students to read expository material and use what they have read as they think and learn.

Chapter 6 focuses on assessment in reading and writing. It begins with a description of the principles that should guide teachers in monitoring the literacy development of children who are deaf. The assessment process is described in detail, and both informal approaches and standardized test information are explained.

In Chapter 7, the role of parents in the language and literacy development of their children is highlighted, and the importance of family–school partnerships is discussed.

Since writing the first edition, I have left Lewis & Clark College, where I spent twelve years. In my new home at Kent State University, the dynamic group of faculty members in the College and Graduate School of Education, and most especially the faculty in the Department of Educational Foundations and Special Services, have had an energizing influence on me. I particularly want to thank Harold Johnson, who told me that the college was looking for a new department chair and asked if I would be interested in applying.

I also want to thank Pamela Luft, who provided an insightful and careful review of this second edition. Pam's expertise on deafness, language, and literacy as well as her wealth of experience in teaching deaf children and teachers-in-training enabled her to offer me the most invaluable advice about every aspect of the book. It was truly my lucky day when she and Harold Johnson became my colleagues at Kent State.

I am grateful to my editor, Stephen Dragin, who guided me as I created this second edition, and his assistant, Bridget McSweeney.

My graduate assistant, Christine Civiletto, offered endless hours of assistance. We both agreed as we put the final touches on the manuscript, that if there are two other people as compulsive as we are, we do not know who they are. Chrissy is already a wonderful researcher, and she will make an extraordinary psychologist.

During the years I have been involved in teacher education, the lines between student and colleague have thankfully blurred; in fact, many of my former students are my most treasured colleagues and friends. Because their ideas appear in this book, I want to thank just a few of you—Valorie Burke (Hutchinson School District, MN), Sister Mary Griffin (Bishop Ryan School for the Deaf, PA), Lynn Woolsey (The Ohio State University), Jill Bailey (Northwest Regional Program, OR), Lindy Twiss (Tumwater School District, WA). Many of my friends entered my life as colleagues and stayed as friends; thank you for all you have contributed to my continued understanding of language, literacy, and deafness—Judy Parmelee (Utah School for the Deaf Extension Consultant Division), Wendy Bond (Columbia Regional Program, OR), Shirin Antia (University of Arizona), George Shellem (New Jersey Department of Education), Barbara Strassman (The College of New Jersey), Cheri Williams (University of Cincinnati), Kathy Kreimeyer (Arizona School for the Deaf), and Marti Gaustad (Bowling Green State University). Wherever I travel, I seem to have a welcome mat, great conversation, and many laughs.

There are five women in my life who seem to defy neat categorization—friend, colleague, daughter, mom, grandmother, mentor, supporter, chastiser, caretaker. Three have the name, or a derivation of the name, Frieda. My grandmother, Frieda Schiller, became deaf as a young child. She yelled at me when I was naughty, looked after me while my mom worked, and played cards with me when no one came outside to play even though we were never able to communicate in the same language. My mentor, Dr. Frieda Hammermeister, was my advisor and major professor at the University of Pittsburgh, and she helped me to understand the deafness that my grandmother had lived with all her life. My daughter, Alison Fredda Schirmer, was named after my grandmother, and she is the spirit of intelligence and independence that my grandmother so desperately wanted to be. My mom, Bella Edberg, grew up as the only daughter in a family with a deaf mother, so she took on enormous family responsibility. She helped me to fly in directions she could only dream about, and I thank her for her selflessness. My friend, Barbara McCormick, entered my life as my secretary and she stayed on as my extra mom. She toiled on the first edition, and I continually see her in this edition. Barb's house is my home away from home.

I certainly do not want to leave out the special men in my life. I miss my dad, Jack Edberg, every day of my life. Whoever wrote the words to the song about the wind beneath my wings must have been thinking about my dad. My son, Todd, was named after a young deaf boy I taught in my first teaching position at the West Virginia School for the Deaf and was the first child to call me mom. Todd's vulnerability and courage are so like his namesake's. While others have thrown me to the proverbial sky, my husband, Jack, has always been standing on earth making sure that I got caught safely each time I came close to the ground. Maybe there's a song for him, too.

1 Language Development and the Goals of Language Instruction

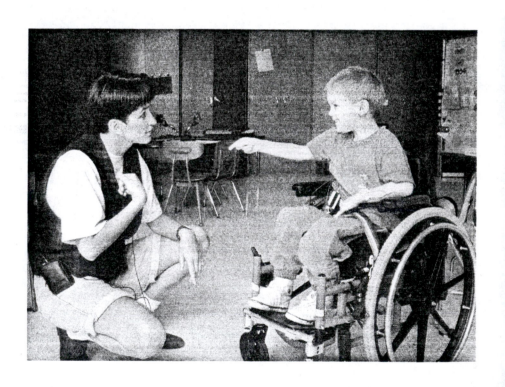

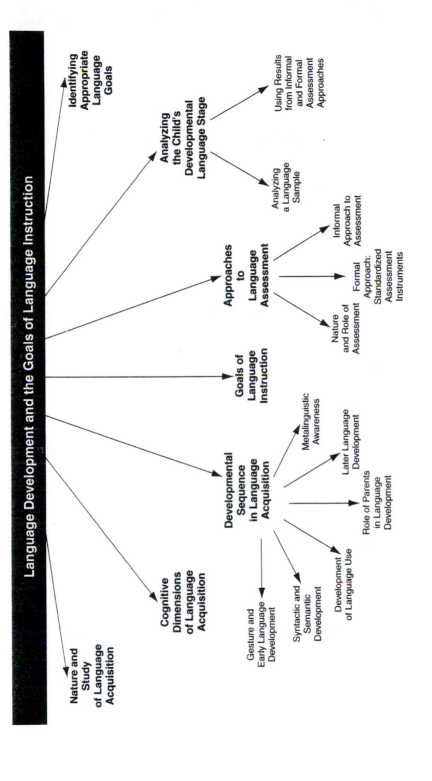

Language Development and the Goals of Language Instruction

- Nature and Study of Language Acquisition
- Cognitive Dimensions of Language Acquisition
- Developmental Sequence in Language Acquisition
  - Gesture and Early Language Development
  - Syntactic and Semantic Development
  - Development of Language Use
  - Role of Parents in Language Development
  - Later Language Development
  - Metalinguistic Awareness
- Goals of Language Instruction
- Approaches to Language Assessment
  - Nature and Role of Assessment
  - Formal Approach: Standardized Assessment Instruments
  - Informal Approach to Assessment
- Analyzing the Child's Developmental Language Stage
  - Analyzing a Language Sample
  - Using Results from Informal and Formal Assessment Approaches
- Identifying Appropriate Language Goals

For many years, descriptions of child language acquisition consisted of lists of developmental milestones. These were basically simple catalogues of sequential steps observed in the developing child's language. For example, Menyuk (1971) described the sequence of development from babbling during the first year of life to single-word utterances to short sentences by the third year. Another example is the 1970 Denver Developmental Screening Test, which used developmental milestones as an evaluation technique.

Since Roger Brown's seminal study (1973) of Adam, Eve, and Sarah, child language research has demonstrated a complexity of the language acquisition process not evident in these earlier descriptions. More important for teachers of youngsters who are deaf, we can learn to use information from this body of research to improve the language learning opportunities for the children in our classrooms.

In this chapter, I will begin by discussing what is currently known about the acquisition of linguistic knowledge in all children, and specifically in the child who is deaf, and what this information means for our goals for classroom instruction. I will then discuss the role of language assessment and describe methods and techniques for using informal approaches as well as formal instruments. Finally, I will explain how the classroom, itinerant, or consultant teacher or language specialist can use assessment information to determine each child's language development stage and to identify appropriate individualized language goals for children who are deaf.

Nature and Study of Language Acquisition

The first known study of child language acquisition was conducted by Psammetichus I, a pharoah of ancient Egypt. According to Herodotus, a Greek historian who lived at the time of Sophocles, Psammetichus I wanted to prove that the Egyptians were the original human race by showing that the Egyptian language was the natural language of humans. He gave two infants to a shepherd to raise, ordered the shepherd to use no speech with the children, and told the shepherd to notice the children's first spoken words. Psammetichus I found that the children did not spontaneously use the Egyptian language, and he unhappily concluded that Egyptians were not the original human race.

Through the centuries, individuals continued to be intrigued by child language acquisition, but systematic study did not begin until the late nineteenth century. Between the 1870s and 1920s, child language was usually studied from the perspective of parents, and data were recorded in the form of diaries. Indeed, most of these studies were conducted by psychologists, and the diaries they kept were observations of their own children. Ingram (1989) noted that interest in child language acquisition at this time was part of a larger interest by psychologists in child development.

Between the 1920s and 1950s, while diary studies continued, studies designed to sample language behaviors became very popular. These studies were strongly influenced by the behavioral theory of learning. Language studies based on behavioral theory had several characteristics in common. The researchers who conducted these studies examined the language of relatively large numbers of children who were chosen in a way that they could be considered representative of even larger numbers of whole populations. These researchers also chose particular language behaviors to test or observe and the procedures they used were precise and consistently followed. The researchers of this era were particularly interested in the average sentence length of children at different age levels, acquisition of speech sounds, and vocabulary development.

From the late 1950s through the 1960s, language acquisition studies using longitudinal language sampling procedures came into prominence. In these studies, language samples of a small number of children were systematically collected over a long period of time. Most of these studies were strongly influenced by the transformational theory of grammar, so they focused on the child's acquisition of syntax.

In the 1970s, researchers shifted their attention away from syntax and toward semantics. In the 1980s, there was again a shift as attention was directed to the study of language use, particularly the development of pragmatics and conversation. In the 1970s and 1980s, an explosion of research interest into the relationship between language acquisition and the child's linguistic and nonlinguistic environment also occurred.

In addition to these new research interests, studies of American Sign Language (ASL) were conducted. Before this time, people assumed that sign language was a visual–gestural representation of English, yet researchers found that ASL had a rule structure distinct from English that represented a linguistically rich language (e.g., Klima & Bellugi, 1979; Stokoe, 1971). Early studies by Stokoe in the 1960s were largely ignored until the 1970s when English sign systems were being developed, and many individuals consider his early work to be the foundation of subsequent ASL research.

From the 1990s to the present, language acquisition study has encompassed a broad range of topics. Some of the areas of study that continue to have important implications for teachers of children who are deaf are investigations into adult–child interaction, second language learning, ASL, language and cognition, metalinguistics, language and literacy, and development of language throughout the life span.

We know a great deal more today about child language acquisition than the ancient Egyptians did. Each study has added new information to a constantly increasing body of knowledge. It is my intent in this chapter to use information from this rich body of knowledge that I believe is most pertinent to the teachers of youngsters who are deaf and apply it in a way that will enable teachers to develop a multifaceted picture of the language development abilities of each deaf child.

I want to emphasize that much of the information in this chapter comes from research in linguistics and child language acquisition. Some studies have been conducted with children who are deaf, and I have tried to cite each of these whenever appropriate. However, it is undeniable that most of the research on this topic has been focused on children who can hear. I include this body of research because it tells us a great deal about the process of language development, and as teachers of children who are deaf, we can rely on our experiences and intuitions when applying this body of knowledge to the children we are teaching.

Cognitive Dimensions of Language Acquisition

Considerable discussion has taken place in the literature regarding the relationship between language acquisition and cognitive development. A thorough explanation of the issues involved in this discussion would go considerably beyond the purview of this chapter. Instead of giving equal emphasis to competing theories, I have decided to present a brief conceptualization of the cognitive dimensions of language acquisition.

According to Reed (1996), cognition is defined as the acquisition and use of knowledge. With this definition in mind, the relationship between cognition and language acquisition can be seen as an interdependent one. In this view, language acquisition occurs as a result of the interaction between the child's innate cognitive abilities, cognitive strategies, and conceptual knowledge.

This interaction can be illustrated with the analogy of the growth of a plant. The seed of the plant is the child's innate cognitive abilities. It provides the child with the cognitive capacity to make sense of linguistic information. The root system is the child's developing conceptual knowledge as he or she interacts with the environment. This root system, or conceptual knowledge, supports language acquisition and grows as the child's language develops. The plant seeks out nourishment by sending its roots in the direction of water and its leaves in the direction of light. These movements by the plant can be likened to the child's own cognitive strategies that nourish language acquisition such as focusing, analyzing, organizing, classifying, and problem solving.

Rice and Kemper (1984) described language growth in the following way:

> The child draws upon the conceptual roots and the innate kernel to establish the first green shoots of language. As the roots develop, they provide further nourishment to strengthen the delicate young conceptual roots. In turn, as the roots firm and expand, they provide support and nourishment for the developing plant. The initial kernel continues to contribute to growth, perhaps through the timed release of growth hormones that stimulate root and leaf development. The stem, branches, and leaves of a plant are shaped by the plant's ecology and evolution. So, too, the syntactic structures, semantic content, and pragmatics of language are responsive both to the child's environment and heredity. . . . Plant growth is governed by geotropic and heliotropic responses to gravity and light. In the same way, the growth of language is shaped by general cognitive strategies and heuristics. These strategies interrelate previous experiences and knowledge with present and future situations. (p. 121)

The child who is deaf begins life with a language seed that is full of cognitive potential. This child needs a fertile environment that will enable the language seed to grow into a mature language plant.

Developmental Sequence in Language Acquisition

Brown (1973) considered the order of progression in knowledge of a first language to be approximately invariant across children learning any language. Is there evidence that the developmental sequence observed in children with normal hearing is applicable to the child who is deaf?

The child with a hearing loss has the same cognitive potential for learning the meaning, structure, and use of language as the hearing child. Through the child's interaction with fluent speakers and signers, language is learned. So it seems logical that children who are deaf would internalize language in the same order of progression as hearing children. Since the 1970s educators (Holmes & Holmes, 1981; Kretschmer & Kretschmer, 1979) have recommended that the language of deaf children be compared to the developmental regularities observed in normally hearing children and that the results of these comparisons be used to create language curricula. Evidence to support this recommendation can be found in the literature.

A number of researchers have examined the language development of children who are deaf along dimensions of syntax, semantics, and pragmatics. They have found stages and sequences of language development in oral and signing deaf children comparable to those found in hearing children (Caselli, 1983; Crowson, 1994; Curtiss, Prutting, & Lowell, 1979; Petitto, 1987; Prinz & Prinz, 1985; Robinshaw, 1996; Schirmer, 1985). The implication is that as teachers of youngsters who are deaf, we need to understand the universals of language development.

Gesture and Early Language Development

Much of the traditional research in prelinguistic development has focused on the child's perception and production of speech sounds. Studies of the relationship between babbling and language acquisition were interesting but not very illuminating to those of us teaching children who are deaf. Research that helps us understand prelinguistic development in deaf children centers on how prelinguistic children use gestures symbolically to represent functions and meanings and how gestural development is related to language acquisition. An example of a symbolic gesture is the young child pointing to an object that is out of reach while looking at his or her mother.

At this point, conclusions from the research on the expression of communicative intent through the symbolic use of gesture in children who are hearing and deaf (Acredolo & Goodwyn, 1988; Bates, Bretherton, Snyder, Shore, & Volterra, 1980; Bates, Thal, Whitesell, Fenson, & Oakes, 1989; Bretherton, Bates, McNew, Shore, Williamson, & Beeghly-Smith, 1981; Carroll & Gibson, 1986; Goldin-Meadow & Morford, 1985; Mohay, 1982; Thal & Bates, 1988; Volterra, 1981; Volterra & Erting, 1990) support the following views:

1. Both infants who are hearing and infants who are deaf use symbolic gestures to communicate.
2. Symbolic gestures appear approximately at the same time as spoken words in hearing children.
3. Symbolic gestures seem to be used for requesting before they are used for labeling.
4. Gestures and words are both used first in routinized activities.
5. Gestural communication is an important stage in the acquisition of language.

Gesture has also been an important area of study for researchers focusing on deaf children who do not have either a spoken or sign language. This type of communication is sometimes called *homesign systems* or *self-styled communication systems*. Across cultures around the world, deaf individuals with no spoken or sign language have been found to communicate with gestures, and deaf children that use homesign exhibit regularities in their communication development that are similar to children learning a conventional language (Goldin-Meadow, Butcher, Mylander, & Dodge, 1994; Goldin-Meadow, Mylander, & Butcher, 1995; Morford, 1996; Morford & Goldin-Meadow, 1997).

Syntactic and Semantic Development

Much of what is known about the development of the structure and meaning of language has come from observations of children communicating with adults and with each other. Children acquire language by moving through predictable stages of syntactic and semantic development. A thorough discussion of all the issues involved in normal language development is beyond the scope of this book, but the reader is encouraged to explore this topic by examining other texts (e.g., Gleason, 1997; Owens, 1996). I will, however, discuss in detail these predictable stages of development because they are pertinent in understanding the language acquisition process in children who are deaf.

Syntactic Development

What is typically referred to as syntactic development really involves *morphology* and *syntax*. As children learn the form of language, they are discovering the rules that govern how morphemes (the smallest meaningful unit of grammatical form) are combined into words (morphology) as well as how words are combined into sentences (syntax).

Stages of syntactic development have been well documented (Brown, 1973; deVilliers & deVilliers, 1979; Tager-Flusberg, 1997; Wells, 1981) and have been used to examine the deaf child's acquisition of spoken English and American Sign Language (Schirmer, 1985; Wilbur, 1987).

Framework of Language Development.   The framework presented in Figure 1.1 represents an order of language development that has been found to be fairly constant across children. The stages are divided by mean length of utterance (MLU) in morphemes rather than by chronological age because, although the rate at which children acquire language has been found to be highly variable, almost every new kind of language knowledge increases the length of utterance. Children whose mean length of utterance is the same tend to do the same things with the morphemes they use. Indeed, the young child seems cognitively limited in the number of morphemes per utterance and uses this limit in consistent syntactic, semantic, and pragmatic ways to express meaning. Beyond four morphemes per utterance, the child is able to make constructions of such variety and complexity that length is no longer a good indicator of development.

The following are the six stages of language development in the framework. The mean length of utterance divisions are based on Brown's stages (1973) with the addition of a single morpheme stage that Brown did not include. (Mean length of utterance is defined as the average number of morphemes the child produces per utterance. The procedure for calculating MLU is provided later in this chapter.)

Stage 1: 1.00 MLU in morphemes
Stage 2: 1.00–1.99
Stage 3: 2.00–2.49
Stage 4: 2.50–3.12
Stage 5: 3.13–3.74
Stage 6: 3.75+

Within each stage is a developmental order of syntactic forms. The framework does not encompass all aspects of syntactic development. Furthermore, development of specific forms and relations does not start and stop within the boundaries of each stage; however, these processes appear in child language most strongly at the particular stage identified in the framework. The child may begin to use a particular form at an earlier stage and may not gain mastery until a later stage. (For a complete description of the framework, the reader is directed to Schirmer, 1989.)

Seeking age norms for the stages of syntactic development is tempting, and some researchers have found age ranges for specific forms. As a teacher of deaf children, keep in mind that rate of acquisition in hearing compared to deaf peers provides relatively little helpful information for instruction. On the other hand, knowing what syntactic features the child is using and whether the order of acquiring these forms is similar to peers is important for planning instruction.

Semantic Development

Semantics is defined as the meaning or content of language. As children learn the content of language, they are discovering the rules that govern the meaning of words, phrases, and sentences.

Researchers have focused on the semantic properties of words and morphemes and on the semantic roles that each word plays in a phrase or sentence so that they can examine hearing and deaf children's development of meaning (Bloom & Lahey, 1978; Brown, 1973; Luetke-Stahlman, 1988; Marvin & Kasal, 1996).

The ways in which children combine semantic categories within sentences become more complex as they are able to produce longer utterances. At the same time, they are able to create utterances of increasing syntactic complexity as well as to add new semantic categories to their repertoires. In Figure 1.2, a taxonomy of semantic categories and their definitions are given. Examples are provided in Figure 1.3.

Development of Language Use

When authors use the term *language use,* they often use it interchangeably with the term *pragmatics.* However, I view pragmatics more narrowly as only one component of use. When we examine how children are acquiring language, we need to recognize that children are learning three different but related areas of use—functions, context,

FIGURE 1.1   Framework for Assessing Early Syntactic Development

Identifier	Descriptor	Verb	Adverb
			here *there*
			in *on*
Personal pronouns (first & second person)	Number	Present progressive without auxiliary	
Plural (regular) *a* *the*		Imperative	
Personal pronouns (third person)	*some*	Present progressive with auxiliary	
Indefinite pronouns (*it, this, that*)		Copula	
	many	Past (irregular)	*now*
	all	Third person present indicative (regular and irregular)	*too*
Personal pronouns (plural)	Possessive (*'s*)	Past (regular)	
Indefinite pronouns (*something, somebody, someone*)	*more* *another* *other(s)*	Embedded sentences —infinitive —*wh*- —relative clause	

FIGURE 1.1   Continued

Negative	Question	Conjunction	Stage	MLU
	Intonation		1	1.00
not *no*	*what* *where*		2	1.00–1.99
	who *when*	*and*	3	2.00–2.49
	how *why*		4	2.50–3.12
can't *didn't* *don't*	Yes/no question		5	3.13–3.74
		and then *because* *so* *but* *or*	6	3.75+

FIGURE 1.2   Taxonomy of Semantic Categories

Entity—any thing or person having a distinct, separate existence

Nonexistence—the child makes reference to the disappearance of an object or the absence of an object or action in a context in which its existence might be expected

Recurrence—the child either comments on or requests the recurrence of a thing, person, or process

Rejection—the child opposes an action or refuses an object that is in the context or imminent within the situation

Demonstrative—the child introduces an entity using *a, the, that, it, here, there*

Object—someone or something either suffering a change of state or receiving the force of an action

Denial—the child negates the identity, state, or event expressed in another's utterance or in his or her own previous utterance

Attribution—property, characteristic, distinctive feature, or quality of something or someone

Possession—objects within the domain of specific persons

Action—perceived movements

Locative—the place or locus of an action

State—the child makes reference to a state of being

Quantity—the child designates the number of objects or persons

Notice—the child refers to attention to a person, object, or event, and must include a verb of notice such as *see, look, listen, watch, hear*

Time—the child makes reference to time (ongoing, imminent, future, past)

Coordinate—the child refers to two events or states that are independent of each other but are somehow bound together in space or time

Causality—the child expresses an implicit or explicit cause and effect relationship (that is, one event or state depends on another event or state for its occurrence)

Dative—the child designates the recipient of an object or action (e.g., *for, to*)

Specifier—the child specifies a particular person, object, or event

Epistemic—the child describes a relationship between two states, or one event and one state, that refers to certainty or uncertainty about an event or state (e.g., "seems like")

Mood—the child expresses an attitude about an event (e.g., *can, must, should*)

Antithesis—the child expresses a dependency between two events or states and the dependency is a contrast between them

Adapted from Bloom & Lahey (1978) and Luetke-Stahlman (1988).

FIGURE 1.3   Examples of the Semantic Categories

Entity:	baby/(holding a doll) ball chair/(looking at the ball on the chair) what's this ↑
Nonexistence:	all gone/(bird lands then flies away) no/(turns picture over so he can't see it) there's no pocket in this jacket/
Recurrence:	more/(holding up an empty glass) can I have another cookie ↑
Rejection:	no/(Mom wants her to put her toys away) don't touch my papers/
Demonstrative:	the man fell down/ I have a VCR at home/
Object:	push me/ drink juice/ Dad is washing his car/
Denial:	no/(child is holding a toy telephone and is asked, "Is that Mommy's telephone?") I'm not tired/(in response to an adult comment, "You're just tired.")
Attribution:	hot/(eating soup for lunch) my pants are dirty/
Possession:	Mommy/(holding up Mommy's book) that's my truck/ Ann's room is big/
Action:	run/(watching her sister running) she's riding her bike/
Locative:	book table/(looking at the book on the table) the kids are swimming in the pool/
State:	you have none/ I feel sick/
Quantity:	two cow/(pointing to 2 animals) I have a lot of friends/
Notice:	watch me/ did you see that ↑
Time:	I going home now/ Lisa will join us later/
Coordinate:	give me the ball but not the bat/ I got a sweater and earrings and money for my birthday/
Causality:	I fell down and hurt my knee/ Bobby can't go because he's being punished/
Dative:	I saved this seat for you/ give some juice to Christa/

(continued)

FIGURE 1.3   Continued

Specifier:	I don't want that cookie/ Addie picked this one for Karlita/
Epistemic:	it's getting cloudy so I think it will rain/ Joe fell off the bleachers . . . is he hurt ↑
Mood:	I can do it/ Lori should give back the money/
Antithesis:	my feet are cold but I have socks and slippers on/ you go to the movies and I'll stay home with Lindy/

and conversation (Prutting, 1982; Roth & Spekman, 1984). I will discuss pragmatics within the topic of language functions, as it is the function language serves for relating to others.

As the reader considers the information in this section, it will become obvious that considerably less is known about how children acquire the ability to use language than about children's acquisition of syntax and semantics. Yet, if use is the overall organizing aspect of language (Owens, 1996), then it is at least as important for children who are deaf to learn the rules governing the use of language within communicative contexts as it is for them to learn the content and form of language.

Functions or Communicative Intents

Language Functions.   *Language functions* refer to the individual's intentions and expectations of the linguistic act. The function of language for individuals to relate to others and satisfy their own needs is called the interpersonal or *pragmatic*. The function of language within individuals for learning about the world is called the intrapersonal or *mathetic*.

In a study of his son's language acquisition from the age of nine months through twenty-four months, Halliday (1975) found six early developing functions and one later developing function. These functions and their definitions can be found in Figure 1.4. He observed that these functions fell into two distinct groups, with the pragmatic intent arising most directly from the instrumental and regulatory functions and the mathetic intent arising from a combination of the personal and heuristic. The seventh function, the informative, was found to emerge considerably after the others.

Although I discuss pragmatic development as if it were separate from syntactic and semantic development, these components are in reality interrelated. Children's acquisition of questions is an example that highlights the relationship between syntactic, semantic, and pragmatic development. Several researchers have found the order of acquisition of wh- question forms to be related to the child's increasing ability to understand semantic concepts (Bloom & Lahey, 1978; Brown, 1973; Lee, 1974). As Schwabe, Olswang, and Kriegsmann (1986) noted, "The consistent sequence of acquisition of wh- forms reflects the child's ability to request information about in-

FIGURE 1.4   Definitions of Halliday's Language Functions

Instrumental—"I want" or requesting; the function that language serves of satisfying the child's material needs, of enabling him or her to obtain the goods and services that he or she wants

Regulatory—"Do as I tell you" or controlling; the function of language for controlling the behavior of others

Interactional—"Me and you" or interacting with others; the function language serves for the child to interact with those around him or her, particularly with individuals who are important to the child

Personal—"Here I come" or communicating feelings; the function of language for expressing the child's own uniqueness, expressing his or her awareness of self as distinct from the environment, and ultimately developing personality

Heuristic—"Tell me why" or questioning; the function language serves for exploring the environment

Imaginative—"Let's pretend" or creating; the function of language whereby the child creates an environment of his or her own through story, make-believe, let's pretend, and ultimately poetry and imaginative writing

Informative—"I've got something to tell you" or declaring; the function of language for communicating information to someone who does not already possess that information

Adapted from Halliday (1975).

creasingly abstract semantic notions" (p. 42). In other words, questions do not exist in a semantic-syntactic vacuum; they serve as functional linguistic devices for the child, such as Halliday's heuristic or "tell me why" function.

It has been observed that the ability to use pragmatic functions increases with age and stage of language development, and that children use new forms to express old functions and old forms to express new functions (James & Seebach, 1982).

Inner Speech and Sign.   The difference between pragmatic and mathetic functions of language is most clearly captured by Vygotsky's concept of *inner speech*. Vygotsky (1962) viewed external speech as speech for others, the turning of thought into words. He viewed inner speech as speech for oneself, speech turned into inward thought. Vygotsky's conceptualization of inner speech is frequently contrasted with Piaget's (1926) concept of egocentric speech. Piaget believed that young children engaged in egocentric speech because they were incapable of taking the perspective of others. According to Piaget, this type of speech disappeared as the child became able to engage in more socially oriented speech. In contrast, Vygotsky believed egocentric speech was a stage of development preceding inner speech; thus one changed into the other.

The research on inner speech, particularly on its purpose for cognitive self-guidance and self-communication, has been reviewed by a number of researchers (Berk & Garvin, 1984; Diaz, 1986; Frauenglass & Diaz, 1985; Frawley & Lantolf, 1986; Pellegrini, 1984). They have found some support for Vygotsky's theory of inner speech, though great individual variation in both the development and production of inner speech.

It seems that if hearing children experience inner speech, then deaf children who use sign language would experience inner sign. To test this hypothesis, Jamieson (1995b) conducted a study with six deaf children, three with deaf mothers and three with hearing mothers, between four years-nine months and five years-five months of age. She found that both groups of children used inner speech, which Jamieson referred to as *private speech,* with the children of deaf parents using a signed form and the children of hearing parents using a spoken form. She also found that the deaf children of deaf parents used more mature forms of inner speech and with greater frequency than the deaf children of hearing parents. Similarly, Mayer and Moskos (1998) conducted a longitudinal study on the spelling development of deaf children who were between the ages of five and nine at the outset. They concluded that when deaf children learn to spell, they use an inner eye, Mayer and Moskos's term for the inner speech of deaf children, to convert their visual–gestural signs into the linear–alphabetic orthography of English.

Context or Presuppositions

Context refers to the environment of the linguistic act, both situational cues and information about the communication partner. (Much of the literature refers to the communication partner as the listener. However, the term *listener* has a connotation that excludes individuals with hearing loss, so the term *communication partner* will be used.) As children are acquiring the ability to use language, they are learning how to use information from context to determine appropriate linguistic forms. Context includes information learned from situational cues and about the communication partner.

Situational Cues.   When children use *situational cues* to determine the form of their message, they are taking into account how formal or informal the communication setting is. For example, a conversation with a teacher during an Individualized Education Plan (I.E.P.) meeting would be more formal than a conversation with the same teacher during recess.

Situational cues also refer to the child's need for perceptual support. Perceptual support is the extent to which the child needs to have direct experience of a topic in order to communicate about it. It includes the ability to communicate about objects not present and events in which one was not a participant.

The Communication Partner.   If the child is to be able to adapt the message to the needs of the *communication partner,* the child must know and be able to use two kinds of information about the partner, prior knowledge and social status.

First, the child makes assumptions about what the partner knows and does not know (in terms of world knowledge, specific knowledge, and prior experiences) about the topic. Based on these presuppositions, the child decides what information to include and what information to leave out because the partner would find it redundant.

Second, the child draws conclusions about the partner's social status. The child learns to consider the partner's gender, age, and role in the child's life. The child may also learn to consider the partner's ethnic background, dialect, and degree of hearing. Based on this information, the child will vary his or her communication style.

At this point, it might be helpful to clarify the terminology being used. Warren and McCloskey (1997) referred to *language* as variation between countries, *dialect* as language variation between regions, *register* as language variation between social situations, and *style* as language variation distinctive of individual speakers. "While most speakers in the United States will spend their lives speaking a single language and often a single dialect, they must master several registers in order to be socially acceptable" (p. 223).

Learning to look for and use information about the communication partner's prior knowledge and social status enables children to become more skilled at adjusting the politeness markers they use and their linguistic forms for conveying formal versus informal register. Warren and McCloskey (1997) found that the ability to vary register develops well into childhood and possibly into adulthood.

Conversation

Conversation depends on the child's ability to learn the discourse rules that speakers/signers and partners use for introducing, maintaining, and terminating a conversation.

To introduce or initiate a conversation, the child must know how to solicit the partner's attention, greet appropriately, and establish eye contact.

To maintain a conversation, the child must be able to ask and answer questions, take turns appropriately, handle regressions, request more information, make repairs, offer new information, acknowledge the partner's information, use eye contact appropriately, and shift topics.

Finally, to terminate a conversation, the child needs to know how to close a topic and use conversational boundary markers such as "It's been great seeing you," "See you later," and "I have to get going."

Conversation is a particularly critical area of research because it represents not only the medium of social exchange but the milieu of language acquisition. In studies of the discourse development of children, it has been found that children at the early stages of language development have already acquired incipient understanding of conversation; by the time they have completed preschool, they have acquired the basic rules of appropriate conversational behavior; and their knowledge becomes increasingly richer through their school years and into adulthood (Brinton & Fujiki, 1984; Foster, 1983; French & Pak, 1995; Miller, Lechner, & Rugs, 1985; Terrell, 1985; Wells, 1986; Wilkinson, Wilkinson, Spinelli, & Chiang, 1984).

In a study of the development of conversational discourse skills in profoundly deaf children between three years-ten months and eleven years-five months of age and who communicated primarily in sign language, Prinz and Prinz (1985) found these youngsters used developmentally appropriate eye contact, conversational attention-getting devices, tactics for conventional turn-taking and for remediating interruptions, and appropriate strategies for initiating, maintaining, and terminating topics.

Role of Parents in Language Development

For children to learn language, they need to have a considerable amount of experience in conversation with adults. In the Bristol study, a longitudinal study of the language development of a group of children over a fifteen-year span, Wells and his associates "found a clear relationship between the children's rate of progress in language learning and the amount of conversation that they experienced with their parents and other members of the family circle" (1986, p. 44).

The nature of the interactions between children and their parents has been examined by a number of researchers, and some interesting findings have emerged.

Motherese

The particular modifications in the language of adults when they are communicating with young children is called *motherese,* or child-directed speech. Another common term used by researchers to describe this special language is *baby talk,* although baby talk tends to connote the use of "baby" vocabulary rather than the characteristics of motherese listed in Figure 1.5. Mothers' language directed to their young children is generally simple, well-formed, and clear. Mothers use higher pitch and more exaggerated stress and intonation than when they are communicating with their older children or with adults. And they typically ask more questions (DePaulo & Bonvillian, 1978; Garton & Pratt, 1998; Grieser & Kuhl, 1988; James, 1990; Snow, 1986).

FIGURE 1.5   Characteristics of Motherese

- Sentences simplified semantically and syntactically
- Sentences well-formed (syntactically "correct")
- Short sentences
- Redundant (i.e., more repetitious)
- About the "here and now" (i.e., talk is about shared perceptions)
- Refers to concrete objects
- Exaggerated stress and intonation
- Clear pauses between utterances
- Sentences simplified phonologically
- Higher pitch
- Greater number of interrogatives
- Greater number of imperatives
- More restricted vocabulary
- Selective use of content words and fewer function words
- Slower (i.e., fewer words per minute)
- Highly intelligible

Some consider the term *motherese* to be a misnomer because not only mothers modify their language to young children but also all caretakers, and even older children. Yet others have found differences between the language modifications of mothers, fathers, and older siblings. Results have indicated that mothers are more attuned than fathers to the developmental level of their children (McLaughlin, White, McDevitt, & Raskin, 1983) and that children under the age of five do not adjust the characteristics of their language when addressing younger children (Tomasello & Mannle, 1985).

While there is general agreement about the characteristics of motherese, there is less agreement on whether motherese indeed facilitates language development. In the motherese hypothesis, researchers propose that the special properties of caretaker speech play a causal role in language acquisition (Gleitman, Newport, & Gleitman, 1984). Although some researchers support the motherese hypothesis and other researchers dispute it, there are two points of agreement. First, as Gleitman, Newport, and Gleitman state, in a general sense, the motherese hypothesis must be so "for it is the only explanation for the fact that language learning is variable—that French children learn French and Turkish children learn Turkish" (p. 76). Second, language acquisition is an interactive process. The language input from the environment may, indeed, be critical to the process, but the child also plays a crucial role. The child must take the initiative to interact with others and actively process the incoming language information (Fivush & Fromhoff, 1988; Furrow & Nelson, 1986; Garton & Pratt, 1998; Gleitman, Newport, & Gleitman, 1984; Hirsh-Pasek & Golinkoff, 1993; Hoff-Ginsburg, 1986, 1990).

Several researchers have looked specifically at the characteristics of motherese used by mothers with their deaf children and found that they sign more slowly, use simpler sentence structures and exaggerated movements, and incorporate repetition (Masataka, 1992, 1996). Evidence also indicates that hearing mothers are more verbally controlling in conversational interactions with their deaf children (Jamieson, 1995a). In an important study, Reilly and Bellugi (1996) videotaped deaf parents signing with their deaf infants and toddlers and found an intriguing difference in the importance of affect over grammar for these parents when compared to hearing parents. In ASL, the absence of simple facial gestures can change the meaning of a statement. For example, to ask a wh- question, the signer must use a furrowed brow as one of the grammatical markers, but this same furrowed brow affectively signals anger and puzzlement. Researchers found that 90 percent of the questions asked to the children under age two were ungrammatical in ASL because of the deletion of the furrowed brow, yet when the children reached their third birthdays, the parents shifted to the appropriate grammatical signal.

Adult Responses to Ungrammatical Forms

One of the questions that has intrigued researchers is why children bring their language into closer and closer approximations to the adult model. Why should they learn more complex forms if their simpler language adequately serves their communicative needs?

In the 1960s, research suggested that children are positively reinforced for correct and increasingly more sophisticated forms and "punished" for incorrect forms.

Brown and Hanlon (1970) found, however, that parents seemed to pay no attention to incorrect syntax and approved or disapproved only of the "truth value" of the child's utterance or the child's use of naughty words. More recent research has demonstrated that parents do exhibit sensitivity to their children's well-formed and ill-formed utterances (Bohannon & Stanowicz, 1988; Demetras, Post, & Snow, 1986; Hirsh-Pasek, Treiman, & Schneiderman, 1984) and that the way they expand and extend what the child has said may be particularly important in helping children focus on correct form (Farrar, 1992; Nelson, Welsh, Camarata, & Butkovsky, 1995).

Context of Parent–Child Communication

Almost immediately after birth, mothers and their children begin to interact with one another in ways that are remarkably like conversations. Rosenthal (1982) found three-day-old infants are more likely to start vocalizing in the presence of maternal vocalization than in its absence. Bloom, Russell, and Wassenberg (1987) observed that turn-taking with an adult caused qualitative changes in the vocal sounds made by three-month-old infants. Rutter and Durkin (1987) found that by two years of age, children are playing an active role in maintaining the coordination of vocal interactions with an adult, and that by eighteen months of age, they are using gaze in ways that are much like adult turn-taking patterns.

Some suggest that child language emerges from routines in the child's daily life in which form and content of the language being used is largely repetitive, such as during bathtime and lunchtime. Bruner (1983) called these routinized activities *formats* and found that they often had a playful, gamelike nature, such as in peek-a-boo and hide-and-seek. The language used in these formats is called *scripts*. The active guidance and support the adult gives in these conversations is called *scaffolding*. There is some evidence to indicate that shared script knowledge contributes to language development (Furman & Walden, 1990; Lucariello & Nelson, 1987).

Children learn language through conversation and use language in conversation to learn about the world. As Wells (1986) wrote:

> Almost every situation provides an opportunity for learning if children are purposefully engaged and there are adults around who encourage their attempts to do and to understand and, in collaboration with them, provide a resource of skills and information on which they can draw. In such situations, language provides a means not only for acting in the world but also for reflecting on that action in an attempt to understand it. (p. 65)

This reciprocal relationship between learning language and learning through language will be further discussed in Chapter 2.

Later Language Development

The emphasis that educators, speech and hearing specialists, and linguists have placed on early language development is self-evident in the amount of research and number of textbook chapters devoted to this topic. It is exciting to watch young children learn language. Their progress is relatively fast, and what they are learning is fairly easy to observe and measure. Yet we know that children do not stop learning language when they have attained basic knowledge of its form, content, and use. And as teachers of youngsters who are deaf, we also know that the child's ability to continue developing in language is critically important to cognitive and literacy development.

Later Syntactic and Semantic Development

In the early stages of language development, children acquire most of the morphologic and syntactic rules of their language, and they develop the ability to express basic semantic relations. In later language development, children add new morphologic and syntactic structures, expand and refine the ones they already use, and express increasingly complex semantic concepts.

Syntactic Development.   The study of later syntactic development has probably received the least amount of attention by linguistic researchers. Based on available data (Lee, 1974; Nippold, 1998; Owens, 1996), the syntactic structures that appear in later language development are listed in Figure 1.6. Currently, we know very little about later language acquisition in American Sign Language (ASL) although, as in early language acquisition, the course of development appears to be similar to English (Wilbur, 1987).

The *personal pronouns* that appear in early language development (see Figure 1.1) include *I, me, my, mine, you, your, yours;* followed closely by *he, him, his, she, her, hers;* and then *we, us, our, ours, they, them, their, these,* and *those.* In later language development, the child gains use of *indefinite pronouns.* The first ones to appear are *it, this,* and *that;* followed by *something, somebody,* and *someone;* and then *nobody* and *no one.* Considerably later *anything, anybody, anyone, everybody,* and *everyone* appear. The child also begins to use *reflexives* consistently (*myself, yourself, himself, herself, itself, themselves,* and *oneself*).

The child also adds to the kinds of *descriptors* he or she uses. *Another, nothing,* and *none* appear, followed later by the many different descriptors that express quantity, such as *any, every, both, few, each, several, least, much,* and place in time, such as *next, first,* and *second.*

Verbs emerging in later language development include *modals (can, will, may* + verb), *do* + verb, and *past progressives,* followed by *could, would,* and *should* + verb. The child then demonstrates the ability to use passives. Some of the last forms to appear are *must* + verb, *shall* + verb, *have* + verb, complex embeddings, gerunds, and *complex auxiliary combinations,* such as modal + *have* + verb + *en* and modal + *be* + verb + *ing.*

Adverbial clauses become evident in later language development, along with other subordinate clauses. Adverbial clauses of *time* (e.g., *when*), *reason* (e.g., *because*), and *purpose* (e.g., *to*) appear considerably earlier than adverbial clauses expressing *condition* (e.g., *if*).

The child continues to gain mastery of the conjunctions that appear in the latter stages of early language development and does not usually begin to use other conjunctions to express finer modulations of meaning for quite a while. These later

FIGURE 1.6   Syntactic Structure in Later Language Development

Identifier	Descriptor	Verb	Adverb
Indefinite pronouns (*nobody, no one, nothing*)		Modals (*can, will, may* + verb)	Adverbial clauses (of time, of reason)
		Past progressive *do* + verb	
Reflexives			Adverbial clauses (of purpose)
	Quantity	*could, would,*	
	Place in time	*should* + verb	
Indefinite pronouns (*anything, anybody, anyone, everything, everybody, everyone*)		*must* + verb	
		have + verb	Adverbial clauses (of condition)
		Complex embeddings	
		Complex auxiliary combinations	
		Gerunds	
		Passives	

FIGURE 1.6   Continued

Negative	Question	Conjunction	Stage
isn't *won't*			7
	Tag questions		8
			9
Later developing contracted negatives (e.g., *wasn't,* *hasn't, aren't,* *couldn't)*			10
			11
	whose *which*	Conjunctions expressing finer modulations of meaning *(although,* *though,* *however,* *therefore)*	12

developing conjunctions include *while, when, until, before, after, for, as, as if, if, although, though, however, therefore,* and *unless.*

The new question form that appears in later language development is the *tag question* (e.g., "You are going, aren't you?"). However, keep in mind that the child is developing the use of yes/no questions commensurate with the use of more complex verb forms (e.g., "Do you see it?", "Should we go to the movies?", and "Have you been eating?"). Note that many of these syntactic and morphologic structures are English-specific. In the section on assessment, I will discuss how to use this information to analyze the language of a child whose first language is ASL. Some children are exposed to both English and ASL, and they are likely to demonstrate some mixing of the two languages at points in their development. Furthermore, many children are not exposed to a full language model in either English or ASL because the adults in their lives use speech only and the child receives limited information through speech-reading and auditory training, or the adults in their lives use pidgin sign. In the section on assessment, I will also discuss issues involved in analyzing the language of these children, and I will present information that teachers can use to analyze the language of children acquiring ASL.

In addition to these forms, the child should be able to recognize the "goodness" of sentences, that is, whether sentences are grammatical or ungrammatical. You would not necessarily expect the child to know what morphologic or syntactic rules were being violated, however, as even adults often have difficulty with this metalinguistic task. The child should also be producing utterances that more and more closely resemble adult models.

Semantic Development.   The child's continued semantic development largely involves the learning of new words, new meanings for words already known, elaborated meanings, and interrelationships between word concepts (vocabulary growth). It also involves changes in the child's ability to relate word concepts (word association), explain word meanings (word definition), and understand nonliteral language (figurative language).

Vocabulary Growth.   Growth in vocabulary occurs throughout the individual's lifetime. One of the major sources of lexical learning is reading. Children add not only words that are longstanding in the language, but throughout their life span they will also add words that are new to the language. Children learn shades of meaning for words they already know, and they learn how some word meanings can be consolidated into one word with an elaborated meaning. They gain full understanding of abstract concepts and subtle meanings of words gradually through their school years (Nippold, 1998; Owens, 1996).

Word Association.   The developmental change in the way that children associate words has been called the syntagmatic–paradigmatic shift. Until the age of approximately seven, in a word association task children will respond to a stimulus word with a word related in syntax. That is, they respond with a word that would likely follow the stimulus word in a sentence. For example, in a syntagmatic association, the child would answer "juice" to the stimulus word *drink*. After the age of seven (usually between five and nine), the child becomes more likely to respond to a stimulus word with a word that is semantically related and of the same grammatical category. For example, in a paradigmatic association, the child would answer "cold" to the stimulus word *hot* (Owens, 1996; Pan & Gleason, 1997).

Word Definitions.   Defining a word involves metalinguistic processes. The youngster must be able to reflect on word meanings and use words to talk about words. When defining a word, young children are likely to describe its appearance or its function. Gradually, youngsters become able to produce synonyms, explanations, and categorical relationships. Word definition tasks have been included in IQ tests for many years because of the research correlating the ability to produce word definitions with intelligence (Nippold, 1998; Pan & Gleason, 1997).

Figurative Language.   Along with vocabulary growth in later language development, the child develops the ability to understand figurative or nonliteral language. We currently know a great deal more about children's comprehension of metaphors, similes, slang, and proverbs than we do about their emerging ability to produce figurative language. Although children begin to understand and use simple figures of speech in early language development, the ability to analyze the meanings of figurative language does not occur until late childhood or early adolescence. This ability to interpret nonliteral language increases with age and seems at least partly dependent on the amount of experience the youngster has had with the various forms of figurative language. The youngster's skill in comprehending figurative language also appears to depend on how relevant the expressions are to the child's personal experiences and whether the expressions appear in isolation or in context (Nippold, 1998; Owens, 1996).

Later Development of Language Use
Throughout their school years, children acquire a range of communicative abilities that allow them to interact socially with increasingly greater skill. As Cooper and Anderson-Inman (1988) noted, "To talk is to interact with the world. Through this interactive process, children make connections with the world and also with themselves" (p. 243).

Functions or Communicative Intents.   In later language development, children learn to express many new communicative intents. Figure 1.7 shows how most of these new language functions (Menyuk, 1988; Owens, 1996) can be conceptualized as growing out of the original seven functions postulated by Halliday (1975). This list is not meant to be exhaustive, and, undoubtedly, the reader will be able to add later developing functions to the ones included.

Context or Presuppositions.   The child's ability to take into account situational cues and information about the communication partner becomes more sophisticated over time. One example of this is the child's use of *indirect requests* (Wilkinson,

FIGURE 1.7   Language Functions in Later Language Development

Instrumental ("I want")
—express personal needs
—cajole
—persuade
—request a favor
—request help
—request permission

Regulatory ("Do as I tell you")
—direct the behavior of others
—dissuade
—threaten

Interactional ("Me and you")
—share problems
—express feelings for others
—describe anticipated reactions
   of others
—criticize
—disagree
—compliment
—promise
—express support
—offer help

Personal ("Here I come")
—express emotions
—complain
—justify

—express opinions
—blame

Imaginative ("Let's pretend")
—tell stories
—role-play

Heuristic ("Tell me why")
—request information
—request clarification
—probe
—solve problems
—predict

Informative ("I've got something to tell you")
—describe
—compare/contrast
—discuss cause and effect
—instruct others
—suggest

Humor

Dissembling

Ambiguity

Persuasion

Negotiation

Sarcasm

Wilkinson, Spinelli, & Chiang, 1984). A young child who is visiting a family friend might just get up and play on the interesting-looking piano in the family room. This same child, who is now a little older, might ask, "Can I play your piano?" Several years later, this same youngster, who is now an adolescent, might look longingly at the piano and comment, "What a beautiful piano. I bet it is wonderful to play." This last statement is an indirect request.

In later language development, children gain mastery over the special registers needed to relate to peers, to members of the same gender and to the opposite gender, to others who share hobbies or interests, to people with similar cultural backgrounds, and to close friends and intimates (Ely, 1997).

Youngsters also learn that school discourse is different from home discourse. One of the common types of classroom exchanges that we never see at home is *"question-answer-evaluate,"* sometimes called *question–answer routines*. For example, the teacher asks, "John, what is the capital of Oregon?" John answers, "Salem." The teacher responds, "That's right. Mary, where is the Columbia River?" As this exchange demonstrates, the teacher controls the dialogue, the child who is called on is supposed to give a brief answer, and the teacher's next question does not necessarily follow logically from the child's answer (Stephens, 1988). Question–answer routines have been found to be particularly difficult for deaf children with learning problems (Bullard & Schirmer, 1991) because the child expects communication to be conversational in nature and has difficulty following the logic of a question–answer routine.

Another difference between home and school language is the contrast between the amount of language produced by the adult and the child. Classroom discourse is marked by a high proportion of teacher language and a relatively small proportion of individual child language. Furthermore, unlike dialogue with parents and peers, dialogue with teachers typically means that teachers control choice of topic, take longer turns, monitor who takes turns and how long their turns are, and determine when the topic should be changed or terminated (Cazden, 1988; Wells, 1986).

In adolescence and early adulthood, young people learn that work settings require a language register that is different from the registers used at home and in school. Furthermore, most work settings demand knowledge of a particular professional jargon (Obler, 1997). Each week in *Newsweek*'s Periscope section, the magazine lists several "buzzwords" used by a given profession; these words, meant to be a cross between jargon and slang, are humorous examples of how professional terminology maintains exclusivity among members.

Conversation.   Several factors contribute to children's conversational ability in later language development. First, conversational ability develops as children become more aware of the conversational norms of their culture (Menyuk, 1988). Second, children become more skilled at engaging in conversation when they are able to take another person's perspective (Owens, 1996). Finally, parents seem to "teach" the rules of discourse by gradually allowing the child to take over responsibility for initiating, maintaining, and terminating conversations as the child's skills increase (Wanska & Bedrosian, 1985).

Clearly, many rules for introducing, maintaining, and terminating a conversation in ASL may be quite different from the rules in English. For example, for ASL users, conversational terminations at social gatherings can take an hour or longer (Lane, Hoffmeister, & Bahan, 1996). In ASL conversations, it is appropriate to wave or tap someone on the shoulder to get his or her attention, and in deaf culture, one is supposed to walk between two signers carrying on a conversation without excusing oneself (Lentz, Mikos, & Smith, 1988).

Children who are deaf need to develop the ability to use appropriate conversational rules in both languages. Conversational ability develops gradually and continues throughout the individual's lifetime. And, as we all can attest, not all adults seem equally skilled at carrying on a conversation.

Metalinguistic Awareness

The ability to reflect upon language is called *metalinguistic awareness*. During the period of early language acquisition, children's knowledge of language is intuitive. Children's ability to think consciously about language and to use language to talk about language signals a shift in their cognitive abilities (Menyuk, 1988). Garton and Pratt (1998) explained metalinguistic awareness using the following analogy:

> Using language is analogous to "using" glass in a window to see the view. We do not normally focus any attention on the glass itself. Instead we focus our attention on the view. The glass serves the purpose of giving us access to the view. But we can, if we choose, look at the glass and may indeed do so for intrinsic interest or for a particular reason. (p. 149)

Metalinguistic awareness develops gradually in most children, beginning in their preschool years. Initially, they demonstrate this awareness by spontaneously making repairs in their own speech or sign, noticing others' errors, and "playing with" words that sound the same or look alike on the hands. By the time children are in first grade, they usually are able to think about the properties of words, they can make grammaticality judgments about sentences, and they have a rudimentary ability to reflect on the basic components of effective communication (Garton & Pratt, 1998; Owens, 1996).

The development of metalinguistic abilities accelerates during the emergence of reading and writing (Ely, 1997). Garton and Pratt (1998) suggested that reading and writing foster attention to words and sounds, syntactic structures of phrases and sentences, forms of paragraphs and longer discourse, and meanings and intents.

The development of metalinguistic awareness in children who are deaf seems to follow the pattern observed in normally developing children who are hearing but at a delayed rate (Gartner, Trehub, & Mackay-Soroka, 1993; Zorfass, 1981). As teachers of children who are deaf, we need to pay particular attention to metalinguistic development because of the relationship between metalinguistic awareness and the child's ability to benefit from our language teaching strategies. In some traditional approaches to teaching language, we ask children to learn sentence patterns. The child with well-developed metalinguistic abilities may be able to reflect upon language well enough to manipulate parts of sentences, but children at early stages of language development would find this a formidable task. I will elaborate on this issue in the next chapter.

Goals of Language Instruction

When we think about goals of language instruction, we are really formulating two types of goals. One type is the set of yearly goals we create for individual children who are deaf. These goals are the specific language structures, meanings, and uses we expect the child to develop understanding of or use of by the end of the academic year. These goals are an outgrowth of our assessment of each child's current language abilities.

The other type of goal we formulate is a more encompassing goal because it represents our philosophy of child language acquisition. How we assess our children, how we choose our teaching strategies and methods, and how we measure their progress will all flow from our beliefs about the goal of language instruction.

The goal of language instruction for children who are deaf is to provide them with a learning environment rich in opportunities to use language for meaningful interaction with others, for reading and writing as well as speaking/signing and listening/ receiving sign, and for thinking about the world. Deaf children are not cognitively or linguistically deficient. Their language does not need to be remediated unless they have concomitant learning problems. An environment abundant with linguistic experiences will enable them to figure out the underlying rules of language for themselves, which will ultimately give them power over their own linguistic systems.

Approaches to Language Assessment

Nature and Role of Assessment

When we assess the language development of children who are deaf, our task is to collect information about their current language abilities, interpret this information, and make instructional decisions based on this information.

Assessment can serve many purposes. Teachers and language specialists need to be able to assess the language of children newly identified as having a hearing loss, children entering an educational program for the first time, children leaving a program, or children undergoing I.E.P. review. We also need to know how to use assessment to monitor children's progress, to evaluate the effectiveness of our language curricula, and to make placement decisions.

Ideally, language assessment is a collaborative effort between the teacher, parents, language specialist, and child. It is my view that language assessments of children who are deaf should be led, whenever possible, by each child's teacher. When the teacher is responsible for carrying out the assessment, or part of the assessment, understanding of the child's language is significantly deeper than when the teacher is given all of the diagnostic information from others. I have observed that teachers who personally assess the language of the children in their classrooms are better able to embed language objectives into learning opportunities and are more aware of their children's ongoing language development.

Process of Language Assessment

Figure 1.8 presents a model of the process of language assessment. It gives teachers and clinicians a unifying structure for carrying out a cohesive and comprehensive language evaluation and provides leeway for determining which instruments and procedures will produce the needed information about specific children. (For complete information about the model, see Schirmer, 1984.)

The assessment moves in a left to right progression: The stop points are the places for deciding whether enough data have been gathered, and the boxes represent the kinds of information needed at this point in the assessment. The ovals describe the

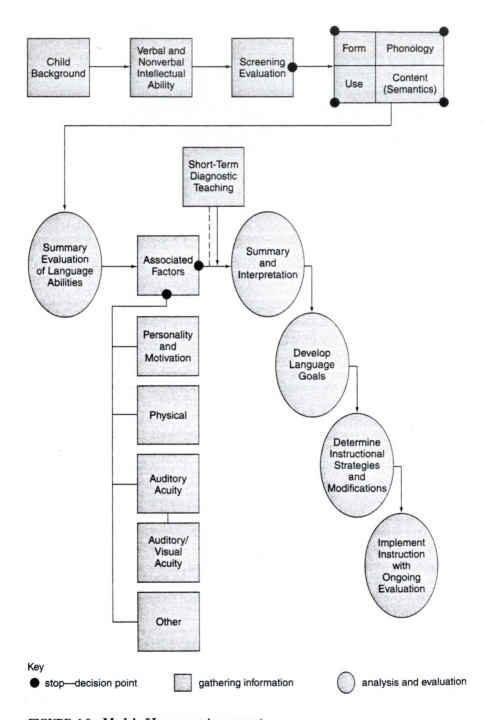

Key

● stop—decision point   ▢ gathering information   ◯ analysis and evaluation

FIGURE 1.8   Model of Language Assessment

© American Speech-Language-Hearing Association. Reprinted by permission.

kinds of analysis and evaluation that should be conducted on the information already gathered. The following list describes the assessment process:

1. Information about the child's background is obtained, if this information is not already known.

2. The child's intellectual functioning is evaluated to identify the child as at an above-average, average, or below-average level because language ability is correlated with intellectual ability. Again, this information may already be available in the child's records and need not be reevaluated. (In my experience, achievement scores predominate in the cumulative files of children who are deaf, but results of intelligence testing are considerably more rare.)

3. A screening evaluation is administered to determine overall language ability and to decide on the need and direction for further evaluation. This step is not necessary when the individual doing the assessment is already quite familiar with the child.

4. The next step involves the assessment of specific language abilities. The model lists the four areas of form, content, use, and phonology. However, the component skills within each area are not provided in the model. The reader is asked to refer to the discussion of component skills earlier in this chapter. Each test or procedure reveals information about the child's language abilities. It is up to the teacher or clinician to determine when enough information has been obtained or when a preceding evaluation has pointed to new areas that need further exploration.

5. When language evaluation is complete, a summary of the child's abilities should be prepared.

6. Factors that might be associated with the child's language should now be evaluated. Information regarding auditory acuity is almost always available; however, when other associated factors, such as visual acuity, seem to be impeding the child's language development, a referral for an outside evaluation may be needed. One factor that should always be considered at this point in the assessment is the child's home and school linguistic environments, taking into account the consistency of linguistic input and any conflicts in the languages used at home and school.

7. At this point, it is often valuable to conduct diagnostic teaching. This allows the teacher to evaluate the child's language in a teaching situation and to try specific methods, techniques, and materials.

8. The information is summarized and interpreted, language goals are developed, instructional strategies and modifications are determined, and instruction is implemented with ongoing evaluation.

The model provides a process for language assessment but does not tell the teacher or clinician which kinds of tests or procedures to use. In the next two sections, the two approaches to assessment, formal and informal, will be described.

Formal Approach: Standardized Assessment Instruments

Formal approaches to assessment involve obtaining a quantitative measure of a student's performance. One type of quantitative measure is the standardized test. In *standardized tests,* which are also called *norm-referenced tests,* the child's performance is compared to the performance of peers (that is, a large group of children at the same age or developmental level).

Standardized assessment instruments offer the advantage of providing objective information about the child's language—that is, information that has not been particularly influenced by the skill or bias of the examiner. Also, standardized tests provide data regarding reliability, validity, representativeness, and standard error of measurement that the teacher can consider in evaluating the accuracy and usefulness of the child's test results. One of the major drawbacks to using standardized assessment instruments is that they measure the child's comprehension or use of decontextualized language. Many tests measure deaf children's metalinguistic abilities more than their linguistic abilities (Ray, 1989). Another drawback is the poor validity and reliability found in many standardized tests of language (McCauley & Swisher, 1984), particularly tests that are developed for deaf children, because these norms tend to be based on a relatively small group of children.

Special Considerations in Using Standardized Tests with Youngsters Who Are Deaf

In the late 1980s, Abraham and Stoker (1988) found that relatively few standardized tests of language had been developed specifically for youngsters who are deaf or had included deaf youngsters in the normative sample, and this is still true. We clearly, then, need to be very careful about choosing and administering a norm-referenced language test.

One of the problems we encounter is the verbal directions. Standardized tests are meant to be administered exactly according to directions. If they are not, the norms are rendered useless (Salvia & Ysseldyke, 1998). However, the verbal directions may be confusing to the child who is deaf, or it may not be possible to interpret them into sign word-for-word, particularly for the ASL child. As Ziezula (1982) stated about testing of individuals, "If the individual being tested cannot fully comprehend the tasks required of him/her, the validity of the results must be questioned" (p. 2).

Another problem with standardized tests, noted by Ziezula, is that test items can discriminate against an individual with a hearing loss, although these items appear to be more prevalent in tests of intelligence, personality, and vocational interest.

These previous considerations all relate to the test. We also need to consider the child. During testing, the child should be benefitting from the kind of amplification he or she uses daily in school. The child should be in good health, with no allergic condition or middle ear infection influencing hearing level. The testing environment should be comfortable, with lighting that enables the child to clearly see the speaker/signer. In addition, the examiner should be fluent in the child's native language (Thompson, Biro, Vethivelu, Pious, & Hatfield, 1987).

Choosing a Standardized Language Test

Beginning with the first Binet–Simon intelligence scale developed in 1916, there has been widespread interest in psychological and educational measurement. Thorum (1981) found that the period between 1920 and 1940 was marked by rapid development of assessment methodology and the publication of achievement, intelligence, aptitude, interest, and personality tests. During World War II, the focus was on developing standardized tests to measure individual aptitudes, potentials, and skills. The 1950s brought standardized tests firmly into the public schools, with language assessment instruments becoming popular in the 1960s. The explosion of language tests from the 1970s to the present leaves us with a seemingly endless number of tests to sort through.

It is a challenge for most of us to choose appropriate standardized tests of language for the deaf children we teach. Unless we have the resources and time to actually read and personally evaluate the hundreds of tests on the market, we need to rely on other sources of information regarding these tests.

One of the oldest and most prestigious resources is the Buros Institute of Mental Measurements, which publishes *Tests in Print* and the *Mental Measurements Yearbooks. Tests in Print* lists and briefly describes every commercially available test published in English. *The Mental Measurements Yearbook* lists and provides evaluative reviews of tests that are new or revised since publication of the last yearbook. These references are available in most libraries.

Textbooks on assessment provide us with a second resource. In recent years, a number of texts have been developed specifically to describe the process of assessment and to evaluate the most widely used tests. A few of these texts are Cohen and Spenciner's *Assessment of Children and Youth* (1998), Salvia and Ysseldyke's *Assessment* (1998), and Taylor's *Assessment of Exceptional Students* (1997).

Our professional journals provide a third resource for test information. Many of our journals such as the *American Annals of the Deaf, The Volta Review, Journal of Childhood Communication Disorders, Journal of Speech and Hearing Disorders,* and *Language, Speech, and Hearing Services in Schools* include examinations of test use, evaluations of testing procedures, and reviews of tests.

In the Appendix: Standardized and Criterion-Referenced Tests, I have listed, described, and briefly reviewed the language assessment instruments I found to be most commonly used with youngsters who are deaf. These instruments were published for the first time or substantially revised within the last fifteen years, and they received relatively positive reviews in the literature.

Informal Approach to Assessment

Informal assessment involves gathering information through observation, analysis of student work, curriculum-based assessment, teacher-made criterion-referenced tests developed to assess the student's Individualized Education Program, and alternative assessment procedures, such as performance assessment (requiring the student to do a task), authentic assessment (requiring the student to apply knowledge to a real-world or simulated setting), and portfolio assessment (requiring the student to submit products that reflect learning over time) (Taylor, 1997).

Informal approaches in language assessment offer the advantage of providing information about the child's understanding and use of language within natural communicative settings. Informal approaches have the best potential for providing a link between assessment and instruction. The disadvantage to these approaches is that the accuracy and completeness of information gathered about the child's language abilities depend heavily on the skill of the teacher or clinician.

Language Sampling

A *language sample* is a segment of a child's language performance regarded as representative of his or her linguistic ability. It has been argued that language sampling techniques should be used for assessing the language of children who are deaf because "language and intelligent behavior occur within a context; changes in context produce changes in language" (Ray, 1989, p. 38).

Obtaining a Language Sample.   Obtaining a language sample from a child with a hearing loss requires an interested, responsive, and minimally directive adult. For the sample to be considered representative, at least fifty utterances should be obtained, and it is preferable to obtain one hundred. Of course, children at the earliest stages of development may not be producing fifty utterances. For these children, I suggest collecting as much of their language as possible.

The following activities have been used with success to collect language samples. Some are more appropriate for younger children and some for older youngsters. A sample can be obtained in less than an hour with younger children and less than thirty minutes with older children, in one setting or over several days in a variety of settings. Classroom aides can do a wonderful job collecting language samples while the teacher is instructing the children. The reader will undoubtedly be able to add to this list of activities:

1. Use toys, such as a dollhouse, to play with a young child.
2. Show the child a wordless storybook or a set of sequential pictures, and ask him or her to describe the action.
3. Tell the child a story, and ask him or her to retell it.
4. Place a brown paper bag in front of the child, and have him or her ask questions to find out what is inside.
5. Have all the ingredients for a sandwich available, and ask the child to tell you how to assemble it.
6. Engage the child in conversation about his or her weekend, vacation, or trip to a store.
7. Record the child's language during instructional activities.

Using videotape provides a record so that an accurate transcription can be made later. However, sometimes it is not possible to use videotape, and in these instances two other strategies can work fairly well, although the transcription will not be as accurate as one obtained through video. One strategy is to keep an ongoing written transcription, though this approach clearly influences the nature of the teacher–child interaction unless a third party is doing the writing, such as an aide during instruction. A second strategy is to subvocalize into an audiotape recorder, which is only possible if the teacher or aide is hearing.

Transcribing the Language Sample.   When transcribing the language sample, I suggest using the form in Figure 1.9. This form was based on one developed by Bloom and Lahey (1978). The following conventions for recording child language data also rely heavily on Bloom and Lahey.

1. Utterance boundary is signified by a slash [/]. I do not use a period, because a period is a convention for written language, and it is important to distinguish an oral or sign utterance from a written sentence. It is sometimes difficult to determine when a

			Page No. _____		
Student's Name _____			Age _____ MLU _____		
Stage _____					
Teacher's Name _____			Date(s) _____		
Activity/ Context	Teacher's Utterance	Student's Utterance	Student's Behavior/Meaning		Analysis

FIGURE 1.9   Form for Transcribing a Language Sample

child has completed one utterance and started another. Linguists use the guideline that the boundary is determined by the length of a pause before the next utterance and by its apparent terminal contour. I also often encounter the problem of the child who connects every utterance with *and* or some other conjunction. Lee (1974) used the rule that one *and* (or any other overused conjunction) connecting two independent clauses was allowed per sentence. Her example was:

> I came home and my dad was there . . ./
> (and) he saw my dog and he started laughing . . ./
> (and) the dog got scared and he started to bark . . ./
> (and) my dad made me take him out/ (p. 75)

2. Questions should be followed by a rising arrow instead of a question mark [↑].

3. An unintelligible utterance or part of an utterance should be indicated by enclosing it in brackets.

4. When a child repeats an adult utterance, the child's utterance is written in full even if the repetition is exact.

5. Conversational route can be indicated through arrows or by leaving space between participants' utterances.

6. ASL glosses should be written in all capital letters with complex glosses connected by hyphens (e.g., WENT-AROUND-THE-BLOCK).

7. Symbols should be designated for distinguishing between sign, oral, simultaneous, and gestured utterances. These symbols should be explained in a key on the first page of the transcription.

Many deaf students use a mix of English and ASL, pidgin sign, and gesture. The transcription systems that have been developed for ASL (e.g., Baker-Shenk & Cokely, 1994; Wilbur, 1987) do not take into account the mixtures of forms, meanings, and uses that these children will produce. However, Johnson and Rash (1990) did develop a method for transcribing the language of children who switch modalities between sign and English; in this method, each utterance is described along the dimensions of context, inflection, sign gloss, spoken component, and phonetic transcription. Whatever transcription format the teacher uses, my suggestion is to keep it as simple and straightforward as possible. Even though many transcription formats were developed for the purpose of conducting research on ASL and are complex, using a complex system when analyzing the language of a deaf child for the purpose of developing language goals and planning instruction is not necessary. Follow the guidelines listed here in creating the final transcript to be used for analyzing the child's language:

1. Maintain the integrity of the child's sentence unit, or utterance boundary, as nearly as possible. Because mean length of utterance is used to measure language growth, it is important to determine when the child has completed an utterance.

2. Record the child's exact utterance. This is often difficult because, as adults, we tend to reformulate an utterance into appropriate grammatical form.

3. Make a note of the utterances that are elliptical. Grammatical ellipsis is an omission of one or more words redundant with the prior utterance. For example, if the teacher asks, "How old are you?" and the child responds, "Five," the child's utterance is elliptical. The child may have knowledge of the full structure, "I am five," but is not required or even expected to use it in this context. Thus, the single-morpheme *five* may not be representative of the child's linguistic ability. (When you count the number of utterances the child has produced, do not include elliptical utterances or utterances that are identical to previous utterances toward the total of fifty or one hundred that you will use in the analysis.)

4. Include the context or activities in which the child is engaged, the child's behaviors, and adult utterances in the transcription. This is particularly important when the child is at the one- and two-morpheme stages because much of the child's actual meaning at these stages of development is inferred. Notations regarding behavior and context can be extremely valuable when analyzing the child's utterances. Also, if the adult's utterances are not notated, you cannot be sure when the child's utterance is elliptical.

Analyzing the Child's Developmental Language Stage

Once the teacher or clinician has obtained a language sample and administered selected standardized tests, the data need to be analyzed. My suggestion is first to analyze the information gained through informal approaches, formulate tentative conclusions, and then use the results from formal testing to modify findings and to reach final conclusions.

Analyzing a Language Sample

The language sample is a snapshot of the child's current language abilities, which you can bring into focus by analyzing along the dimensions of syntax, semantics, and use. The first step is to analyze the child's syntactic and morphologic forms, which you can write directly on the form you used for transcribing the language (Figure 1.9).

Start by calculating the child's mean length of utterance. First, count free and bound morphemes. A *free morpheme,* such as *man* or *play,* can occur alone, whereas a *bound morpheme,* such as the *ly* in *manly* and the *ed* in *played,* must be attached to another morpheme. Compound words, proper names, ritualized reduplications (e.g., *trick or treat, thank you*), irregular past, catenatives (e.g., *wanna, gonna*), and internal word changes to indicate plural (e.g., *feet, people*) are counted as single morphemes. Auxiliaries, plural (-*s*), possessive (-*s*), third person singular present indicative (-*s*), regular past (-*ed*), present progressive (-*ing*), contractions, participles and gerunds (-*ing*), and comparative forms (-*er*, -*est*) are counted as separate morphemes.

The rules for counting morphemes in ASL would obviously be somewhat different from the preceding rules for counting morphemes in English. For a thorough discussion of sign morphology, the reader should examine works by Isenhath (1990) and Wilbur (1987). As a general rule, however, a separate morpheme is counted each time a handshape, location, or movement signals a unit of meaning.

Once you have counted the child's morphemes, mean length of utterance is calculated by dividing the number of morphemes by the number of utterances. You should also note the child's *upper bound,* which is the longest utterance the child produces. The upper bound tells you about the child's willingness to take risks, to try new language features that add to the length of an utterance.

The mean length of utterance gives you an expectation about what forms and meanings the child will likely be expressing.

Now turn to the two formats for syntactic and morphologic development. Figure 1.1 presents a framework for early syntactic development and Figure 1.6 for later syntactic development. You know that the acquisition of forms does not stop and start within the boundaries of each stage, so no matter how long the child's mean length of utterance is, you need to use both frameworks for analyzing the child's utterances.

Each utterance is analyzed separately for forms the child is using. The analysis is written next to the utterance on the transcription. For example, if the child produced "doll falling," *present progressive without auxiliary* (for "falling") would be written in the analysis column.

When you have completed the analysis for syntax and morphology, the second step is to use Figure 1.2 for analyzing the child's semantic development. Again, each utterance is analyzed separately, but this time you are analyzing the child's use of semantic categories. For example, the child's utterance, "doll falling," is now analyzed as *entity, action.* In the analysis column, *entity, action* is written below *present progressive without auxiliary.*

When all utterances have been analyzed, forms and meanings appearing in the language sample are tallied. It is helpful to write the tallies directly onto enlarged photocopies of the frameworks and the taxonomy.

The tallies provide a picture of the child's current syntactic, morphologic, and semantic abilities. At each stage of development, it is clear which forms and meanings the child is using consistently, inconsistently, and not at all.

The next step in the analysis is to examine the child's abilities in the area of language use. Figure 1.10 presents a checklist of language functions, presuppositions, and conversational rules. The checklist simply offers a column for checking whether the child demonstrates, does not demonstrate, or sometimes demonstrates a particular skill or whether there was no opportunity to observe the skill. It is valuable, however, to include comments in this column regarding your impressions of the child's abilities.

FIGURE 1.10   Checklist of Language Functions, Presuppositions, and Conversational Rules

(Scale is from 1 to 5, with 1 representing "not observed" in the child's language, 3 representing "uses sometimes" or "uses appropriately some of the time," and 5 representing "uses appropriately at all times.")

	1	2	3	4	5

Language Functions

Instrumental—requests, expresses personal needs, cajoles, persuades, requests a favor, requests help, requests permission

Regulatory—controls, directs the behavior of others, dissuades, threatens

Interactional—interacts with others, shares problems, expresses feelings for others, anticipates reactions of others, criticizes, disagrees, compliments, promises, expresses support, offers help

Personal—communicates feelings, expresses emotions, complains, justifies, expresses opinions, blames

Imaginative—creates, pretends, tells stories, role-plays

Heuristic—questions, requests information, requests clarification, probes, solves problems, predicts

Informative—declares, informs, describes, compares/contrasts, discusses cause and effect, instructs others, suggests

Presuppositions

Situational Cues—takes into account how formal or informal the context is, needs perceptual support, makes indirect requests

The Communication Partner—takes into account the partner's background knowledge, is able to use different language registers

Conversational Rules

Introducing a Conversation—solicits conversational partner's attention, greets appropriately, establishes eye contact

Maintaining a Conversation—asks questions, answers questions, turn-takes appropriately, handles regressions, requests more information, makes repairs, offers new information, acknowledges the partner's information, uses eye contact appropriately, shifts topics

Terminating a Conversation—closes a topic, uses conversational boundary markers

If the child uses ASL, or any mixture of ASL with English, pidgin, and gesture, you should complete all the steps above and also add the ASL acquisition checklist in Figure 1.11. This checklist focuses specifically on the features of ASL. At present, no standard format for presenting ASL linguistic forms has been developed, so the checklist presented here is only one possible format. The reader is encouraged to review ASL texts, such as *Signing Naturally* (Lentz, Mikos, & Smith, 1988) and *Learning American Sign Language* (Humphries & Padden, 1992), particularly for information on classifiers.

At this time, no framework is available that delineates the developmental progression of ASL acquisition in children even though some research on the features of ASL that are acquired earlier than others has been conducted. For example, Bonvillian and Siedlecki (1996) found that highly contrasting locations, such as forehead, chin, and on and in front of the trunk, were acquired first, and other types of locations, such as those involving complex handshapes in which point of contact is relatively small and the signing hand crosses the body's midline, were acquired much later. The lack of a developmental ASL outline gives greater importance to using all of the instruments, not just the ASL acquisition checklist. The frameworks for assessing early and later language development (Figures 1.1 and 1.6) are based on studies of language acquisition across cultures, and though the forms are English-specific in the frameworks, when using them with ASL, you can analyze the child's use of the equivalent form in ASL. For example, present progressive is a verb tense in ASL marked by movement that shows continuing action; if the child uses the present progressive form, you should analyze it as such. The same holds true for the pronouns, descriptors, negatives, question forms, conjunctions, and many of the verb forms. The taxonomy of semantic categories (Figure 1.2) is also applicable to ASL because children acquiring ASL use the same semantic categories as children acquiring spoken languages.

Using Results from Informal and Formal Assessment Approaches

The two approaches to language assessment—informal through language sampling and formal through standardized tests—should then be combined to give you a complete representation of the deaf child's current language abilities. Once you understand the child's current level of language functioning, you can develop language goals.

Identifying Appropriate Language Goals

Language goals are identified by comparing the child's current language abilities with the forms, meanings, and uses you would expect to appear at the child's stage of development. In other words, language goals are developed based on what has already appeared and what would be expected to appear in the child's language.

FIGURE 1.11   ASL Acquisition Checklist

	Consistently Present	Inconsistently Present	Not Present
Articulation			
Hand shape			
Palm orientation			
Location			
Place and manner			
Movement/hold			
Noun/verb distinction			
Fingerspelling			
Nonmanual signs			
Morphology			
Verb Inflections			
Intensifier			
Manner			
Aspect			
Tense			
Number			
Distribution			
Time			
Noun Inflections			
Intensifier			
Size			
Plural			
Quantity			
Quality			
Order			
Shape			
Spatial relationship			
Pronoun			
Regular			
Indexing/determiners			
Possessive			
Classifiers			
Syntax			
Indexing			
Simple sentence			
Complex sentence			
Command			
Verb agreement			
Subject–object agreement			
Topic/comment			
Existential "have"			
Comparative			
Conditional			
Yes/no question			
Wh- question			
Negation			
Conjunction			
Idiom			

The following case study of a child who is deaf illustrates how information from the assessment and analysis procedures previously discussed can be used in creating appropriate language goals.

A CASE STUDY

Chaulanda is a profoundly deaf child, seven years-three months old who used a mixture of spoken English and sign. Her MLU (mean length of utterance) was calculated to be 5.71. I will not try to show the full analysis of Chaulanda's language, but I will highlight a few of the major goals I developed and discuss how I decided on them.

When I examined Chaulanda's use of questions, using Figures 1.1 and 1.6, I found that she used *what, who,* and *when* questions consistently. She used no *where* questions, no *how* questions, and only two *why* questions. She asked many *intonation* questions, such as "You play basketball?" but no fully formed *yes/no* questions. If Chaulanda were developing ASL, "You play basketball?" would be analyzed as a fully formed *yes/no* question if she raised her eyebrows, put her head down between her shoulders, and tipped her head forward, ASL grammatical markers for *yes/no* questions. She also used no *tag* questions in the language sample. Her MLU placed her well beyond Stage 6, so I had expected her to be consistently using the Stage 2 and 3 forms, using at least a few of the Stage 4 and 5 forms, and perhaps starting to use the later-developing form, tag questions. When I compared her development of questions with other forms on the frameworks, I found a similar pattern. She was consistently using the syntactic and morphologic forms from Stages 2 and 3, but her use of forms beyond Stage 3 was sporadic.

I chose the goals with this pattern of development in mind. Since Chaulanda's stage of language development seemed to be clearly beyond Stage 2, the Stage 3 question form *where* became an important goal and one I would target for classroom emphasis. I also considered it appropriate to add *how* and *why* questions because she was already using a few *why* questions, and *how* questions typically appear in child language at about the same time. My last goal for question forms was *yes/no* questions because this form usually appears next in child language, and Chaulanda gave evidence of being ready to begin using this form through her consistent use of intonation questions. I did not include *tag* questions because at this point they seemed considerably beyond her stage of development. When she began to develop the use of *yes/no* questions, I would probably add tag questions as a goal.

I identified goals for Chaulanda from each of the other categories (Identifier, Descriptor, Verb, Adverb, Negative, and Conjunction) in the same way. At this point in Chaulanda's language development, these goals were all English-specific.

When planning language goals, the teacher first concentrates on the forms from stages earlier than the child's stage of development (as determined from the child's mean length of utterance) that do not appear or do not appear consistently in the language sample. These become the first and most important goals. The next step is to look at the forms in the child's current stage of development that he or she is using inconsistently or not at all. These also become language goals. The final step is to determine which of the forms from the later stages of development would be expected to appear next in the child's language, and these are added as appropriate goals.

If Chaulanda was acquiring ASL as a first language, I would need to use the frameworks a little differently. Instead of looking for the English inflections and word order, I would be looking for the syntactic and morphologic structures in ASL that express the same grammatical intent. For example, when analyzing Chaulanda's language for her use of questions, I would examine the ways she expressed wh- questions, *yes/no* questions, and *tag* questions in ASL, and I would expect these forms to appear in the approximate order presented in the frameworks.

If Chaulanda was acquiring both ASL and English at the same time, it would be important for me to be aware of the possibility that she might mix the languages, utterance to utterance or within the same utterances, by alternating between ASL and English. Research on bilingualism indicates that this mixing is normal. In assessing her language, I would need to analyze the ASL features and English features within each utterance. The language goals I created for Chaulanda would include goals for ASL and goals for English.

If Chaulanda was exposed to incomplete models of English or ASL, she might produce a mix of English, ASL, home signs, and gestures. I would, first of all, need to analyze the English features and ASL features she expressed and use this analysis to develop appropriate goals in both English and ASL. Second, I would look at Chaulanda's home signs and gestures in terms of what she was trying to express semantically and pragmatically. The goals for syntax that I chose for Chaulanda would include forms in ASL and English that are used to express these meanings and functions that Chaulanda was already expressing in her home signs and gestures.

Given that Chaulanda did not interact with individuals using ASL, she could not be expected to have acquired ASL, so I did not use the ASL acquisition checklist (Figure 1.11). Although many of her signs were conceptual in nature, they did not represent the linguistic manifestations of ASL. Without meaningful, conversational interactions with individuals fluent in ASL, Chaulanda was no more likely to acquire ASL than the hearing children in ancient Egypt would acquire Egyptian when no one used that language with them. It might be argued that there are features of ASL in sign systems used simultaneously with English, and if I had used the ASL acquisition checklist, I may have noted that Chaulanda was, indeed, using some ASL markers. Then the teacher could have helped Chaulanda build on these emerging linguistic features. Certainly, if Chaulanda begins to associate with deaf peers and adults who use ASL, her future teachers will want to analyze her acquisition of ASL and develop appropriate ASL goals for her.

Once I had analyzed Chaulanda's syntactic and morphologic development and created goals for these areas, I analyzed her semantic development. I used Figure 1.2 to determine which semantic categories she used with consistency and which she used inconsistently or not at all. When I identified semantic goals for her, I included not only those categories she used inconsistently, such as *time,* and those she seemed ready to begin using, such as *mood,* but I also included goals related to vocabulary growth within the categories she was already expressing.

When I analyzed Chaulanda's development of language use, I found she demonstrated many skills appropriate to her age and language development level. One of the goals I identified was in the area of conversational turn-taking. Chaulanda was able to participate in short conversational turns but had some difficulty giving more than brief responses to her conversational partner. I included extended turn-taking as an appropriate goal, realizing also that this particular goal would provide the teacher an instructional context (that is, conversational role-playing) for many of Chaulanda's syntactic, morphologic, and semantic goals.

The goals for Chaulanda that I have discussed represent just a few of the ones identified for her. I used information from the other sources in the assessment, such as standardized test results, to modify and extend the goals initially identified through the language sample.

Final Comments

Using a model of language acquisition based on what is currently known about normal language development, the language abilities of a child who is deaf can be analyzed and described. Individual language goals are based on the discrepancies found between forms, meanings, and uses currently appearing in the child's language with those expected to appear according to the child's language development stage. These individual language goals can include both English and ASL. Language goals can then be used to provide a learning environment that enhances the child's cognitive capacity to create for him- or herself a deep-level, abstract, and complex language or languages. In the next several chapters, I will be describing aspects of this learning environment.

Suggested Readings

Garton, A., & Pratt, C. (1998). *Learning to be literate* (2nd ed.). Oxford, England: Basil Blackwell.

Gleason, J. B. (1997). *The development of language* (4th ed.). Boston: Allyn and Bacon.

Salvia, J., & Ysseldyke, J. E. (1998). *Assessment* (7th ed.). Boston: Houghton Mifflin.

Sternberg, M. L. A. (1998). *American sign language dictionary.* New York: HarperCollins.

Taylor, R. L. (1997). *Assessment of exceptional students* (4th ed.). Boston: Allyn and Bacon.

Valli, C., & Lucas, C. (1995). *Linguistics of American Sign Language* (2nd ed.). Washington, DC: Gallaudet University.

CHAPTER

2

Language Development within the Classroom Setting

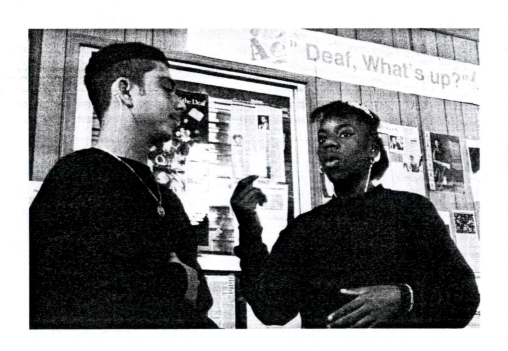

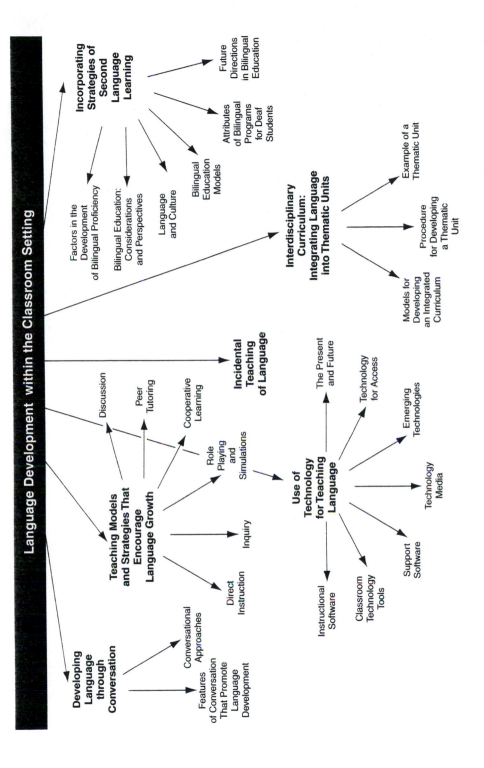

Language Development within the Classroom Setting

Incorporating Strategies of Second Language Learning
- Factors in the Development of Bilingual Proficiency
- Bilingual Education: Considerations and Perspectives
- Language and Culture
- Bilingual Education Models
- Attributes of Bilingual Programs for Deaf Students
- Future Directions in Bilingual Education

Interdisciplinary Curriculum: Integrating Language into Thematic Units
- Models for Developing an Integrated Curriculum
- Procedure for Developing a Thematic Unit
- Example of a Thematic Unit

Incidental Teaching of Language

Teaching Models and Strategies That Encourage Language Growth
- Discussion
- Peer Tutoring
- Cooperative Learning
- Role Playing and Simulations
- Inquiry
- Direct Instruction

Use of Technology for Teaching Language
- The Present and Future
- Technology for Access
- Emerging Technologies
- Technology Media
- Support Software
- Classroom Technology Tools
- Instructional Software

Developing Language through Conversation
- Conversational Approaches
- Features of Conversation That Promote Language Development

47

The teacher of deaf youngsters who has taken the time to assess each student's current language abilities is confronted with the question of how to encourage each child's continued language development. In the past, teaching methods developed for use with youngsters who are deaf relied heavily on the notion that their language needed to be straightened out. Teachers were therefore advised to use strategies that focused almost exclusively on English syntax, such as the Fitzgerald Key (Fitzgerald, 1949; Pugh, 1955) and Apple Tree (Caniglia, Cole, Howard, Krohn, & Rice, 1975). (See McAnally, Rose, and Quigley, 1998, for a thorough description of traditional language methods.)

Current knowledge of language acquisition has led to dramatic changes in the way language instruction in the classroom is viewed. It is widely recognized that labeling and drilling the deaf child on surface structure features has no lasting or significant influence on the child's internalization of the language itself, whether that language is English or ASL. The alternative is to create an environment replete with opportunities to interact with others using the language for meaningful communication. As Harrison, Layton, and Taylor (1987) noted, "developmental language programs for deaf children must be constructed around the notion that the acquisition of language and the concurrent understanding of the function of language occur through topical communicative exchanges which are the product of shared activities" (p. 230).

In this chapter, I will discuss language as a curricular foundation on which the full school day is built and not as a subject area that comprises one class period per day. Hopefully, this chapter will help the reader take the language goals that he or she carefully and explicitly developed for each child and embed those goals within a myriad of daily learning experiences.

The first approach I will discuss is conversation because it should be the foundation of any language program for deaf children. I will also present specific teaching models and strategies that encourage language growth, strategies that incorporate language goals incidentally in learning activities, approaches that develop an interdisciplinary curriculum linking language to subject areas, and strategies that promote second language learning.

Developing Language through Conversation

Two lines of reasoning support the use of conversational strategies for teaching language to children who are deaf. First, because language develops within conversational contexts, strategies that come as close as possible to replicating natural conversational interactions between parent and child and child and child can provide deaf children with an authentic environment for learning language (Clarke, 1983; Clarke & Stewart, 1986; Stone, 1988).

Second, because children who are deaf often demonstrate problems in developing conversational competence, language teaching strategies that incorporate conversational skills are needed by many deaf children (Griffith, Johnson, & Dastoli, 1985; Newton, 1985; Weiss, 1986). Based on these two lines of reasoning, one could make the observation, as Holdgrafer (1987) did, that "in effect, conversation is a goal of language intervention as well as a general strategy for teaching language" (p. 71). Furthermore, for Kretschmer and Kretschmer (1995), language instruction best takes place in communication-based classrooms where the goals are "conversations that are comprehensible, meaningful, interesting, and relevant to children and conversations that are focused not on learning about language but on learning language and content through language" (p. 14).

Features of Conversation That Promote Language Development

Conversation has been defined as "the initiation and maintenance of topics while interchanging reciprocal roles of speaker and listener in smooth and coordinated turn-taking" (Holdgrafer, 1987, p. 71). Given that conversation is crucial to language development, it is important to ask if certain specific features of conversation are considered particularly critical and, therefore, should be integrated into a conversational teaching strategy.

Prinz and Masin (1985) found that adult recasting of deaf children's utterances facilitated their language development. Prinz and Masin defined *recasting* as a particular kind of adult response to a child's preceding utterance. Recasting occurs when the adult response is signed or spoken in a different syntactic structure than the child just used while maintaining the central meaning expressed by the child.

Prinz and Masin conducted their investigation with six children from nine months to six years of age at the outset of the study. Two children had deaf parents who primarily used ASL in the home, and the other children had hearing parents who used manually coded English or pidgin sign. Their teachers used pidgin sign, which the authors described as "combining semantic and syntactic aspects of both ASL and signed English" (p. 360). Parents and teachers were given training on how to recast the children's utterances into the specific syntactic structures that the researchers had targeted. The study lasted for five months, and during that time each child received at least twenty hours of intervention. Prinz and Masin found that the targeted syntactic–semantic structures in ASL and English appeared in the spontaneous communication of the children in the study. The implication of this finding is that recasting is one of the conversational features between adult and child that supports language development.

Wood and associates (Wood & Wood, 1984; Wood, Wood, Griffiths, Howarth, & Howarth, 1982) found that several conversational features worked in combination to encourage deaf children to be conversational partners with their teachers. Personal contributions, in the form of comments or statements, and phatics (phrases such as "Oh, that's interesting" and "I see," head nodding in response to the child's contribution, or repeating the child's comment) by the teacher resulted in greater conversational participation, elaborated answers, and greater asking of questions by the child. Asking questions, particularly stringing questions together, and requiring the child to repeat phrases resulted in little spontaneous conversational participation by the child.

Wood and associates also found, however, that simply asking teachers to become more responsive to the deaf children's responses produced better conversations but not the lively or purposeful discussions the researchers had observed in other classrooms because the teachers these researchers observed had some difficulty always understanding the children's meaning. Wood and associates concluded:

> [A] very great strain is put on the teacher's conversational skills as she struggles to interpret short, ambiguous utterances. If she goes straight into repair to "sort things out," she may be increasing the problems facing both her and the child. In such a situation it is perhaps not surprising that a teacher's reaction to such a high degree of uncertainty may be to keep control through questioning whence she can judge the appropriateness of the child's responses. (p. 61)

Luetke–Stahlman (1993) described a number of strategies that teachers have used successfully with hearing children, yet she could find no studies using these strategies with deaf children. She divided these strategies into two categories— *environmental* and *linguistic*. Environmental strategies include setting up the physical environment so that the child has a need to use language, making sure that the child has opportunities to socially interact both verbally and nonverbally, and identifying moments in which the child is motivated to use language. Linguistic strategies include providing a language model that is somewhat more complex than the language the deaf child currently produces, asking questions that encourage the child to use targeted grammatical forms, expanding and recasting the child's utterances in conversation, engaging in self-talk so that the child can observe the adult using language, and adding new vocabulary and explanations when responding to the child.

Conversational Approaches

Several conversational approaches have been used with children who are deaf. With the first approach, the teacher uses naturally occurring opportunities during the school day to have conversations with the children. Clarke and Stewart (1986) suggested that teachers of deaf children exploit opportunities for short and meaningful conversations with individual children throughout the school day and orchestrate opportunities for longer conversations with small groups of children.

Rogers, Perrin, and Waller (1987) found that naturally occurring opportunities for conversation are the result of a special kind of relationship between teachers and students. They observed that children become enthusiastic conversational partners over time when their teachers consistently respond with interest to the topics they initiate, encourage them to share their thoughts, and allow them time to complete what they wanted to discuss without interruption.

The second approach the teacher can use is the one developed by Stone (1988) for use with children who are deaf. At the center of this approach are *conversational scenarios*. Conversational scenarios are "role-playing situations which contain appropriate dialogue. They are planned by the teacher and presented to the child in such a way that a realistic conversation takes place between teacher and child. The child's part in the conversation requires the use of a specific conversational skill which has not been mastered. Acquiring this skill is the teacher's objective" (p. 28).

Unlike the first approach in which the teacher capitalizes on opportunities during the school day to engage the children in conversation, Stone's approach requires careful planning and a setting aside of time for the scenarios to be role-played. There are five essential elements to any scenario:

1. The situation and topic are familiar to the student.
2. The teacher makes sure that the student understands the situation before beginning.
3. As the dialogue proceeds, there is a conversational need for the targeted conversational skill to arise.
4. The teacher does not tell the child what to say, rather the situation and conversation bring about a need for use of the targeted skill.
5. The situation and conversation are carried to a logical conclusion. (Stone, 1988, p. 29)

Scenarios begin with the teacher "setting the stage." For example, the teacher might provide the following description to a child who is working on the skill "initiating a conversation":

> Let's pretend that your grandmother came for a visit last weekend. She took you to the zoo. On Monday, you come to school and tell your friend Valorie about it. I'll be Valorie and you be yourself.

The teacher and child then role-play the scenario. But what happens when the child makes a mistake? Stone considered it important that the teacher intervene only when the mistake is related to the specific skill targeted for the scenario. Errors involving other conversational objectives can be noted by the teacher for future scenarios. But when the mistake is pertinent to the scenario's objective, the teacher should intervene. The following four intervention strategies are recommended by Stone:

1. *Teacher Clarification.* In this strategy, the teacher offers a statement that clarifies what the child just expressed. The following dialogue is one example of teacher clarification. The teacher and student are role-playing the scenario just described; the teacher is the friend, Valorie, and the student is herself, Lillian. Lillian is a deaf child who communicates orally in spoken English.

LILLIAN: Hi, Valorie.

VALORIE: Hi, Lillian.

LILLIAN: I saw different animals at the zoo with my grandma.

VALORIE: (Pauses, looks confused, then smiles). Oh, you mean your grandma visited and took you to the zoo?

LILLIAN: Yes. My grandma visited, and she took me to the zoo.

2. *Role Switching.* In this strategy, the teacher and student switch roles so that the teacher can demonstrate the conversational skill. They then switch back to their original roles. Using the same scenario, role switching might look like this:

> **TEACHER:** Let's switch. I'll be Lillian and you be Valorie.
>
> **TEACHER (as Lillian):** Hi, Valorie.
>
> **CHILD (as friend):** Hi, Lillian.
>
> **TEACHER:** My grandma visited last weekend. She took me to the zoo.
>
> **CHILD:** Neat.
>
> **TEACHER:** Okay. Let's switch back. You be yourself, and I'll be Valorie.

3. *Requesting Clarification.* In this strategy, the teacher makes a comment or looks at the child in a way that makes it obvious to the child that his or her utterance was not appropriate. The teacher then pauses, giving the child time to clarify it. In the scenario, instead of using teacher clarification or role switching, the teacher could have used requesting clarification in the following way:

> **LILLIAN (the child):** Hi, Valorie.
>
> **VALORIE (the teacher):** Hi, Lillian.
>
> **LILLIAN:** I saw different animals at the zoo with my grandma.
>
> **VALORIE:** Excuse me? What did you say?
>
> **LILLIAN:** My grandma visited. She took me to the zoo.
>
> **VALORIE:** Oh, your grandma visited. That's neat. Tell me what you saw at the zoo.

4. *Prompt.* This strategy is used in conjunction with role switching. The difference is that the teacher steps out of the role play and points out to the child the place in the conversation where the child is making a mistake. Using the scenario with Lillian and Valorie, prompting would look like this:

> **LILLIAN (the child):** Hi, Valorie.
>
> **VALORIE (the teacher):** Hi, Lillian.
>
> **LILLIAN:** I saw different animals at the zoo with my grandma.
>
> **TEACHER:** That was ok, but there's another way to say it. Let's switch. I'll be you, and you be Valorie.
>
> **TEACHER (as Lillian):** My grandma visited last weekend. She took me to the zoo.
>
> **CHILD (as Valorie):** Neat.
>
> **TEACHER (as Lillian):** Okay. Let's switch back.

Role switching and prompting obviously interrupt the flow of the conversation, and Stone recommended they be used only when the other two strategies do not give sufficient feedback to the child.

A third conversational approach is the use of *scripts*. As described by Whitesell and Klein (1995), scripts "are generic, contextualized language structures that people use in their daily lives. Scripts capture a culture's knowledge and the typical communication that occurs in ordinary life situations (e.g., in a restaurant, in a doctor's office, or at a birthday party)" (p. 118). The script framework that Whitesell and Klein used with their deaf and hard of hearing students included the following components: scenes with action variables that describe the things that the people will do, typical roles, typical props, and scripted language. They found it valuable to add activities before and after script enactments to provide background knowledge and to learn what interested the children. For example, they found that viewing a film or sharing books was particularly helpful as well as motivating.

Instructional conversations are a fourth approach. Perez (1996) maintained that there is an important difference between social and instructional conversations. Instructional conversations focus on concepts and academic content; the teacher creates the context or the activity for the conversation, and the child is an equal partner in topic development and discussion. Perez used this approach with hearing students learning English as a second language and found that "through repeated instructional conversations around concrete, class-selected activities, the children explored the relationship between their prior experiences and their developing understandings, their roles within the school groups and their families, and between their developing languages" (p. 180).

A combination of naturally occurring conversations with targeted language goals, or *scaffolded conversation*, is a fifth approach. In a scaffolded conversation, the teacher is aware of the child's language goals and provides opportunities within the conversation to support the child's use of particular structures, meanings, and uses. The scaffold is a support structure, temporary in nature, that assists the child in using new forms and meanings. Skarakis-Doyle and Murphy (1996) used this approach with a five-year-old deaf child and found that it facilitated her language acquisition.

Teaching Models and Strategies That Encourage Language Growth

The terms *model* and *method*, often used interchangeably in the literature on teaching, both refer to a design for a particular kind of teaching activity. The design is described in terms of its theoretical underpinnings, goals, procedures, and strategies for carrying it out. The term *model* implies that the description is a somewhat idealized version that is open to interpretation. The term *method* implies that the description is actually a prescription to be followed relatively closely.

I have chosen to use the word *model* because I believe that the terminology should emphasize the teacher's self-efficacy, flexibility, and reason. I agree with McNergney, Lloyd, Mintz, and Moore (1988), who wrote that a teacher is a professional "who decides how to apply his or her specialized knowledge and skills to solve particular problems and does so with a reasonably high degree of self-determination" (p. 37).

In this section, several models will be described. The reader will be familiar with most, if not all, of these models from course work in educational psychology and methods of teaching school subjects. The purpose of discussing these models is neither to repeat the information in those courses nor to discuss the research supporting or not supporting the effectiveness of any model for teaching subject matter and for encouraging the development of thinking skills. The purpose, instead, is to present these models in light of how well each one can encourage the development of language in children who are deaf. These content area instructional models can be used simultaneously to teach content and language. As such, they reflect an interdisciplinary approach to instruction that I discuss in detail later in this chapter.

Teaching strategies will also be discussed with the same purpose in mind. A *strategy* is a careful plan for meeting teaching objectives and overcoming obstacles. According to this definition, a number of strategies are used within any teaching model.

The models and strategies discussed here are either commonly used or are relatively new models or strategies that offer exciting opportunities for language development. The reader can use these particular models and strategies as seeds for creating a mixed garden of classroom learning activities. As Joyce (1987) observed, "A highly skilled performance in teaching blends the variety of models appropriately and embellishes them. Master teachers create new models of teaching and test them in the course of their work, drawing on the models of others for ideas that are combined in various ways" (p. 420).

For each of the models, actual scenarios of teaching lessons are provided. Note that for the purpose of readability, dialogue in all scenarios is written in English although many of the teachers and youngsters use ASL or pidgin sign. Indeed, all of these models can be used to encourage the development of both ASL and English. Whether the teacher uses ASL, spoken English, simultaneous speech and sign, or pidgin sign with or without voice, hopefully the teacher recognizes the importance of providing a consistent language model to the child who is deaf.

Direct Instruction

The term *direct instruction* has come to have both a broad and a narrow definition. In the broadest sense, direct instruction is any form of structured teaching. Gersten, Woodward, and Darch (1986) referred to this definition of direct instruction as little "d" little "i." When defined narrowly, as Direct Instruction with big "d" big "i," it consists of the following features:

1. Teach an explicit step-by-step strategy. (When this is not possible or necessary, model effective performance.)
2. Develop mastery at each step in the process.
3. Develop strategy (or process) corrections for student errors.
4. Gradually fade from teacher-directed activities toward independent work.
5. Use adequate, systematic practice with a range of examples.
6. Use cumulative review. (p. 19)

For some teachers, direct instruction denotes the even narrower definition of scripted lessons developed for the commercially available DISTAR programs in reading, math, and language.

As a teaching model, the definition developed by Baumann (1988a) is appropriate. According to Baumann, in direct instruction the teacher tells, shows, models, demonstrates, and explains the skills, processes, and strategies to be learned. What are the opportunities for language development within a direct instruction lesson? On one level, it would appear that direct instruction provides a lot of opportunity for receptive language but limited opportunity for expressive language. After all, the teacher dominates the interaction between teacher and child, and virtually no child-to-child interaction is built into this model. However, providing frequent student opportunity to respond is a vital component of the model. Although responses can be brief, teachers of deaf youngsters with language goals in mind can encourage responses that require the youngsters to express themselves in elaborated ways. The following scenario illustrates some of the ways that language development can be nurtured within a teaching lesson implementing a direct instruction model.

SCENARIO

In a self-contained classroom for deaf and hard of hearing students, Ms. Dimitrov was teaching a lesson on state capitals to a group of fifth grade students who used simultaneous communication in sign and spoken English. She began by orienting the students to the topic.

MS. DIMITROV: What have we been discussing in social studies?

JILL: United States.

MS. DIMITROV: Tell me more. What about the United States?

JILL: We learned about the fifty states . . . different states.

MS. DIMITROV: Right, we've discussed the names of the fifty states and where they are on a map. What else did we learn?

JANE: Parts of the country. You know.

MS. DIMITROV: I do? Tell me what you know. Tell me about parts of the country.

JANE: You mean like New England, like that?

MS. DIMITROV: Yes.

JANE: Okay. Well, there is New England states. They're in the northeast part of the United States. I think Maine, Vermont, New Hampshire, Massachusetts, Rhode Island, Connecticut . . .

This orientation phase went on a bit longer while Ms. Dimitrov activated the youngsters' background knowledge by reviewing previous learning. She could have asked closed questions, questions requiring one- or two-word answers, and accomplished this phase in less time. But by asking open-ended questions, questions requiring elaborated answers, and expanding on the children's responses, she combined her content goals with language goals. After she obtained answers from all four youngsters, she continued her introduction of the lesson by telling the students what they would be learning that day.

MS. DIMITROV: Today we'll learn something new about the states. We'll be learning about state capitals. Here's a map of the United States. The capital is marked with a star. Sometimes the capital is the biggest city in the state. Sometimes it's the most well-known city. But sometimes it's a small city. Let's start with Oregon. The capital of Oregon is Salem. Here it is on the map. Jodi, what's the capital of Oregon?

JODI: Salem.

Ms. Dimitrov continued the presentation phase of the lesson by explaining the new information, using the map as a visual representation of the information, and frequently checking for understanding. But because Ms. Dimitrov was just as interested in the children's language development as she was in their subject matter knowledge, she modified her procedure sometimes and asked questions requiring longer responses and discussions between students. These responses encouraged particular syntactic forms, semantic categories, and functions that were language goals for individual children.

MS. DIMITROV: Jack, you said the capital of Washington is Olympia. But I think Seattle is the biggest city in Washington.

JACK: I think Seattle is bigger than Olympia.

MS. DIMITROV: I think so, too. But why is Olympia the capital?

JACK: Sometimes the capital is a small city.

JODI: Olympia is close to Seattle.

JANE: Maybe the capital is a small city. But near a big city.

MS. DIMITROV: Look at the ones we already found on the map. Tell me about them.

JACK: Salem is a small city. But near Portland. Sacramento is a small city. Near San Francisco.

JILL: No it's not. Sacramento is a big city.

JACK: Not big like San Francisco . . .

When Ms. Dimitrov finished presenting ten state capitals in this way, she provided the students with practice on the new information.

> MS. DIMITROV: Take out your white boards and markers. I'll fingerspell the name of the state. You write the capital. When I give the signal, hold up your board. . . .

When the students completed this activity, Ms. Dimitrov gave each one a blank map of the United States. She then listed ten states on the chalkboard. For seatwork, the students were supposed to write the names of the capitals in the appropriate places on their individual maps.

During the practice phases, first guided practice and later independent practice, Ms. Dimitrov recognized that there was less opportunity to incorporate language goals. But whenever the chance arose, she encouraged the youngsters to discuss the characteristics of the state capitals as well as to memorize their names, thus nurturing the development of semantic categories such as attribution and causality and functions such as description and compare/contrast.

Inquiry

As a model of teaching, *inquiry* provides students with a learning experience similar to the kind of investigation scholars and scientists engage in when they are exploring phenomena, generating principles and theories, and organizing knowledge (Joyce & Weil, 1996). It is generally agreed that inquiry involves six major steps:

1. *Identifying and Defining the Problem.* Often this step involves generating a question. When the teacher presents the students with a puzzling occurrence, Orlich and associates (1998) refer to the model as guided inductive inquiry. In guided inquiry, the teacher plays "the key role in asking the questions, prompting the responses, and structuring the materials and situations" (p. 304). In unguided inquiry, the teacher allows the students to think of their own questions and situ-ations, and the students take "responsibility for examining data, objects, and events. Because the teacher's role is minimized, the students' activity increases" (p. 304). Of course, the increased student activity also encourages increased student language interaction.

2. *Forming Hypotheses.* In this step, the students propose educated guesses regarding the answer to the question they generated in step 1. They develop a statement of research objectives.

3. *Gathering Data.* This step can involve experimentation, reading, surveying others, or other methods of collecting evidence relevant to the problem.

4. *Analyzing and Interpreting Data.* In this step, the students examine the data, organize it in a way that makes sense, and use it to test their hypotheses.

5. *Formulating Conclusions and Making Generalizations.* Based on their results, the students determine whether the hypotheses are supported or not. They then construct an explanation and, if possible, generalize their results to other situations or events.

6. *Replicating.* This step involves obtaining new data which may lead the students to revise their conclusions.

A seventh step in the inquiry model is added by some authors. Joyce and Weil (1996) call this step an *analysis of the inquiry process*. Pasch, Moody, and Langer (1995) describe this step as one in which the students examine, analyze, and discuss their own thinking processes.

What are the opportunities for language development within an inquiry lesson? Inquiry clearly provides abundant opportunity for receptive and expressive language not only between the teacher and the students but also among the students. The following scenario demonstrates some of the ways that an inquiry lesson can incorporate language goals.

SCENARIO

Ms. Parmelee has been teaching a unit on the physical properties of matter to a class of high school juniors, some using ASL and some using simultaneous communication, at the state school for the deaf. For today, she planned an inquiry lesson on the concept of specific gravity.

> **MS. PARMELEE:**   I brought in two cans of pop, one diet and one regular. I have two containers of water. I'm going to drop a can into each container of water. Watch carefully . . .

Ms. Parmelee dropped the cans into the water and much to the surprise of her class, one can floated and one can sank.

> **MS. PARMELEE:**   Do you have any questions?
>
> **MINNIE:**   Why did one can float and one can sink?
>
> **ANNA:**   Are they different? What's different?
>
> **GEORGE:**   One is diet. Why did the diet pop float? Look at the weight on the can.
>
> **MS. PARMELEE:**   They're both twelve ounces.
>
> **ALPHONSE:**   Let me hold them. Okay. They look the same size. Something's wrong . . .

Ms. Parmelee let them discuss the possibilities a few more minutes and then she wrote "Problem" and "Question" on the overhead projector.

> **MS. PARMELEE:**   What's our problem?
>
> **ANNA:**   Two cans of pop look the same but one floats and one sinks in water.
>
> **MS. PARMELEE:**   What question do we want to answer?

GEORGE: Why does the diet pop float and the regular pop sink in water?. . .

Ms. Parmelee wrote "Hypothesis" under George's question.

MS. PARMELEE: We've talked about hypothesis before. What hypothesis do you want to make?

ALPHONSE: My hypothesis is I think that the aluminum for the diet can is less than the aluminum for the regular can.

MINNIE: But they weigh the same.

ALPHONSE: Maybe not. The weight on the can is the pop. It tells how much pop is inside.

MINNIE: Okay. I agree. That's my hypothesis, too.

ANNA: My hypothesis is that the regular pop has sugar in it so it sinks. The diet pop has no sugar so it floats.

ALPHONSE: But diet pop has something in it.

GEORGE: I don't remember the name but it's not the same as sugar.

ANNA: Okay. Wait a second. My hypothesis is that the regular pop has sugar in it so it sinks. The diet pop has that weird name in it but it's not so much inside. There's less inside. So it floats.

GEORGE: I have the same hypothesis as Anna.

MS. PARMELEE: How do we find the answer to our question?

MINNIE: We need a scale. I want to weigh the two cans.

ANNA: I think we need to get some sugar and some of the other sweetener. Then we can compare them. Like how much you need to make a drink sweet . . .

The students developed several more ideas and then gathered the materials they needed. During the experiments, they discussed their findings. They ultimately figured out that aspartame, an artificial sweetener, weighs less than sugar.

Throughout this lesson, Ms. Parmelee encouraged the youngsters to discuss their questions and possible solutions and to pay careful attention to what the other students were contributing to the discussion. Sometimes she rephrased a statement or expanded a comment, not only to provide clarification or further information but also to emphasize specific language goals regarding syntax, semantics, and use. Because she had analyzed each student's language earlier in the year, she had these goals in mind and was able to encourage the development of particular language features within the context of this science discussion. For example, she was able to embed into the dialogue several indefinite pronouns and adverbial clauses, the semantic categories epistemic and antithesis, and the heuristic functions of problem solving, probing, and predicting, which were language goals for several youngsters in the class.

Role Playing and Simulations

In *role playing* and *simulations,* students recreate and act out a problem, event, or situation. Although simulations are designed to reflect reality, they are safe for the children who participate (Orlich et al., 1998; Rockler, 1988).

Role playing and simulations have their roots in the pretend play of young children. Yawkey and Hrncir (1983) noted that "pretend play provides a basis for using objects and situations 'as if' they are other things" (p. 265). These two researchers found that for the preschool child, imaginative play serves an important function in language development. They observed four links between role playing and language development:

1. Role playing encourages the use of various forms of communication because "the child uses language to become the chief observer, participator, and actor" (p. 265).

2. Role playing encourages the development of social language because in pretend play children re-enact social situations from their own world. They learn to express not only many of the functions of language, such as the instrumental and interactional, but also the "words flowing among and between the child actors expand social relationships with others" (p. 266).

3. Role playing encourages creative expression because the activity itself is free of real-world constraints. Thus, children can use a box for a car and describe to one another the features of the car.

4. Role playing encourages concentration. Yawkey and Hrncir found that children's increased concentration and attention to the actions, situations, and ideas they developed in their pretend play required extended communication among themselves.

Role playing in preschool and kindergarten classrooms is usually used spontaneously by the children rather than planned by the teacher. However, some children rarely engage in role playing. Levy, Schaefer, and Phelps (1986) conducted a study in which they encouraged role playing by all the children in a preschool classroom by (a) centering the curriculum around a common theme, (b) stocking the housekeeping center with props that supported the theme and having the teacher explain the use of the props to the children, and (c) having the teacher model appropriate play behaviors by assuming one of the roles at first and later facilitating the children's play within the housekeeping center.

Levy and her associates found that the language of the boys in the study increased significantly beyond the growth that would be predicted through maturation alone. The lack of significant difference in the girls' language was explained by the investigators' observation that before intervention, the children who engaged in pretend play in the housekeeping center were primarily girls and rarely boys. The implication of this finding is that teachers can create an atmosphere conducive for pretend play among children who would not otherwise normally engage in pretend play and that, furthermore, the pretend play for these children encourages the development of their language.

When used as a model of teaching for children beyond the kindergarten level, role playing consists of nine basic steps:

1. The teacher introduces the problem and explains role playing.
2. The teacher analyzes and assigns the roles.
3. The teacher decides how the situation will be acted out.
4. Concurrent with the third step, which involves the actors, is the fourth step, which involves the observers. In this step, the observers determine what they will look for during the role play.
5. The problem is actually enacted.
6. The simulation is discussed, analyzed, and critiqued. This step also involves decisions regarding the next simulation.
7. Step 7 combines and repeats steps 5 and 6, using new participants and revised action. This step can be repeated several times.
8. All the students participate in a discussion of the problem and make plans for ways they can solve similar problem situations in their own lives.

What are the opportunities for language development within a role-playing and simulation lesson? The discussions that take place prior to and after the simulations and the actual role play itself obviously provide much opportunity for the use of expressive and receptive language. The following lesson provides some of the ways that role playing and simulations can incorporate language goals.

SCENARIO

Mr. Esch has been spending quite a lot of time discussing feelings with his class of seventh grade students at the state school for the deaf. He has decided to try a role-playing lesson on two emotions with which all of the youngsters are having difficulty. For this lesson, Mr. Esch uses ASL and expects the students to use ASL.

MR. ESCH:　We've been talking about different emotions. What are some of the feelings we've discussed?

RONI:　One was jealousy.

JANET:　A different one was disappointment.

ROSITA:　I think we talked about frustration.

MR. ESCH:　Right. Today I want to discuss anger . . .

Mr. Esch went on to ask the students what anger meant to them, what situations made them angry, and how they handled their anger. Then he set the stage for the role playing.

MR. ESCH: I've noticed that when one of you gets angry, it is hard on you, and it's hard on the people around you. You need to figure out how to control your own anger, and you also need to figure out how to deal with someone else's anger. We can discuss our feelings, and then you know in your head how you're supposed to behave. But when something makes you mad, you forget and just blow up. Another way is to role-play. In a role play, each person takes a role, pretends the situation is real, and practices how to behave in the situation. Patrick, what's a role play?

PATRICK: I don't know.

MR. ESCH: Roni?

RONI: Role play means that we make believe a situation that makes us angry. Then we try not to blow up.

MR. ESCH: Right. You practice how to react to the situation. For the first role play, I'll be one person, and I need one other person. Patrick? Okay. Patrick and I will decide on a situation. But the rest of you have an important role, too. You need to watch us carefully and figure out if our behavior is helping or hurting. These are the two emotions we're working on . . .

Mr. Esch wrote "Handling My Own Anger" and "Dealing with Someone Else's Anger" on the chalkboard. Then he and Patrick stepped outside the classroom and decided on a simulation. Mr. Esch came into the room, sat in a chair, and pretended to write. Patrick walked up to him.

PATRICK: Mr. Esch. I want to talk with you about my test.

MR. ESCH: I'm very disappointed, Patrick. You didn't study and got an F.

PATRICK: (Becoming angry) I tried to study, but I didn't understand the math. It's not fair. I missed two days of class.

MR. ESCH: (Becoming angry) If you didn't understand the math, you should have come to see me. You have to take responsibility.

PATRICK: (Very angry) It's not my fault. (He crumples the test paper and throws it in the trash. Then he stomps out of the room.)

MR. ESCH: Okay. That's the end of the role play. What do you think?

JANET: Was that a real situation?

PATRICK: It happened one time to me. Not with Mr. Esch.

JANET: Both of you got mad.

MR. ESCH: What went wrong?

ROSITA: First, I think you made Patrick mad because you said he didn't study. But he did. He didn't understand the math. But he did try.

MR. ESCH: That's a good point. And then Patrick got mad.

RONI: I noticed that Patrick got mad. Then you got mad. Then Patrick got madder.

MR. ESCH: What would be a better way to behave?

PATRICK: I don't know. Maybe I could explain more. Why I didn't understand the math.

MR. ESCH: That would probably help. I felt you were blaming me.

ROSITA: Take responsibility for yourself.

MR. ESCH: (Pointing to the chalkboard) We've talked about "Handling My Own Anger." But how did I deal with Patrick's anger?

JANET: Not good. You got angry.

MR. ESCH: What would be a better way to behave?

ROSITA: I think you should have explained and not got angry.

MR. ESCH: Rosita, you can be Mr. Esch in the next role play. Then you can show how Mr. Esch should behave. Who wants to be Patrick?. . .

The students complete two more simulations, alternating roles and trying out different solutions. After the last simulation, they discussed situations in their own lives and how they could handle them in the future.

The discussions inherent in this teaching model provide the same opportunities for infusing language goals as other models in which discussion is used. The actual role play itself can provide the teacher with a fairly structured setting for encouraging the appearance of particular language features. Even though the simulation is not scripted, by setting the stage for the role play, the teacher can make it necessary for the players to use specific syntactic forms, semantic categories, and language functions. For example, if Mr. Esch asks Patrick during the role play, "What will you do for the next test?" Patrick is encouraged to use a verb form expressing future tense, to express time and mood semantically, and to use the heuristic function.

Cooperative Learning

Cooperative learning involves a set of teaching strategies that are designed to structure student-to-student interaction in the classroom in a way that fosters cooperation rather than competition or individualization. In every classroom, learning goals are established. How students view these learning goals marks the difference between competitive learning, individualized learning, and cooperative learning.

In writing about cooperative learning in general education classrooms with special needs students, Johnson and Johnson (1986) noted that in competitive learning, the goals can be achieved by one or only a few students, so some students work hard to do better than the others in the class and some work relatively little because they feel they have no chance at all. In individualized learning, students work in isolation to achieve learning goals that have no relationship to the goals of anyone else in the class. In cooperative learning, the goals are shared by classmates, and they can only be accomplished if everyone works equally hard.

Cooperative learning looks like traditional group work, but cooperative learning is distinguished by the following essential elements, according to Johnson, Johnson, and Holubec (1993):

1. *Positive Interdependence.* In cooperative learning, group work is structured so that students need each other to complete the group's task. In traditional group work, one member can do most of the work and make most of the decisions, and some members can do relatively little. In cooperative learning, the performance of each group member is the concern of every group member, and responsibility for leading the group is shared.

2. *Face-to-Face Interaction.* In cooperative learning, students must interact with one another. In traditional group work, youngsters in the same group can work on separate parts of a project and never interact with other members of the group.

3. *Individual Accountability.* In cooperative learning, every member of the group is responsible for learning the information at a level of mastery appropriate to the individual student. In traditional group work, only the final product is assessed, and individual students are not held accountable for how much they contributed or for how much they learned.

4. *Interpersonal and Small-Group Skills and Group Processing.* In cooperative learning, the social skills needed to work harmoniously with others in a group are taught by the teacher, and the students are given opportunities to analyze how effectively they are using these skills to work together. In traditional group work, it is assumed that students already know how to work with others.

What are the opportunities for language development when using cooperative learning strategies? The face-to-face interaction essential to cooperative learning provides extensive opportunity to use language expressively and receptively with peers. The following lesson illustrates how language goals can be incorporated within cooperative learning.

SCENARIO

In a public school classroom, Ms. Twiss teaches a multiage group of elementary-level students who are deaf or hard of hearing. The students communicate simultaneously in sign and spoken English. For the science unit on animal species, she decided to divide the class into groups of three and assign one species to each group. She set up the groups heterogeneously so that within any group at least one student was at a lower ability level and at least one was at a higher ability level.

She developed one set of questions and discussed the questions with the whole class. She gave each student material about the species written at a level that the student could read independently. For one child, this meant that the material was largely in picture form. Ms. Twiss then assigned roles to group members. In each group of three, one student was a summarizer–checker whose responsibility was to make sure every person in the group understood the information, one student was a recorder whose responsibility was to write the answers to the questions, and one student was an encourager–observer whose responsibility was to encourage each group member to contribute to the process, and to monitor how well the group was working together.

Ms. Twiss explained to the students that when they finished writing their answers to the questions, every group would make a report to the class. She told them that each student in the group would be responsible for delivering part of the report. She also explained that the class would probably have extra questions to ask and that each member of the group needed to be able to answer any question. Finally, she told them that the group would receive a grade based on the group's presentation.

When Ms. Twiss finished her explanation, the groups moved their desks together and started to work. One of the groups consisted of Sydney, Oudi, and Susan.

SYDNEY: I have the questions. Our species is kangaroo.

OUDI: Wait. I'm the recorder. I need a pencil.

SYDNEY: Okay. Right. I'm the summarizer–checker. Susan's the encourager–observer.

SUSAN: Good job!

SYDNEY: What's the first question?

OUDI: What does the species look like?

SUSAN: I have a picture. It has short front legs and big back legs.

SYDNEY: In my paper it calls them limbs. The front ones are called fore limbs. The back ones are called hind limbs.

OUDI: What do you want me to write?

SYDNEY: Short fore limbs and big hind limbs.

OUDI: Let me see how that's spelled.

SUSAN: It has a long tail.

OUDI: So I'll list three things, right?

SUSAN: It has a pouch, too.

MS. TWISS: You need to make sure each person adds information. I don't think Oudi has contributed.

SYDNEY: Look in your paper, Oudi, and see if it says anything different.

OUDI: That's all I can find. I guess I can say it has fur.

MS. TWISS: Susan, you should encourage Oudi to find more information in his paper.

SUSAN: What else does it say?

OUDI: That's all.

> MS. TWISS: Sydney, you should summarize what you found out and make
> sure everyone knows the information.
>
> SYDNEY: Okay. A kangaroo has two short fore limbs, two big hind limbs,
> a long tail, a pouch, and fur. What's the next question?
>
> OUDI: Where does this species live?. . .

The face-to-face interaction between students in cooperative learning
groups, such as in the preceding scenario, provides the same kinds of opportunities for language development as discussion provides in the other teaching models.
It also provides a particular opportunity to focus on language goals that relate to
conversational skills. For example, the student-to-student interaction in cooperative learning groups allows youngsters to practice turn-taking, asking and answering questions, requesting more information, acknowledging someone else's
information, and shifting topics appropriately.

Peer Tutoring

Peer tutoring is "one child teaching another child of approximately the same age and
skill level" (Cooke, Heron, & Heward, 1983, p. 1). It is similar to cross-age tutoring
in which older and more knowledgeable students tutor younger students, but peer tutoring is easier for classroom teachers to manage because they can set it up within individual heterogeneous classes whereas cross-age tutoring requires the cooperation
of several teachers across grade levels whose schedules may differ considerably
(Kauchak & Eggen, 1997).

Peer tutoring has typically been used for drill and practice on functional academic skills such as spelling words and math facts (Delquadri, Greenwood, Whorton,
Carta, & Hall, 1986). However, it has also been used successfully in learning activities that require lengthy student responses. For example, peer tutoring can be used in
answering comprehension questions, as the following scenario illustrates.

SCENARIO

In Ms. Twiss's class, the students have been studying about Australia. Ms. Twiss
has divided the class into student pairs and given each pair the same set of eight
questions.

> MS. TWISS: I have given you eight questions. Each person has to pick four
> questions. You need to find the answers and then teach the answers to your
> partner.
>
> WILLIAM: Do we write the answers?

MS. TWISS: You should write notes to yourself, but you don't need full sentences.

LINDA: How do we divide the questions?

MS. TWISS: You need to cooperate. Maybe Diane wants to answer number one. But you want to answer number one. You have to look at the other questions and decide. Diane can answer number one, but you want number five. So Diane says okay. Now set up your desks with your partner. You have twenty minutes to answer your questions, then twenty minutes to teach the answers to your partner. At eleven o'clock you'll have a quiz.

LIZ: (To Averil) I think first we need to read all the questions.

AVERIL: Okay. I'm going to mark the ones I like. You mark the ones you like.

After reading the questions, Liz and Averil decided that Liz would find the answers to numbers 1, 5, 6, and 8, and Averil would answer 2, 3, 4, and 7. They spent the next fifteen minutes finding the answers and making notes to themselves.

MS. TWISS: It's time to start teaching your partner the answers.

LIZ: I have number one, so I'll start. What is the size of Australia, and where is it located? It's 2,948,366 square miles. It's southeast of Asia. It's between the Pacific Ocean and the Indian Ocean. I'm not sure if we need to know this, but it's a continent.

AVERIL: Do you think it's fine to write three million square miles?

LIZ: I don't know. In the book it says the exact amount. You have number two.

AVERIL: What is the population, where do most people live, and what languages do they speak?. . .

Peer tutoring allows for the same kind of student-to-student interaction as in cooperative learning, and the same kinds of language goals can be incorporated into peer tutoring lessons. In particular, alternating between being tutor and tutee allows for the development of skills involved in extended turn-taking and taking into account the communication partner's background knowledge.

Discussion

One of the strategies used in many teaching models is *discussion*. Wilen (1990) made the observation that discussion "should mean an educative, reflective, and structured group conversation with students," but that, realistically, to teachers it "generally means a recitation or review of basic information about a content-related topic" (p. 3).

Pasch and associates (1995) pointed out that many teachers confuse having a discussion with asking questions. In questioning, "communication travels from teacher to student, back to teacher, and is redirected to another student, forming a pattern like a many-armed spider, with the teacher at the center. In a discussion, the patterns of communication are much more diverse. While the initial stimulus may come from the teacher, additional comments may travel from student to student, with students adding questions or comments as desired" (p. 234).

Orlich and associates (1998) found the following elements to be essential to discussion:

1. A small number (preferably four to eight) of students meeting together.
2. Recognition of a common topic or problem.
3. Introduction, exchange, and evaluation of information and ideas.
4. Direction toward some goal or objective (often of the participants' choosing).
5. Verbal interaction—both objective and emotional. (p. 261)

It is this last point, verbal interaction, that makes discussion a rich language milieu. Virtually all language functions, presuppositions, and conversational rules can be incorporated as language goals within discussion, as the following scenario demonstrates.

SCENARIO

Mrs. O'Hara has been teaching a unit on the neighborhood to a class of second graders at the school for the deaf. The children are sitting in a semicircle on the floor, and Mrs. O'Hara has put photographs on a portable easel. Mrs. O'Hara uses simultaneous communication but often repeats phrases in ASL.

MRS. O'HARA: Let's look at the pictures of our school and the neighborhood around it.

PATTY: Dorm. Sleep in the dorm.

AWILDA: Cafeteria. School building. Playground.

RICARDO: Track. PE building. Library.

MRS. O'HARA: Great. You found lots of places in our picture. Now, what if Dr. Finn, the superintendent, had enough money to buy something new for the school, such as a building or a special classroom? What suggestion would you give him?

AWILDA: I think a new dorm.

MRS. O'HARA: Tell us why.

AWILDA: The girls' dorm is old and smells and small and the bathroom, you know, is old.

JOANNIE: My room is nice. My mom bought me posters, and I put them on the wall. She got them at Saturday Market.

MRS. O'HARA: That's interesting, but you're off the point, Joannie. What about using the money to build a girls' dorm? What do you think?

JOANNIE: I think that's a good idea because then they could build apartments. I visited my cousin, and at her school they have apartments not dorms.

MRS. O'HARA: A girls' dorm is a good idea. What's another?

RICARDO: Pool outside.

PATTY: That's dumb.

MRS. O'HARA: It's not a dumb idea, Patty. But maybe you don't like the idea. Why not?

PATTY: Because in October, November, December, January, February, March, April, it's cold.

MRS. O'HARA: Patty thinks that the outside pool wouldn't be used much. Because in the summer, you go home. And when you're at school, it's usually cold.

RICARDO: I want a pool outside.

MRS. O'HARA: That's fine. That's our second idea. What's another?

PATTY: Computers.

ANN: We have computers. Look.

PATTY: One.

ANN: But we have a computer room. Upstairs.

PATTY: I want computers. In the classroom.

MRS. O'HARA: How many in each classroom?

PATTY: One, two, three, four, five.

MRS. O'HARA: Oh, you want a computer for each person.

JOANNIE: Not me. I hate computers.

MRS. O'HARA: Computers for each classroom is a third idea . . .

Mrs. O'Hara continued the discussion for a few more minutes, encouraging each child to contribute at least one idea. During this discussion, as well as other discussions in which the students engaged, Mrs. O'Hara incorporated goals of language use for each child. For example, knowing that one of the children's goals included complains, justifies, expresses opinions, and blames, which are language functions from the personal category, Mrs. O'Hara encouraged this particular child to express these functions within the discussions.

Use of Technology for Teaching Language

Technology is a tool. For many years, technology referred to paper, pencils and pens, books, chalkboards, chalk, maps, pictures, rulers, and other concrete items. Later, technology included media such as filmstrips, slides, 16mm films, overhead projectors, models and kits, and games as well as audiocassettes and records. In the 1980s, educational technology included all of these things plus computers and videocassette recorders (Nelson, Prosser, & Tucker, 1987; Seidman, 1986). The schools of the 1990s added interactive systems such as interactive videodisc systems and hypermedia (Blanchard & Rottenberg, 1990; Buttery & Parks, 1988; Colman, 1989; Hansen, 1989; Hosie, 1987; Howe, 1985).

Today's schools include "low-tech" and "high-tech" tools. What is state-of-the-art one day seems to become obsolete the next. As we consider ways to use technology for teaching language, we should keep in mind the difference between a tool and a gadget. A gadget has practical uses, but its major attraction is its novelty. A tool has long-range potential. As teachers of children who are deaf, we need to consider using technology when it serves as a tool to enhance and extend the learning of language.

The difference between these two terms is well illustrated by a dialogue between two of my colleagues who teach courses in Kent State University's teacher education programs. When asked what technology he uses in his instruction, Dr. Michael Schwartz wrote, "I teach these courses using books, ideas derived from them, my own understanding of those ideas, some wit and whatever wisdom I can summon. I also use a piece of chalk on a blackboard from time to time." Dr. Albert Ingram responded by writing, "Instructional Technology as a field is a lot more than just the current round of hardware and software. The goal is that it be a linking discipline that helps translate knowledge of human learning into effective instruction that consists more of techniques, processes, and ideas than of hardware and software. I tell teachers that they can do great instructional design using nothing more than a pencil and a pad of paper."

Although much has been written about the potential of technology to transform classrooms, studies have shown that teachers are slow to assimilate media into their instruction (Muffoletto, 1994; Seidman, 1986). Ainsworth (1987) observed that schools "make use of these technological appliances rather like a mother may use telephone directories to boost a child at the dinner table. They serve a function, but not the one for which they are best suited" (p. 26). In other words, teachers may be using the equipment but not the technology.

It is not my objective to discuss the capabilities of currently available technologies and the applications of these technologies to classroom instruction. The literature is replete with articles and texts on this topic. My objective here is to look at how the media can be used to help develop the language and literacy of children who are deaf.

Our field has always viewed media as a critical component of teaching deaf children because we have recognized the importance of supplementing the amount of informational input to the child with a hearing loss, particularly through the visual channel. Indeed, from the mid-60s to mid-80s, a conference on educational media and the deaf was held yearly.

No consensus has emerged regarding the categorization of technology in education. In the first edition of this book, I used the following categories: learning about the technology, learning from the technology, learning with the technology, learning about thinking with the technology, and managing learning with the technology. Orlich and associates (1998) categorize technology as traditional instructional tools, telecommunications for distance learning, telecommunications in cyberspace, and personal computers. However, the organizing system of Roblyer, Edwards, and Havriluk (1997) seems most appropriate for the present. They divide the arena of educational technology into instructional software (drill and practice, tutorial, simulation, instructional games, problem solving), classroom technology tools (word processing, spreadsheet, database), support software (gradebooks, worksheets, test generators, printing and presentation graphics, desktop publishing, statistical packages, IEP generators), technology media (interactive videodisc and CD-ROM, hypermedia, distance learning), and emerging technologies (personal digital assistants, artificial intelligence, virtual reality, voice and handwriting recognition, multimedia-based simulations).

Instructional Software

The earliest uses of computer software involved *drill and practice activities,* which are less beneficial in language learning because the instructional approach involves practicing isolated skills. The purpose of drill and practice is to develop automaticity (Bloom, 1986). With this in mind, these programs can be used to help deaf children remember particular grammatical features or learn sight vocabulary.

Tutorial software "uses the computer to deliver an entire instructional sequence similar to a teacher's classroom instruction on the topics. This instruction is usually expected to be complete enough in itself to stand alone; the student should be able to learn the topic without any help or other materials from outside the courseware" (Roblyer, Edwards, & Havriluk, 1997, p. 89). Tutorials on subject areas, such as the principles of light and reflection, can provide children who are deaf with incidental language learning, that is, through reading and responding to the material, the child is using language. But the use of tutorials for learning language is questionable because language is best learned through meaningful, conversational interaction and not through lectures on grammatical structures and forms.

A computer simulation is a model that replicates a real-world (or even imaginary) activity, phenomenon, or system. *Simulations* tend to fall into two categories—simulations that teach by showing the physical characteristics or mechanisms of an object and simulations that teach how to do something by showing the sequence of steps or placing the students in hypothetical situations (Alessi & Trollop, 1991). Simulations can be used for learning language incidentally because they require critical thinking, analysis and synthesis of information, and problem-solving skills.

Instructional games (e.g., adventure, arcade, board, card, combat, logic, sports, role-playing, quiz, word) are typically drill and practice or simulation activities with game rules (Forcier, 1999). They tend to be used as a reward rather than an instructional tool for content material or language.

Software focusing on problem-solving skills has the same benefits and drawbacks as the other types of instructional software. Even though the problem-solving activities may lead the deaf child to use language receptively and expressively, they involve no direct conversational interaction that can support and extend language learning.

Regardless of how well designed instructional software is, teachers of deaf children need to be aware of the potential mismatch between the language used in the program and the English language ability of the child. They can both frustrate the deaf child and encourage guessing rather than thinking.

Classroom Technology Tools

Word processing is a powerful tool for writing development, and many of the strategies that I discuss in Chapters 5 and 6 incorporate this technology. For deaf children, writing provides a milieu for interaction in English, and word-processing techniques provide a simple way to make changes in compositions and communication. Children can draft a composition, share it with the teacher or a peer, use feedback for revising and editing, and make changes with relative ease using word-processing software.

Spreadsheets and *databases* tend to be used more often by teachers to manage their own information than by students. Spreadsheets are software programs that organize and manipulate numerical information. Spreadsheet software is the numerical corollary to word-processing software. "A spreadsheet helps users manage numbers in the same way that word processing helps them manage words" (Roblyer, Edwards, & Havriluk, 1997, p. 134). Database software, on the other hand, combines words and numbers. This type of software program enables the teacher to store, organize, and manipulate textual and numerical information. Both spreadsheets and databases can be used in teaching content area material, such as comparing the infant mortality rate of South American countries, tracking plant growth over several weeks, or charting the major events during a particular historical time. Similar to instructional software, the benefits to language development may be incidental, depending on how much discussion is integrated into the learning activities.

Support Software

The two types of support software that can be used effectively in instruction are *desktop publishing* and *presentation graphics*; both allow students to add style and visual distinction to their written work. Desktop publishing is a kind of word-processing software that allows the user to manipulate the form and appearance of the printed page. Presentation graphics allow the user to manipulate print and color and to incorporate pictures and other visual depictions. These software programs can be used as tools for language acquisition when they are integrated into writing instruction, which I will discuss in the chapters on literacy.

Technology Media

Interactive videodisc and *CD-ROM* are basically combinations of optical technology with personal computers. "Laser videodiscs store text, audio, video, and graphics data in analog format" (Roblyer, Edwards, & Havriluk, 1997, p. 180). CD-ROMs are made of the same material as videodiscs, are smaller in size, and can store a great deal more information. A myriad of products are currently available including curriculum packages, simulations, databases, movies and documentaries, interactive multimedia presentations, interactive storybooks, and reference materials. The opportunities for teaching language are as diverse as the kinds of materials being developed. Deaf students can read articles and books, gather information from multiple sources, engage in a simulation, develop a multimedia report, and within these activities, use language for learning, thinking, and communicating.

Hypermedia is software that connects elements, such as audio, video, photographs, graphics, animation, and text, within the computer system in a nonlinear manner via hypertext links. Hypermedia is an authoring system that enables students to incorporate a variety of elements into their writing. The higher level thinking skills these systems encourage as the students analyze the available information and synthesize it into their work and the smooth way that hypermedia blends with the nature of the writing process as writers move back and forth between planning, drafting, and revising make hypermedia an excellent teaching tool.

MacGregor and Thomas investigated the effects of a *computer-mediated text* (CMT) system on the reading and writing performance of forty-five deaf children in grades four through six. The researchers were particularly interested in studying the influence of (a) the electronic dictionary that the students could access at any time during their reading of passages on the CMT system, (b) extrinsic motivation in the form of post-passage vocabulary and comprehension questions, and (c) intrinsic motivation in the form of a vocabulary game. They found that vocabulary knowledge was facilitated with this CMT system and that post-passage questions were more motivational than the games. The investigators concluded that the strengths of the CMT system "were its interactive nature, the capability for immediate feedback, and the provision of student-controlled vocabulary knowledge acquisition" (MacGregor & Thomas, 1988, p. 284).

Videodisc computer systems are another example of technology that is interactive. One of the first interactive videodisc systems developed specifically for use with students who are deaf was produced by the Media Development Project for the Hearing Impaired at the University of Nebraska in the late 1970s. The first system they developed included a videodisc of a captioned film, teacher guide materials, vocabulary instruction, filmstrip-type sequences, and interactive quiz sections that students could respond to by manually writing the answers on paper or by using a computer keyboard (Propp, Nugent, Stone, & Nugent, 1981).

Tomlinson-Keasey, Brawley, and Peterson (1986) studied the effectiveness of an interactive videodisc system to teach English language skills to deaf students in junior high school. Although the investigators found no significant differences between the progress of students using the system and students engaged in regular classroom instruction, the investigators believed that the system was motivating to deaf students learning English syntax.

"HandsOn" was an interactive videodisc system developed as a bilingual approach to teaching English to deaf students who are fluent users of ASL (Copra, 1990; Hanson & Padden, 1989). In this system, stories signed in ASL were recorded on videodiscs. By using the computer, the child could access the ASL story alone, access English text above the video simultaneously with the ASL story, or access the English text without the ASL story. At any point, the child could move back and forth between the ASL video and English text.

Prinz (1991) conducted a study on the combined use of a computer program, called the *ALPHA Interactive Language Program,* with videodisc still and action pictorial sequences. The system was designed so that the language lessons presented by the ALPHA program on the computer could be supplemented with real-life pictures on the videodisc player. Furthermore, the youngster using the system was supposed to be accompanied by a teacher or speech–language pathologist who interacted with the child in speech and/or sign. The adult's role was to comment on, clarify, and expand on the child's language during the sessions. Prinz reported that the five- to twenty-year-old deaf subjects in the study demonstrated significant gains in reading and writing new words and sentences. He also reported that there was some evidence to support the observation that the youngsters showed strong gains in general language skills.

Distance learning involves the delivery of instruction when the teacher and students are separated over distance and/or time and can involve combinations of one- and two-way audio, video, and computer linkages. Instruction delivered via distance learning can entail two-way interactive video instruction at one end of the spectrum to asynchronous web-based instruction at the other end. In addition to the delivery of instruction through distance learning, the Internet offers a spectrum of interactive environments for distance education and communication including e-mail, chat groups, conferencing, listservs, newsgroups, and bulletin boards. Also, the World Wide Web offers a plethora of information and is available in many classrooms and in virtually all public libraries. A study conducted by the National Center for Education Statistics found that 67 percent of public schools in the United States planned to connect their classrooms to computer networks in the near future (Gonzalez & Hamra, 1995). School districts are investing heavily in technology. An example of state involvement is Ohio, which initiated a program called SchoolNet in the mid-1990s designed to bring technology into all Ohio classrooms. The benefit for language development is that deaf children and youth who are in classrooms with computers that are networked can engage in discussions that are timely, relevant, and not restricted by space and time. They can also seek out information easily and share this information with others through writing and face-to-face communication in the classroom. The following scenario illustrates how one type of software can enable deaf and hearing students to work collaboratively in real time over distance.

SCENARIO

MS. WOOLSEY: Our next unit will be Africa. Another class is also doing a unit on Africa. They're 7th graders also, but they go to a different school in Cleveland.

BILL: How can we work with students at a different school?

HAROLD: Are they coming here? Are they deaf?

MS. WOOLSEY: They're not coming here. And they're hearing kids. Let me show you where you'll meet them.

Ms. Woolsey brings the students to one of the classroom computers and clicks on the Palace software icon. The software allows her to create a building that looks like the school building, and a set of classrooms. It also allows her to manipulate icons that represent the students and to attach each student's name to an icon. Next, she shows them how they can connect to and disconnect from the software, move from room to room, type comments so that they appear to others in the room, type comments in whisper mode so that they only appear to the person with whom they want to communicate, and add and remove props. Then, she gives each student an opportunity to practice using the software by providing a list of places in Africa and the names of their partners at the other school. Komiko's first "conversation" with her partner via the Palace software is as follows:

BILL: Hi, my name is Bill. How are you?

KOMIKO: I'm fine. This is really fun. Ms. Woolsey came here and explained how to use this software. We can change how we look from day to day, where we sit or stand, and if we have desks or chairs or other things in the room.

BILL: I know. I move over here or near you. We can talk or whisper. We need to talk about report.

KOMIKO: I have the list of places for our report. We can pick from Angola, Ghana, Mali, or Madagascar. The others have been taken.

BILL: I like Angola.

KOMIKO: Okay. That's fine with me. What do we need to find out?

BILL: On my paper have eight things we do. (1) where is Angola, (2) what is climate, (3) what is population, (4) what is language, (5) history, (6) problems, (7) ways to solve problems, (8) how other countries can help.

KOMIKO: Because we have eight things to find out, I think we need to split them up. You can take four and I can take four. We can find out the information, and then come back and talk about it. Is that a good idea?

BILL: Okay. I take odd numbers and give you even numbers. Think okay?

KOMIKO: That's fair.

Bill and Komiko, and the other pairs of students, spend between ten and twenty minutes "talking" with each other via the Palace software three times each week for three weeks. During these discussions, they share the information they're learning and figure out what they need to do next. Komiko helps to provide a consistent English language model for Bill. In between their meetings, they each do their own research and writing. Their last conversation about the report was as follows:

BILL: Finish your parts?

KOMIKO: Yes. I have my four sections. You have the first part, so you start.

BILL: Angola is near Zambia and on the southwest coast of Africa.

KOMIKO: The Climate is moderate because of the Benguela Current.

BILL: No capital letter for climate.

KOMIKO: That's right. Thanks. Your part is next.

BILL: The population in Angola is 10,674,500.

KOMIKO: The languages in Angola are Banta and Portuguese.

BILL: Angola became Independenct on November 11, 1978. Before that, it was controlled by England, Germany, and Portugal. Angola's capital city is Luanda.

KOMIKO: That's really good except how you spelled independent. Health care is a big problem in Angola. The life expectancy for men is only forty years and for women forty-three. Hospitals in Angola are terribly short of supplies. Patients are helped in very poor and dirty hospitals. That would not be accepted in the United States. Angola has little clean drinking water because people use the river. People use it to bathe and as a toilet, too. It has become very dirty.

BILL: Ways to solve the problems are clean the water with chemicals before going into the river. Get better toilet technology. And improve the best medicine, build more hospitals.

KOMIKO: I think we need to change the last sentences. Maybe say this. Angola needs to get better toilet technology, improve the medicine, and build more hospitals.

BILL: I'm making the change. Thanks.

KOMIKO: Other countries can help Angola and give money or things to Angola to help them improve.

BILL: You need to say what things.

KOMIKO: How's this? Other countries can help Angola. They can give money for hospitals, toilet technology, and medicine.

BILL: Great.

Emerging Technologies

Some of the emerging technologies are personal digital assistants, artificial intelligence, virtual reality, voice and handwriting recognition, and multimedia-based simulations. As Roblyer, Edwards, and Havriluk (1997) note, "These technologies share a common thread: They are all designed to simulate something—intelligence, reality, or an assistant—to accomplish their purposes. They also combine hardware and software components" (p. 239). Because they are emerging, they are not widely used in education, and there is no current application for creating a learning environment that enhances the language development of deaf children and youth.

Technology for Access

One category of technology does not fit neatly into the ones I have discussed previously. This is the use of *technology for access*. Although access is the major purpose of this technology, it can also be used to support language development.

Captioned films are films in the areas of education and entertainment that have subtitles specifically created for audiences of persons with hearing loss. *Closed captioned television* is the captioning of TV shows. In closed captioned television, the subtitles appear only when the viewer has set the decoder. Film, television, and video captioning offer the potential for encouraging the reading development of youngsters who are deaf. Two research studies on the influence of captioning illustrate this potential.

Hertzog, Stinson, and Keiffer (1989) conducted a study in which they showed a technical film captioned at approximately the eighth- and eleventh-grade reading levels to deaf college students. Greatest comprehension was achieved when viewing the film was supplemented by teacher instruction at several stop-points during the film. Students identified as "high" readers comprehended more information from the film, with or without supplementary instruction, than students identified as "low" readers. Students identified as "low" readers comprehended less information from the film without supplementary instruction, and mainly benefitted from instruction when the film was captioned at the eighth-grade level rather than the eleventh-grade level.

Hertzog, Stinson, and Keiffer concluded that when a "class is mixed in terms of reading ability, the teacher should try to select captioning that matches the reading level of the poorer readers to ensure that the film will reinforce instruction" (p. 66). Although this conclusion seems to follow logically from the results of the study, it also seems logical that numerous opportunities to watch captioned films on subjects with which the youngsters are familiar will likely result in increased reading ability. In other words, the technology of captioning can provide a medium for the reading of highly motivating material which in turn will help children who are deaf to become better readers.

Koskinen, Wilson, and Jensema (1986) conducted a study on the use of closed captioned TV programs for reading instruction. Eight teachers, with deaf students between the ages of thirteen and fifteen (reading at levels from first to third grade), were given ten one-half hour captioned TV programs on videocassettes, scripts of the programs' captions for each child in their reading groups, and reading lesson suggestions. The investigators compared student retention of sight vocabulary, teacher perception of student comprehension, and teacher perception of student interest for the teachers' regular reading lessons and the captioned TV lessons. Although statistical data were not reported, the investigators reported observing that the students showed improvement in all areas when closed captioned TV was used for reading instruction. They concluded that "the combination of an entertaining picture with written words appears to be a powerful tool for reading instruction" (p. 46).

TTs, text telephones, were developed to provide telephone access to individuals with speech or hearing loss. Originally called TTYs, then TDDs, TTs can be used to enhance the language development of children who are deaf, but relatively few articles have been written on this topic. TT conversations between teenagers who are deaf have been used as the context for examining conversational behaviors (Geoffrion, 1982; Johnson & Barton, 1988; Rittenhouse & Kenyon, 1987); however, no references are available on studies that used TTs to teach conversational skills and other aspects of language use. Yet, as Rittenhouse and Kenyon noted, "One could hypothesize that improved TDD language in deaf children would lead to improved reading and language ability" (p. 212).

Linkages between computers and telephone lines have resulted in computer software that enables deaf individuals to use their computers as TTs. Recent advances have added video capability so that senders and receivers can see one another, as well as read their messages. For children who are deaf, this technology allows them to have phone conversations even if they cannot read and write, and the written message supports the learning of English.

The Present and Future

Technology offers the promise of being a powerful tool for deaf students within learning environments that are rich in opportunities to use language for learning and thinking. We have relatively little information at present to guide teachers' use of these tools with deaf students or their assessments. For example, Johnson (1997) found a paucity of research concerning the use of Internet technologies within educational programs for deaf students. The future uses of technology in classrooms lie with teachers. Perhaps Schrum and Berenfeld (1997) said it best:

> It is essential that educators take the lead in assuring that uses of information technologies are pedagogically sound, organizationally strong, and institutionally supported. We think that the entire world is now available to begin this incredible adventure. We, therefore, encourage educators to do what educators have always done best: plan educational experiences that promote active and engaged learning for all students, and design professional experiences for themselves so that they also continue learning. (p. 158)

Incidental Teaching of Language

When the term *incidental* is used, it generally means that two events are occurring concurrently, one is major and one is minor, and the minor event is fortuitous. I use the phrase "incidental teaching of language" similarly but with a deemphasis on the "minor" aspect. To me, incidental teaching of language means that the teacher of youngsters who are deaf always has a double agenda—content and language. Every instructional event is an opportunity to develop language. The content goal might be the "major" one, but the language goal is never really "minor."

Warren and Kaiser (1986) defined incidental language teaching as "interactions between an adult and a child that arise naturally in an unstructured situation and are used systematically by the adult to transmit new information or give the child practice in developing a communication skill" (p. 291). The difference between incidental language teaching and direct language teaching is the difference between participating in real conversation and practicing language pattern drills. As Staab (1983) noted, "Learners must engage in meaningful activities with other speakers [or signers] who model the appropriate language functions and forms. A meaningful activity is defined as any activity in which speakers [and signers] concentrate on doing something rather than on language. The rules are learned by observation and participation in these activities, while competent language users model the process" (p. 165).

Figure 2.1 presents several learning activities that involve the incidental teaching of language. These examples were created by graduate students preparing to become teachers of deaf children. As part of their practicum and coursework, they had each obtained a language sample from a child who is deaf, analyzed it, and determined appropriate language goals for the child in the areas of syntax, semantics, and use. They were then asked to create instructional activities that incorporated the child's language goals. Each graduate student worked with a different child, so the instructional activities they developed were for children from preschool through high school.

It was explained that the activities would be evaluated on the basis of (a) how whole, meaningful, and relevant the language was to the child, (b) how appropriate the activities were to the child's age, language development stage, and conceptual level, and (c) whether the activities reflected the importance of function over form. Finally, they were told that the only unacceptable activity would be a grammar lesson.

These activities are examples. They are not meant to encompass the range of possibilities but only to demonstrate that if a teacher has a language goal in mind, whether an English or ASL goal, the learning situation can be structured in a way to encourage the receptive or expressive communication of that form, meaning, or use. Creating, adapting, and modifying an activity to meet the unique needs of an individual deaf child is the role of the teacher.

Interdisciplinary Curriculum: Integrating Language into Thematic Units

Interdisciplinary curriculum, as defined by Jacobs (1989a), is "a knowledge view and curriculum approach that consciously applies methodology and language from more than one discipline to examine a central theme, issue, problem, topic, or experience" (p. 8). Depending on one's perspective, interdisciplinary curriculum has been referred to in the literature as "integrating the language arts," "language across the curriculum," "webbing," and "theming" (Donaldson, 1984; Wagner, 1985).

Although the concept of interdisciplinary curriculum did not originate in our field, it would seem that youngsters who are deaf would benefit greatly from this curriculum design for several reasons. First, the common set of concepts that are explored in an interdisciplinary curriculum are expressed through a common set of vocabulary, and the learning of this vocabulary becomes deeper as the nuances of meaning are examined and applied to a variety of contexts. Dillon (1990) noted that

FIGURE 2.1   Examples of Learning Activities Incorporating Incidental Teaching of Language Goals

Goal	Grade Level	Activity
Conjunction *and* Coordinate	Preschool/ kindergarten	This is a "memory game" activity. The teacher arranges at least six items on the activity table, such as empty food containers with labels. The teacher asks the children to pretend they went shopping. The children study the items on the table, and then all close their eyes. The teacher takes two items and puts them in a grocery bag. The children open their eyes and raise their hands if they know what's been purchased. The teacher watches for and guides the use of *and* in the answers.
Possession	Preschool/ kindergarten	For show-and-tell, the children drop their items into a box held by the teacher. The teacher reaches into the box, takes out an object, and asks, "Whose is this?" The child will probably answer "mine," or another child might answer "Susie's."
Plural Number Quantity	Early elementary	The child is learning the concept of set in math. As the child divides various colored items into sets, the teacher asks questions, such as "How many _____s are in this set?" and "Tell me about this set."
Question forms: *who, what, how, where, why, when*	Junior high school	As part of a deaf studies unit, the students interview a deaf adult. The students have to develop a list of questions prior to the interview.
Mood	Junior or senior high school	Once each week, the class reads a newspaper or news magazine article and has a discussion. The teacher encourages the youngsters to express their feelings about events that can affect their lives.
Imperative verb form	High school	The class has been learning how to fix an auto engine. During a review, the teacher gives the name of an engine problem, and the student has to list the steps involved in fixing it. Each student takes a turn.
Instrumental: persuades	High school	During a civics class, the students have been examining issues involved in the upcoming November election. They now have to persuade classmates to vote for a particular candidate or a ballot measure.

"language across the curriculum implies that we focus on what meaning learners make and how that meaning is made, how learners come to know their experience by placing a shape on it through their language, how learners structure their experience by 'languaging' it" (p. 8).

Second, an interdisciplinary curriculum avoids the fragmentation and lack of connection that a typical curriculum fosters. Deaf students can miss much incidental information, particularly when they are in classes with hearing students, and after a unit of instruction, they may have learned bits and pieces of knowledge but be unable to connect one area of learning with another. The use of common terminology and concepts within an integrated curriculum makes it more likely that youngsters who are deaf will be able to access fully the information presented and draw the connections between bodies of knowledge.

Third, an interdisciplinary curriculum makes sense in educational programs for students who are deaf because it is a way to deal with the expansion of knowledge in all areas of study and the difficulty in making parts of the curriculum relevant to the youngsters. As Jacobs observed, "Knowledge will not stop growing, and the schools are bursting at the seams" (1989a, p. 4). Thematic study allows youngsters to explore a few topics in depth. Obviously, hard choices are needed to determine which topics to study and which to leave out, but those decisions are being made anyway by state curriculum departments, program curriculum specialists, and classroom teachers.

Fourth, thematic study encourages youngsters to see real-life applications of the information they are learning. Jacobs noted that "only in school do we have 43 minutes of math and 43 minutes of English and 43 minutes of science. Outside of school, we deal with problems and concerns in a flow of time that is not divided into knowledge fields" (1989a, p. 4). Interdisciplinary curriculum provides a context for seeing associations between bodies of knowledge and making associations to issues in their own lives.

Models for Developing an Integrated Curriculum

How an interdisciplinary curriculum is designed depends largely on how many teachers and classrooms are involved. If one teacher with a class of students who are deaf is the only person in his or her school building who believes in using this approach, the model used will undoubtedly look quite different from the one used by a group of teachers across grade levels who are equally committed to the approach.

Similar to this group approach, at one school for the deaf, the language program at the elementary school was blended with the subject area curricula from science, social studies, math, and the arts. Instruction throughout the school was organized around thematic units. The themes were identified by the teachers, who then divided instructional responsibilities based on their areas of strength (Ramsey & Conway, 1995). This all-school curriculum is only one example of integrated curriculum design. In the following paragraphs, I will briefly present models based on a continuum of designs developed by Jacobs (1989b).

Parallel Disciplines

Parallel disciplines is a model in which topics taught in different subject areas are chosen to parallel one another. The content that has been taught in each of the subject areas is not changed, only resequenced. For example, in social studies the teacher has always taught about Middle Eastern countries in the spring but decides to teach this unit in the fall to parallel the science unit on fossil fuels. According to Jacobs, "Teachers working in parallel fashion are not deliberately connecting curriculum across fields of knowledge; they are simply resequencing their existing curriculum in the hope that students will find the implicit linkages" (p. 15).

For the teacher of children who are deaf, this model provides a relatively easy way to move toward an interdisciplinary curriculum. In the parallel disciplines model, vocabulary development is encouraged because the same vocabulary is taught in each subject area discipline.

Complementary Disciplines

Complementary disciplines is a model in which a topic is explored from the perspective of two or more disciplines that complement one another. For example, a high school teacher might decide to combine the subject areas of health and history for a unit on AIDS and the history of communicable diseases, which would include information on the transmission of HIV as well as an exploration of how societal attitudes toward AIDS are similar to or different from attitudes in the past toward other communicable diseases.

This model provides the teacher of youngsters who are deaf with an opportunity to help students see relationships between concepts in both subject areas and, of course, to express these relationships in class discussions and in their writing.

Thematic Units

Thematic units is a model in which each school subject focuses on the same topic for a unit of study and approaches the topic from the unique perspective of the discipline. Thematic units can be taught periodically throughout the school year and can last from a few days to a quarter or semester, though they generally are three to five weeks in duration. An example of a thematic unit is provided in Figure 2.2.

Because terminology and concepts cut across the subject areas in thematic units, this model helps to build deaf youngsters' vocabulary and knowledge structures and provides opportunities to explore the relevance of ideas to their own lives.

Complete Interdisciplinary Study

Complete interdisciplinary study is a model in which all school learning is themed around common topics. The school day is flexible to allow for more or less amounts of time to be spent on any activity on any given day. Topics chosen are ones that capitalize on student interest and motivation. This model requires enormous flexibility on the part of teachers and administrators, and it carries some risk that state-mandated curricular areas would not be covered. However, this may be the most nurturing cur-

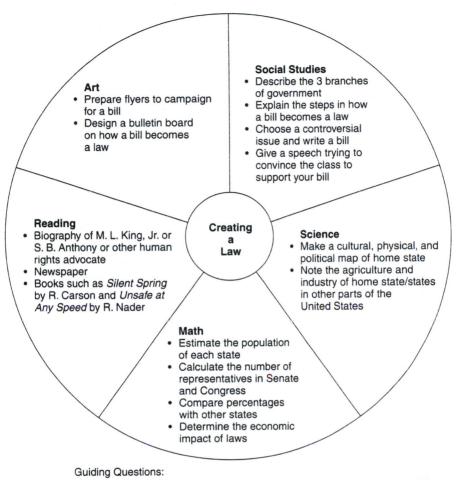

Guiding Questions:

1. What is a law?
2. What is the purpose of laws?
3. Why do some bills succeed and some bills fail to become laws?
4. What is the impact of laws on citizens?

FIGURE 2.2   Example of a Thematic Unit

riculum for language and cognitive development because it is based so directly on the child's own interests, concerns, and questions.

Procedure for Developing a Thematic Unit

The steps presented in a procedure for developing a thematic unit are based on approaches developed by Jacobs (1989c) and Norton (1982). This procedure can be used by teachers at all levels of instruction, and it can be used by one teacher working alone or a group of teachers working as a team. Itinerant and consultant teachers of the deaf can be a resource to classroom teachers as they develop a thematic unit.

Step 1. *Identify a Topic.* The teachers agree on a topic for the thematic unit. The topic should be broad enough to cut across several subject areas yet narrow enough to be explored in depth within the time frame of the unit. According to Jacobs (1989c), topics can be themes, subject areas, events, issues, or problems.

Step 2. *Brainstorm Ideas.* Using the topic as a focal point, the teachers brainstorm questions or subtopics that are associated with the topic. One way to do this is by creating a web. In the center of the web, the topic is written. On lines emanating from the center, subject areas are written, such as social studies, science, math, art, health, and reading. As ideas are generated, they are placed under the most appropriate subject area heading.

Step 3. *Organize Ideas and Add Pertinent Subtopics.* The web that was created from the brainstorming activity is looked at critically at this point. Redundant subtopics are combined, final decisions are made regarding where to place subtopics, and obvious gaps are filled in with new ideas.

Step 4. *Establish Topic Questions to Guide the Unit.* The teachers develop four to five questions that serve to guide the unit as a whole. These questions provide a common purpose for the unit. Jacobs (1989c) viewed these questions as a kind of scope and sequence for the unit. She noted that "the questions are cross-disciplinary in nature and are analogous to chapter headings in a textbook" (p. 59).

Step 5. *Develop Learning Activities That Correspond to the Subtopics in the Web.* These learning activities also need to provide ways to explore the questions developed in step 4. The activities should include a multitude of opportunities to use language in face-to-face communication, in reading, and in writing.

Example of a Thematic Unit

The example in Figure 2.2 was created by a group of teachers who developed this thematic unit for middle school–level youngsters who are deaf. In the past, only the social studies teacher would have taught this unit as part of her government curriculum while the science teacher might have been teaching a unit on the solar system and the health teacher a unit on drug awareness.

The teachers who implemented this unit were still able to teach significant concepts in their own subject areas, but the concepts were complemented as the students went from class to class. The teachers were also able to build on the students' vocabulary by presenting new words for the new concepts being taught in the unit, but now the learning of these new words was reinforced because they were used in a variety of subject area contexts. These teachers were able to offer the students many experiences in writing and reading about the topic. And they were able to encourage face-to-face communication during small-group and whole-class discussions, student speeches, and class presentations. All in all, thematic units such as this one on "creating a law" can provide teachers of youngsters who are deaf with a curriculum design that makes sense both for language learning and content learning.

Incorporating Strategies of Second Language Learning

No discussion of language teaching models and strategies for children who are deaf is complete today without a review of current bilingual education approaches and the theories that underlie these approaches. Within just a few years, bilingual education moved from idea to implementation in many programs across the United States and Canada.

What is bilingualism? Most of us would respond to this question with an answer such as, *bilingualism* is being able to converse in two languages. We might then be asked, what do you mean by converse? Face-to-face? Reading? Writing? Does conversing mean that the individual is able to have an equally thoughtful conversation about abstract concepts in both languages? The problem in defining bilingualism is that there is no precise point of mastery at which a person is bilingual. Rather, most linguists view bilingualism as being on a continuum from native-like control of two languages at one end and production of meaningful utterances in two languages at the other end.

A person's placement on this continuum certainly depends on his or her proficiency in the language syntactically, semantically, pragmatically, and phonologically, but it also depends on his or her ability to vary registers, to think in the language as well as to comprehend and produce it, and to read and write in the language as well as to engage in face-to-face communication (McCollum, 1981).

As we consider the research and practice on bilingualism and bilingual education, we should keep in mind that almost all of the literature focuses on the learning of two spoken languages and the using of two spoken languages in educational settings. Little research on the development of bilingualism in sign and spoken languages and bilingual educational approaches with children who are deaf is available.

Factors in the Development of Bilingual Proficiency

Age of Acquisition
One of the factors that influences bilingual proficiency is age of acquisition. Harding and Riley (1986) observed that there are four major points at which individuals become bilingual—infancy, childhood, adolescence, and adulthood. They defined infant bilingualism as the simultaneous acquisition of two languages, childhood bilingualism as the successive acquisition of two languages, adolescent bilingualism as the acquisition of a second language after puberty, and adult bilingualism as the acquisition of a second language after age nineteen. After reviewing the literature on the age factor

in second language acquisition, Singleton (1995) found that there is no evidence that younger second language learners are either more or less efficient or successful at learning a second language and, indeed, that there are no critical periods during which a second language should or should not be introduced.

Family and Community Languages

Infant and childhood bilingualism are the result of a combination of influences that include language used by the mother, language used by the father, language used in the community at large, and the parents' strategy in communicating with the child. It used to be thought that "one language-one source" was an essential attribute for any linguistic environment. To put this another way, it was believed that children could successfully learn two languages only if there was consistency regarding which language came from which adult. However, studies of families using a mix of languages have shown that children can become bilingual even when parents do not each use a separate language at all times.

In addition to the parents, the community has a strong influence on a child's language development. In fact, Romaine (1989) noted that when a home language is a minority language, children often show preference for using the language that is dominant in the community. "Sociolinguistic studies of minority languages have shown that it is usually very difficult for children to acquire active command of a minority language, where that language does not receive support from the community" (p. 169).

Individual Differences

Children show individual differences in their ability to learn a second language just as they show individual differences in all areas of learning. Individual factors include language aptitude and intelligence, a family environment that encourages conversation and questioning, motivation through friendships in which peers use or do not use a second language, and the ambition to use the second language because it carries or does not carry social, economic, and educational benefits (Baker, 1996; Gardner, 1979; McLaughlin, 1990).

Family and Community Attitudes

Children grow up in families and communities that convey beliefs about language and culture. These attitudes significantly influence children's success or lack of success in becoming and remaining bilingual (Cummins, Harley, Swain, & Allen, 1990).

Communities can frame bilingualism in a positive light, and this attitude can result in increased motivation by citizens to learn a second language. However, bilingualism can also be viewed negatively by a community, and this attitude can result in the disinclination of its members to learn a second language. Sometimes society maintains an outwardly positive attitude toward a minority language because the language is a symbol of ethnic heritage. However, a dichotomy exists between the public and private attitude. Privately, individuals recognize that the minority language is not well accepted since it is not used in the workplace, in schools, by individuals in positions of power, or by the media (Baker, 1996).

Parental attitude toward bilingualism has a particularly strong influence on children's acquisition of a second language. When the attitude of the community and the attitude of the parents are in conflict, parental attitude has been found to enable children to resist the negative pressure of the community (Gardner, 1979).

Ultimately, attitude is at the heart of bilingualism, and attitude change is at the heart of a bilingual education program. Lewis (1981) asserted that "any policy for language, especially in the system of education, has to take account of the attitude of those likely to be affected. In the long run, no policy will succeed which does not do one of three things: conform to the expressed attitude of those involved; persuade those who express negative attitudes about the rightness of the policy; or seek to remove the causes of disagreement" (p. 262). In relation to persuading those who disagree or removing other causes of disagreement, attitudes about minority languages tend to change only when majority individuals learn about the minority language and culture, see that individuals who use the minority language are held in esteem by others, and do not feel threatened by the minority culture.

Bilingual Education: Considerations and Perspectives

Bilingualism and Cognitive Development

For a number of years, it was thought that bilingualism had a negative effect on intelligence. It was believed that there was only so much room in the brain, and if too much room was needed to sort out languages, there was simply less room for other kinds of knowledge. In addition, it was believed that bilingual education resulted in lower academic achievement (Hakuta, 1986).

The relationship between bilingualism and cognition has been extensively studied, and the results are, well, mixed. Baker (1988) found that the history of research into the relationship between bilingualism and intelligence could be divided into three overlapping periods: the period of detrimental effects from the early nineteenth century to the early 1960s, the period of neutral effects from the late 1950s to the early 1960s, and the period of additive effects from the early 1960s to the present. Unfortunately, the methodological problems inherent in much of the research make any clear-cut statement regarding a relationship almost impossible, although Baker argued that the available evidence indicates that bilingualism results in cognitive advantage. Other researchers have drawn the same conclusion (Gonzalez & Schallert, 1999).

Cummins (1979, 1984) argued that an interaction between sociocultural, linguistic, and school program factors underlies the cognitive advantage of bilingualism that some children experience. He hypothesized that there are three broad levels of linguistic proficiency, and each level has concomitant cognitive effects. At the level Cummins called *limited bilingualism,* the child demonstrates low proficiency in both the first and second languages. He believed that negative cognitive effects are the result of limited bilingualism.

At the level he called *partial bilingualism,* the child is at an age-appropriate level in one of the languages. He considered that neutral cognitive effects, that is, neither positive nor negative effects, are the result of partial bilingualism. Cummins referred to this level as the lower threshold level of bilingual proficiency and believed that its attainment is sufficient to avoid any negative cognitive effects.

At the level he called *proficient bilingualism,* the child is at age-appropriate levels in both languages. He believed that positive cognitive effects are the result of proficient bilingualism. Cummins referred to this level as the higher threshold level of bilingual proficiency and considered that its attainment is necessary for long-term cognitive benefits.

He postulated that studies reported to have found cognitive and academic advantages among bilingual children were conducted with children who had attained the upper threshold level of bilingual proficiency and that studies reporting negative cognitive effects were conducted with minority language children who had "failed to develop a sufficiently high level of proficiency in the school language to benefit fully from their educational experience" (1984, p. 60).

Relationship between First and Second Language Acquisition

Much of the information available on child language acquisition is based on the learning of a first language. Teachers of bilingual children need to ask themselves if this picture of the language acquisition process is different for children learning two languages simultaneously in infancy or for the learning of a second language in childhood.

Research has demonstrated some striking similarities in the development of syntactic structures and the kinds of simplifications and overgeneralizations that are made early in the acquisition process for first and second languages (Hakuta, 1987; Kessler, 1984). Nevertheless, the two processes are not identical.

Although acquisition of two languages in infancy is called *simultaneous,* Kessler (1984) found that there is often an uneven development in the two languages. One reason for this difference in development is that the child may actually be exposed to one language more than the other. This is likely to happen, for example, when each parent uses a different language with the child and the child spends more time with the mother than with the father. Uneven development can also occur when the community's attitude is more positive toward one language, so the child is motivated to use this language more often than the other language.

Some evidence indicates that children learning two languages simultaneously pass through a stage in which the two languages are undifferentiated; that is, they function as a single language system that is constructed from elements of both languages and, therefore, is distinct from either language presented to the child (Kessler, 1984; Lindholm & Padilla, 1978; Redlinger & Park, 1980; Vihman, 1982, 1985). However, Genesee (1989) argued that the same evidence used by researchers to support a unitary language system hypothesis can be reexamined and used to demonstrate that bilingual children are able to differentiate between the two language systems from the beginning and that they use their differentiated systems in context-sensitive ways.

For children learning a second language after gaining proficiency in a first language, the process of acquiring the second language is similar but not identical to the stages involved in first language acquisition. According to Hakuta (1987), one aspect that changes the process is the environment. In first language acquisition, the child is immersed in the language virtually all of his or her waking hours, whereas in second language learning, the child may be exposed to the language for a few hours a day or less. In some instances, the setting is quite different from the natural conversational interactions between caretaker and child.

A second difference in second language learning is that at any given stage of development in the second language, the child is more cognitively advanced than he or she was at the same stage of development in the first language. As Saville-Troike (1979a) pointed out, "In general, a child learns his first language to express new meanings he perceives in his environment; in a second language, he usually learns new terms to express concepts he has already assimilated" (p. 116).

A third difference is that knowledge of a first language can cause some interference with learning a second language. Interference occurs when rules from the first language are applied inappropriately to the second language (Kessler, 1984; Saville-Troike, 1979a).

In reviewing the literature, Gonzalez and Schallert (1999) observed that we do not yet know how bilinguals cognitively store information or how the two verbal representation systems relate to one another. The issue becomes even more complex when we consider one language as spoken and the other as visual–gestural. And the picture becomes even more complicated when one of the languages has no written form that can be used to support language development.

Language and Culture

Culture is a pattern of beliefs, values, behaviors, arts, customs, institutions, social forms, and knowledge that are characteristic of a community. Culture is transmitted to succeeding generations through material products, physical interaction with members of the community, and language. In the words of Saville-Troike (1979b), "Children learning their native language are learning their own culture; learning a second language also involves learning a second culture to varying degrees, which may have very profound psychological and social consequences for both children and adults" (p. 140).

Bilingualism presumes biculturalism, but how realistic is this presumption? According to Harding and Riley (1986), "Biculturalism refers to the co-existence of two cultures in the same individual" (p. 42). Yet even when individuals achieve proficiency in two languages, they tend to feel a connection predominantly to one of the cultures.

Biculturalism in deaf bilingual education programs means including deaf culture. The culture of most, if not all, of the child's teachers and parents may not be deaf culture because the teachers and parents are likely to be hearing. In essence, the significant individuals in the child's life must import a culture with which they are relatively unfamiliar.

Bilingual Education Models

Bilingual education models tend to fall into two major categories—models based on the phasing out of the first language as the child gains proficiency in a second language, and models based on the development and maintenance of two languages throughout the child's schooling. The bilingual education models described in the following sections are the three major paradigms discussed in the literature. Keep in mind, there is no single ESL (English as a Second Language) or bilingual education model, and there is no single ESL or bilingual teaching strategy. Almost all of the models and strategies discussed in the literature involve two spoken languages. When we apply these to educating deaf children bilingually, the approaches need considerable modification.

Immersion

In an *immersion* bilingual education model, all or most classroom instruction is in the second language (Aguirre, 1982). A number of researchers distinguish between immersion and submersion programs (Baker, 1996; Cummins, 1979; Romaine, 1989). Both programs look like an immersion model, but the students in the two programs look quite different. In an immersion program, the students are from a dominant culture. The educational goal for these students is enrichment. By learning a second language, they become additive bilinguals. In a submersion program, the students are from a minority culture. The educational goal for these students is assimilation, not enrichment. By learning a second language, the language of the dominant culture, they become subtractive bilinguals. The term *submersion* is thus used by these researchers to describe what really happens to minority students in an immersion program.

According to Cummins (1984, 1987), two factors interrelate to make it extremely difficult for the minority language child to succeed in an immersion program. The first factor involves the amount of support the classroom context offers the child for communicating. In classrooms in which teaching involves meaningful and relevant explanations and discussions, language understanding is supported. However, most classrooms involve the kind of discourse described in Chapter 1—a high proportion of teacher language, question–answer routines that are quite different from conversational questions and answers, and movement between topics that are often unrelated to one another, such as from social studies to science.

In the typical classroom, understanding the language of the teacher well enough to comprehend the subject matter the teacher is explaining can be an enormous challenge to the minority language child. Cummins depicted this factor as a range of contextual support, with context-embedded communication at one end of the continuum and context-reduced communication at the other end.

> They are distinguished by the fact that in context-embedded communication the participants can actively negotiate meaning (e.g., by providing feedback that the message has

not been understood) and the language is supported by a wide range of meaningful paralinguistic and situational cues; context-reduced communication, on the other hand, relies primarily (or at the extreme end of the continuum, exclusively) on linguistic cues to meaning and may in some cases involve suspending knowledge of the "real" world in order to interpret (or manipulate) the logic of the communication appropriately. (1987, p. 62)

The second factor that influences how much the minority language child will benefit from an immersion program is the level of cognitive demand required in classroom communication. Cummins defined cognitive demand as "the amount of information that must be processed simultaneously or in close succession by the individual in order to carry out the activity" (1987, p. 63). He conceptualized cognitive demand as being on a continuum, with cognitively demanding communication at one end and cognitively undemanding communication at the other end. Since most classroom instruction involves the processing of information that is cognitively demanding, it can be surmised that the minority language child would be likely to have considerable difficulty benefitting from instruction in a second language.

Cummins pointed out that surface fluency in a language, a skill level he called *basic interpersonal communication skills,* is adequate for context-embedded and cognitively undemanding communication, such as in informal conversations, but simply not sufficient for the context-reduced and cognitively demanding communication in most classrooms. He determined that classroom instruction requires a level of skill he called *cognitive academic language proficiency.*

Baker (1996) noted that Cummins's theory could be used to explain why minority language children may seem ready for immersion when in reality they have acquired only enough ability in the second language to carry on informal conversations. The "theory suggests that children operating at the context-embedded level in the language of the classroom may fail to understand the content of the curriculum and fail to engage in the higher order cognitive processes of the classroom, such as synthesis, discussion, analysis, evaluation and interpretation" (p. 154).

Two strategies are typical of immersion programs. In one strategy, the teacher uses only the second language; often, the teacher is monolingual and unable to speak the child's first language. Another strategy is sometimes referred to as *ESL pull-out instruction* in which the child receives formal English-as-a-second-language instruction for a period of time each day, which is conducted in the child's first language. During the rest of the school day, the child is in a classroom in which the teacher uses the second language.

How can the immersion model be applied to bilingual programs for deaf children? It depends on the first language of the child. If the deaf child comes to school having developed ASL as a first language, immersion would mean classroom instruction in English with, perhaps, ESL pull-out instruction about English conducted in ASL. If the deaf child comes to school having developed a contact language of sign and English (sometimes referred to as pidgin sign language or pidgin sign English), immersion could mean either ASL-only or English-only instruction in the classroom with pull-out instruction in the other language. In either scenario, the deaf children would be receiving most instruction in a language with which they were not proficient. Therefore, they would suffer the same negative effects as minority language children in submersion bilingual programs.

Transitional

In a *transitional* bilingual education model, classroom instruction is initially in the child's first language. The second language is gradually introduced, and the goal is to mainstream the child full-time into classes where the second language is used for instruction. The educational goal of transitional programs is assimilation, and children in these programs, as in immersion programs, often become subtractive bilinguals.

According to Trueba (1979), transitional programs typically are designed to last no more than three years, and the concept of transition "refers to both the language use (from the home to the school language) as well as the nature of the classroom (from a 'special' to a 'regular' classroom)" (p. 56).

The transitional model would seem to be inappropriate for deaf children because the goal is monolingualism and not bilingualism; however, one of the strategies developed within this model, structured immersion, may be applicable. In structured immersion, students use their native language with each other in the classroom, but the teacher, who is bilingual, generally responds in the second language (Baker & deKanter, 1983).

Maintenance

In a *maintenance* bilingual education model, the child's minority language is given equal emphasis as a language of instruction throughout his or her schooling. The educational goal is pluralism, and children in these programs are likely to become additive bilinguals.

Trueba (1979) noted that maintenance programs can take three forms. In one form, the minority language is used for face-to-face communication, but the dominant language is the language of instruction in the subject areas and is used in reading and writing. In a second form of the maintenance model, reading, writing, and subject-matter instruction are conducted in both languages, but the dominant language is predominantly used for all subjects except culture. In the third form of the model, there is an equal balance in the use of the minority and dominant languages.

Can the maintenance model be applied to bilingual education programs for deaf children? One assumption underlying this model is that children come to school with proficiency in a first language that is maintained as the second language is introduced. Of course, this is not the case with most deaf children. Although the model may seem an inappropriate match, some of the strategies seem quite appropriate for classrooms with deaf children. For example, using English and ASL for differential instruction may be quite beneficial to deaf children acquiring both languages. And having two teachers who each use one language is a strategy that has been used in several educational programs. For instance, classes can be team taught by one teacher using English and another using ASL. In another approach, the teacher uses English while the teacher's aide uses ASL. Any of these strategies can enrich language development in bilingual education programs for deaf children.

Dual Language

In a *dual language* bilingual education model, both languages have equal status, both languages are taught as languages, the teachers are bilingual and use both languages, and half of the students are language minority and half are language majority. As in maintenance programs, the goals are pluralism and bilingualism. The languages are generally compartmentalized so that only one language is used for instruction at any time (Baker, 1996).

This model seems quite appropriate for educational programs with deaf children, though difficult to implement. One of the issues is the language fluency of the teachers. It would be difficult to find qualified teachers who are proficient in both English and ASL as well as knowledgeable enough to teach the rule structures of both languages. In addition to the lack of qualified teachers, dual language programs may work less successfully when the children are not initially fluent in any language, which is often the case in classrooms of young deaf children.

Attributes of Bilingual Programs for Deaf Students

Three attributes are integral to bilingual programs for deaf children.

1. ASL is viewed as the deaf child's first language.
2. Deaf individuals should be empowered within educational programs.
3. Deaf culture should be part of the curriculum.

ASL Is Viewed as the Deaf Child's First Language. Fundamental to any bilingual education program for children who are deaf is the idea that ASL is the first language of deaf children and English is the second language (Paul, 1998; Reagan, 1988; Vernon & Andrews, 1990).

In the past, the decision has been that English is the first language of children who are deaf. Oral/aural approaches, simultaneous communication, manually coded English systems, reading, and writing have all been employed to enable the deaf child to develop English as a first language.

Advocates of bilingual education programs argue that ASL is or should be the deaf child's first language for several reasons. First, ASL is seen as the language of the deaf community because ASL developed through communication between deaf individuals over hundreds of years. Vernon (1987) noted that ASL "is a totally visual language which has evolved into its present grammar and hand configurations because generations of deaf people through trial and error have found these to be the best, that is, they are the easiest to form and to read" (pp. 159–160).

Second, ASL has been promoted as the deaf child's first language because compared to manually coded English systems, ASL is viewed as easier for the child who is deaf to learn. Vernon (1987) found that hand positions and movements from sign to sign in manually coded English were difficult to execute and read, largely because they were based on the grammar and vocabulary of spoken English and not based on the visual modality in which they were being used. He noted that by contrast, ASL's "structure is ideally suited to sight and to the motor and visual functions of human beings" (p. 159).

Third, ASL gives the deaf child entrance into the deaf community. Reagan (1988) called ASL a language of "group solidarity." He observed that ASL "functions as both the deaf community's vernacular language and its principal identifying characteristic. Further, it has been, and remains, the sine qua non for membership in the deaf community" (p. 2).

Fourth, the importance of ASL to deaf individuals can be demonstrated by the fact that although ASL has not until quite recently been used as a language of instruction in the schools, it has flourished among deaf individuals. Unlike most languages that are passed on from parent to child, deaf children have usually learned ASL from peers, older deaf youngsters, deaf teachers, deaf houseparents, and deaf staff members at residential schools for the deaf (Reagan, 1985; Stewart, 1987).

If an educational program for children who are deaf decides to encourage the development of ASL as the child's first language, several issues need to be considered. One issue is that the language of the parents is probably English, the language of the dominant community. The literature is replete with studies on the effects of attitude on the acquisition of a minority language and studies examining the influence of parental attitude on the child's language acquisition. Therefore, bilingual education programs will need to deal directly with parental attitudes toward ASL. And, of course, the issue of parent–child communication when the child is learning a language that is foreign to the parent or a second language to the parent will need to be considered.

Another issue is the role of *pidgin sign,* which some individuals capitalize as in Pidgin Sign English or Pidgin Sign Language. However, other individuals do not capitalize this term because they do not consider it the name of an actual language. Either way, pidgin sign is generally used to describe an individual's use of ASL signs in English word order and with some inclusion of English morphemes. It is often used simultaneously with speech or a mouthing of words with no voice. Instead of pidgin sign, some people use the term *contact signing.* Valli and Lucas (1995) define contact signing as "a kind of signing that results from the contact between American Sign Language and English and exhibits features of both languages" (p. 409).

Pidgin sign can serve important functions both within and outside the classroom. For example, pidgin sign provides a way for individuals who are fluent in ASL and individuals who are fluent in English to communicate with one another. It also allows teachers to present information in sign to their students when the manually coded English system they are using becomes cumbersome. Nonetheless, pidgin sign is not a language in itself, and because it is neither ASL nor English, it cannot provide the deaf child with the richness of forms, functions, and uses from either of those languages.

The complexities involved in the kinds of communication used by hearing and deaf individuals within classrooms of deaf children and in the broader community have led some professionals to argue for a broader definition of ASL that encompasses the ways that individuals actually use sign to communicate (Moores, 1996). But, we must keep two issues in mind as we think about the importance of bilingualism for deaf children. First, deaf children will cognitively try to make sense of the rule structure of the language used by the significant adults in their lives; their own language will reflect this rule structure. If the language used by the adults does not follow the rule structure of a culturally shared language, such as English or ASL, then the language deaf children will develop will be neither English nor ASL. Second, ASL, like all languages, is constantly changing. The rule structure of ASL looks somewhat different than it did fifty years ago, and it will look different fifty years from now. Educators and parents can help deaf children to learn ASL within bilingual education programs, but they cannot prescribe the rules of ASL, mandate that they be used the same throughout the United States, or keep them static.

Deaf Individuals Should Be Empowered within Educational Programs. There is virtually no disagreement among advocates that bilingual education programs will not succeed unless deaf individuals play a major role in design, implementation, and evaluation. However, it is recognized that it may take considerable time to change behaviors and attitudes to the point at which deaf individuals will be full participants in educational decision making.

Vernon and Andrews (1990) reported that discriminatory practices have kept deaf adults out of positions of importance in schools, colleges and universities, and the workplace. And there is certainly a relationship between the overall low academic achievement among students who are deaf and the limited number of deaf professionals.

Deaf Culture Should Be Part of the Curriculum. For youngsters who are deaf to develop positive attitudes toward ASL and the deaf community, advocates consider it critical that deaf culture be a part of any bilingual program. According to Reagan (1988), study of deaf culture should include the heritage and traditions of deaf people, the structure of the deaf community, social behaviors among deaf individuals, the history of deaf culture, and subcultures within the deaf culture, such as Black deaf and Latino deaf. He also recommended the inclusion of cross-cultural study, which should encompass the dominant Anglo-American culture, other minority cultures in U.S. society, and the cultures of deaf people in other countries.

These three characteristics are discussed frequently in the literature on bilingual education programs for deaf children even though they are not the only important aspects of a bilingual program. Indeed, throughout this book teaching models and strategies for language and literacy development are discussed that are crucial to any educational program for children who are deaf.

Future Directions in Bilingual Education

Although many educational programs for deaf children have incorporated features of bilingual educational models and strategies, there has been a lack of research on the effectiveness of these approaches. The rhetoric has been high, and the literature contains numerous articles and essays supporting bilingual education. But the programs that have implemented these approaches have provided little data to help others know what features are and are not effective (Andrews, Ferguson, Roberts, & Hodges, 1997; Saunders, 1997; Strong, 1995).

As I discuss models and strategies for teaching reading and writing to deaf children in the following chapters, I will include variations, depending on whether the teacher is using ASL, simultaneous communication, or spoken English, only when the language of instruction makes an important difference.

Whatever languages are used with deaf children, we know that providing a consistent, rich linguistic environment is crucial. As educators, we need to consider the role of ASL and English in the life of a deaf child. Both languages can serve the child socially, though ASL is certainly the language of social interaction in the deaf community. Yet English remains the language of the dominant community in the United States and will serve the deaf child educationally and economically. Furthermore, English is at present the only medium for reading and writing, though there have been efforts to develop a written form of ASL.

TESOL (Teachers of English to Speakers of Other Languages) (1997) developed ESL standards for pre-K–12 students that are relevant to teachers of children and youth who are deaf. In fact, the preface to the standards includes the following statement about the importance of English that is just as meaningful to deaf students as it is to students learning English as a second or additional language. "Full proficiency in English is critical for the long-term personal, social, and economic development of all students in the United States" (p. 10). The standards revolve around three goals— to use English to communicate in social settings, to use English to achieve academic success in all content areas, and to use English in socially and culturally appropriate ways. These important standards certainly apply to deaf students as well.

Final Comments

The teacher of children who are deaf must be able to create a classroom environment rich in opportunities for each child to develop the forms, meanings, and uses of language in face-to-face communication. This means that the teacher must be able to concurrently accommodate both language goals and academic goals. The agenda is twofold. The first part involves being able constantly to remember each child's individual language goals and embed these goals daily into all learning activities. The second part involves teaching the child subject area information appropriate to the child's academic level, helping the child develop the ability to think critically and creatively, and enabling the child to learn how to learn.

In this chapter, models and strategies used by teachers of deaf children for actualizing this twofold agenda were described. I also discussed issues involved in bilingual education for children who are deaf. While this chapter concentrated on face-to-face communication, the next chapter will focus on the development of reading and writing in children who are deaf.

Suggested Readings

Baker, C. (1996). *Foundations of bilingual education and bilingualism* (2nd ed.). Clevedon, England: Multilingual Matters.

Joyce, B. R., & Weil, M. (1996). *Models of teaching* (5th ed.). Boston: Allyn and Bacon.

Orlich, D. C., Harder, R. J., Callahan, R. C., & Gibson, H. W. (1998). *Teaching strategies: A guide to better instruction.* Boston: Houghton Mifflin.

Parasnis, I. (Ed.). (1998). *Cultural and language diversity and the deaf experience.* Cambridge, England: Cambridge University.

Roblyer, M. D., Edwards, J., & Havriluk, M. A. (1997). *Integrating educational technology into teaching.* Columbus, OH: Prentice Hall.

CHAPTER

3 Literacy Development

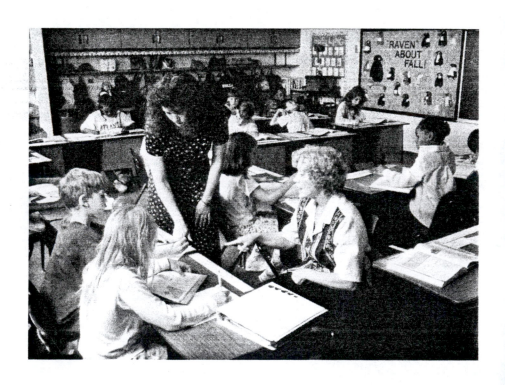

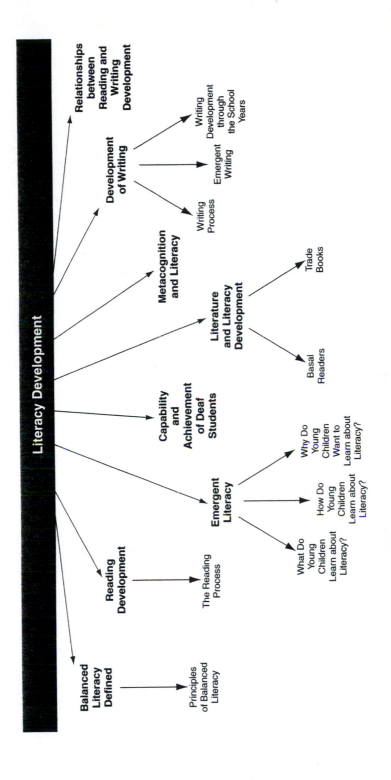

Literacy Development

- Balanced Literacy Defined
  - Principles of Balanced Literacy
- Reading Development
  - The Reading Process
- Emergent Literacy
  - What Do Young Children Learn about Literacy?
  - How Do Young Children Learn about Literacy?
  - Why Do Young Children Want to Learn about Literacy?
- Capability and Achievement of Deaf Students
- Literature and Literacy Development
  - Basal Readers
  - Trade Books
- Metacognition and Literacy
- Development of Writing
  - Writing Process
  - Emergent Writing
  - Writing Development through the School Years
- Relationships between Reading and Writing Development

Holistic approaches to teaching and learning are based on the belief that the whole is different from and greater than its parts, so they emphasize the wholes of subject matter and the integration of parts with wholes (Harris & Hodges, 1981). During the 1980s and 1990s, holistic approaches were the lens through which educators philosophically, pedagogically, and theoretically viewed literacy development. The traditional basal reader, skills, and language experience approaches that had historically dominated reading instruction were reexamined and reformulated to be compatible with holistic philosophy and theory. For teachers of youngsters who are deaf, the changes were profound and yet subtle. They were profound changes because they challenged our assumptions about the roles of teachers and students. They were subtle changes because, in our field, we had always recognized the importance of providing a classroom environment that reflects the value of relevant, meaningful, functional, and authentic learning experiences.

Like a pendulum, these strategies swing back and forth as they gain and lose favor with the education community. The whole language end of the pendulum was a reaction to the emphasis that had earlier been placed on reading and writing skills. Strategies based on a whole language approach reflected constructivist theory whereas strategies based on a skills approach reflected behaviorist theory. Now, the pendulum has returned to the center, and the approach currently receiving favor is called *balanced literacy*. According to Pressley (1998), "Balanced-literacy teachers combine the strengths of whole language and skills instruction, and in doing so, create instruction that is more than the sum of its parts" (p. 1).

This chapter will define balanced literacy and discuss the rationale for using balanced-literacy principles in teaching children who are deaf. Current views of reading and writing development and the kinds of reading materials that can enhance the development of literacy in deaf youngsters will also be discussed. Finally, the instructional implications of the relationship between language, literacy, and cognitive development will be examined. Teaching strategies that incorporate these principles will be presented in Chapters 4 and 5.

Balanced Literacy Defined

Balanced literacy can best be defined in relationship to whole language and skills-development emphasis. From its inception, whole language was difficult to define because it was conceptualized in a number of ways, from a movement to a philosophy, a set of principles to a learning theory, types of materials to teaching strategies, and a curriculum focus to a political perspective. Most definitions were similar to K. Goodman's (1989), who stated, "The term whole language itself draws on two meanings of whole. It is undivided, and it is integrated and unified" (p. 210).

As a movement, whole language began in the late 1970s and was originally built on the developmental theories of John Dewey, Jean Piaget, Lev Vygotsky, and Michael Halliday (Goodman, Y., 1989; McCaslin, 1989). Whole language theory evolved from these early influences in response to research in reading, writing, early childhood, and curriculum, which, in part, explains the difficulty one has in capturing the essence of whole language. Whole language theory is as much psychological, philosophical, cognitive, and linguistic theory as it is educational theory.

Skills-development emphasis has been easier to define than whole language. To most educators, a skills emphasis has meant focusing instruction on specific skills identified as developmentally important in reading and writing. The skills that are emphasized in this approach typically center around word-level recognition, but skills instruction also includes areas of comprehension such as getting the main idea and making inferences. Skills emphasis tended to reflect teacher-directed instructional approaches whereas whole language tended to reflect more student-centered instructional approaches.

Balanced literacy is an approach designed to combine the best features of whole language and skills. Balanced literacy instruction involves spending considerable time teaching skills and supporting students as they apply these skills to reading literature and writing. Using the analogy of baseball, Pressley (1998) wrote,

> Whole language is like little league baseball if players only played games. Their playing of whole games would be substantially impaired by lack of skills. Just as bad, skills emphasis is like little league baseball if it involved mostly infield, outfield, and batting practice. As good as players experiencing such an approach might be at picking up grounders, running down fly balls, and hitting consistently, they would not be baseball players. They would not know how the components articulate as part of an entire game. Baseball, like all sports, involves development of skills and practice in applying those skills in whole games, played at a level appropriate to the developmental level of the players. (p. 283)

Principles of Balanced Literacy

The following principles reflect the essential qualities of balanced literacy, yet they are not meant to be rules, tenets, laws, or truths. These principles are compatible with Halliday's (1984) concept that three types of learning involving language occur simultaneously and interdependently: learning language, learning through language, and learning about language.

Support for these principles can be found in the literature on whole language, skills emphasis, and balanced literacy (Goodman, K., 1989; Harste, 1989; Moorman, Blanton, & McLaughlin, 1994; Pearson, 1989; Pressley, 1998; Pressley & Afflerbach, 1995; Shuy, 1981; Smith, 1978; Spiegel, 1992). Examples of these principles will be provided in Chapter 4 when I discuss models and strategies that promote literacy development.

All Forms of Expressive and Receptive Language Work Together
Reading and writing are interrelated processes; therefore, development in one area enhances development in the other. Balanced literacy classrooms engage children in writing as much as reading.

Focus Is on Meaning of Written Language in Authentic Context

The context of reading and writing in the classroom should reflect real-life settings, and literacy activities should be relevant to the child as much as possible. From the beginning of instruction, children should be engaged in the reading of whole, real, predictable texts that represent quality literature. The goal of instruction is viewed as comprehension of meaning for readers and expression of meaning for writers.

Classrooms Are Communities of Learners in Which Literacy Is Acquired through Use

This principle is based on the belief that in order to learn to read and write, children need ample opportunity to engage in reading and writing and to share their responses with others. Both reading and writing are tools for learning, thinking, growing, and changing. In this view of literacy development, the teacher is a collaborator as well as a facilitator and leader.

Children Are Motivated When Given Choice and Ownership

Becoming a skilled reader can be a difficult and time-consuming process, and children are more likely to work through the complexities when they are motivated. Allowing them to choose what to read and write can build a sense of ownership, which, in turn, supports their understanding that written language can be used in personally and socially satisfying ways.

Processes Are More Important Than Products

The skills involved in reading and writing are crucial and should be taught effectively, whether within or without context. But ultimately, the child's ability to use the skills in the process of reading and writing is the only worthwhile measure of skills instruction.

Literacy Development Is Part of an Integrated Curriculum

Reading and writing should be used to learn and think about subject areas. Teachers of science, social studies, math, health, and other content areas are also teachers of reading and writing.

Reading Behaviors of Skilled Readers Reveal What Instruction Should Accomplish

Skilled readers identify words efficiently while reading, so instruction should focus in part on the development of decoding abilities. Skilled readers also reflect on their comprehension and actively construct meaning by using their own prior knowledge to understand the text. Instruction should also focus on building the child's background knowledge and helping him or her to become a metacognitive reader.

Reading Development

I use the term *development* quite deliberately. Reading is developmental. It is part of the youngster's language development. Although in this section I arbitrarily separate reading from other forms of language for the purposes of describing how children learn to read, reading can no more be truly separated from the development of writing, speech, or sign than semantics can be separated from syntax and use.

In the last two decades the amount of research into literacy has exploded. In this section, I will describe what is currently known about the development of reading in children who are deaf, drawing as well on the research regarding reading development in all children.

The Reading Process

Reading involves an interaction between the reader and the text. The reader brings prior knowledge and experiences that shape expectations for the text. As these expectations are confirmed or disconfirmed, information is integrated and meaning is created. In this view of reading, meaning is not fixed by the author but is constructed by the reader (Dreher & Singer, 1989; Jones, 1982; Strickland, 1982; Wittrock, 1982). The reader's prior knowledge and experiences include general world knowledge, specific knowledge of the topic, past experience with the written genre, ability to understand the syntax and lexicon, and skill in decoding the words (Beck, 1989; Blachowicz, 1984; Hacker, 1980; Jones, 1982).

The complex interaction between reader and text has led some researchers to view this relationship as a transaction rather than an interaction (Chaplin, 1982; Probst, 1988; Rosenblatt, 1978; Weaver, 1994). "Transactional theory proposes that the relationship between reader and text is much like that between the river and its banks, each working its effects upon the other" (Probst, 1988, p. 378).

The reciprocal relationship between the reader and the text can be partly illustrated by the following example of a narrative passage.

> Alison's hair was white with snow in the few minutes she had been waiting for the bus. She checked her watch again, worried about her first day at work.

One reader might interpret this passage to mean that Alison was worried about being late to work on her first day because busses are often delayed during snow storms. Another reader, with less knowledge of public transportation but with more knowledge of human nature, might interpret Alison's worry to be related to her wet hair. Yet another reader might draw on personal experience to view Alison as being absorbed with worry over being able to learn her new job, and only abstractedly gazing at her watch.

To understand how readers construct meaning from text, it is essential to understand what kinds of knowledge they bring to texts. Schema theory provides a way to conceptualize these knowledge structures.

Schema Theory

Schema is a construct used in theories of perception, memory, and learning. According to schema theory, conceptual knowledge is organized cognitively into memory structures called *schemata* (*schemata* is plural, *schema* is singular). A schema can be thought of as a framework that interrelates one's knowledge and experiences about a topic. Schema is thought of as having hierarchical organization with more general concepts stored at the top. Some researchers view this framework as having slots or placeholders for the schema that fit within, or are embedded within, the lower parts of the hierarchy. It is through this framework that new information is interpreted, stored in memory, and retrieved when needed.

For a concept to be comprehended, it must trigger a schema from the individual's memory. The person's prior knowledge and experiences that are organized in schemata in turn influence how the new information and new experience will be understood. In essence, then, individuals store and arrange their knowledge and experiences as schemata that they then use in interpreting new information and experiences.

However, schemata are not static entities; they change as an individual processes new information and experiences. Learning can occur when new information or a new experience fits into an existing schema. This is referred to as *accretion, assimilation,* or *comprehension.* Learning can also occur when the new information or experience does not fit neatly into the schema, and the schema changes, is modified, or is altered. This is called fine tuning or *accommodation.* Finally, learning can take place when a schema is discarded and a new schema developed to accommodate new information and experiences. This is called *restructuring.*

It is important to recognize that sometimes new information or a new experience that does not fit neatly into an existing schema can be ignored, considered irrelevant, unimportant, or even incongruent. (Psychologists have long recognized this phenomenon as *denial.*)

Perceiving, interpreting, and classifying new information and experiences into schemata is an active cognitive process as incoming information evokes associations with an existing schema. When new information or a new experience requires the reorganization of cognitive structures, a schema undergoes qualitative change, and cognitive development has taken place (Anderson, Spiro, & Anderson, 1978; Beers, 1987; Blachowicz, 1984; Hacker, 1980; Lange, 1981; Monteith, 1979; Pearson & Spiro, 1982; Richgels, 1982; Rumelhart, 1980; Thorndyke, 1977; Thorndyke & Hayes-Roth, 1979).

Readers use their schemata to create meaning from text. As Strickland (1982) stated, "Reading is a process that both develops schemata and depends on schemata" (p. 10). Two kinds of schema have been identified as particularly important in the reading process—content schema and textual schema.

Content Schema.   *Content schema* is the prior knowledge readers have about any given textual topic. Content schema includes the reader's general world knowledge, particular information, and personal experiences about a topic. Evidence suggests that background knowledge directly influences reading comprehension of hearing and deaf readers (Anderson, Spiro, & Anderson, 1978; Callahan & Drum, 1984; Gormley,

1981; Marr & Gormley, 1982; Ohlhausen & Roller, 1988; Recht & Leslie, 1988; Stevens, 1980), and, indeed, activating and expanding children's background knowledge prior to reading is conventional wisdom to teachers.

One of the problems faced by youngsters in reading a new story, chapter, article, poem, essay, or any text passage is *schema availability.* Do they already possess a rich schema for the content? Jenkins and Heliotis (1981) noted that "many children who are characterized as poor comprehenders earn this distinction because they lack the requisite background knowledge that authors assume they possess" (p. 37). The following passage was taken from *Look Who's Playing First Base* by Matt Christopher, a book written at the 2.7 reading level as calculated with the Dale-Chall readability formula.

> Art's first pitch missed the plate for ball one. His next missed, too. His third was over. The Maple Leaf then drove the two-one pitch for a single over short.
>
> A bunt advanced him to second base. Art fielded the ball and threw out the hitter. One out.

To comprehend this passage, and a number of other sections of the novel, the youngster would need a fairly complete understanding of baseball terminology and, probably, personal experience in playing the game.

A second, but related, problem in reading a new text is *schema selection.* This problem occurs when the youngster possesses ample background knowledge but does not use it to interact with the text. Pearson and Spiro (1982) found that sometimes children are unaware that they possess relevant schemata. They also found that some children focus on an inappropriate schema because they are misled by a nonsalient feature of the passage or because the text requires combinations of background knowledge. Pearson and Spiro observed that problems in schema selection are often associated with overreliance on bottom-up processing, or decoding of individual words.

One example of how children who are deaf can have difficulty with schema selection is illustrated by a chapter in the novel *Ellen Tebbits* by Beverly Cleary. Near the beginning of one of the chapters, Beverly Cleary writes, "To Ellen Tebbits and Austine Allen spring meant something much more important. It meant no more winter underwear." A few paragraphs later, Ellen, bragging about her ability to ride a horse, says to Austine, "Once I rode bareback." The rest of the chapter deals with Ellen's predicament when she and Austine have an opportunity to go bareback riding, and her boasting is put to the test. The child who focuses early in the chapter on the phrases "no more winter underwear" and "bareback" may misinterpret the actual meaning of these phrases, overestimate their importance for understanding the rest of the chapter, and not even notice the central idea of the chapter.

A third problem is *schema maintenance* and *schema shift.* It has been observed that able readers continue to use a schema as long as it is appropriate, and they are able to shift a schema when the passage calls for it. However, some youngsters have difficulty in flexibly maintaining and shifting schemata as they interact with text. The ability to maintain and shift schemata requires that the youngster be aware of what he or she knows, and does not know, and what to do about it. This awareness of one's own knowledge and thinking involves metacognitive abilities, which will be discussed in greater depth later in this chapter.

Studies with deaf children have found that (a) general world knowledge, particular information about a topic, and personal experiences of a topic have a positive influence on their reading comprehension and (b) improvement in comprehension can be obtained by building background knowledge with thematic organizers and ASL summaries prior to reading (Andrews, Winograd, & DeVille, 1994; Jackson, Paul, & Smith, 1997; Schirmer & Winter, 1993).

Readers use their schemata not only for text content but also for text structure.

Textual Schema.   *Textual schema* is the reader's mental organization of how typical text is structured. Most of the research regarding textual schema has focused on the structure of narrative text. Expository text schema will be discussed later in this section.

Story Schema.   The reader's cognitive representation of narrative text is referred to as *story schema.* Because story schema provides the reader with an expectation of what form a typical story takes, the skilled reader uses this schema to notice important or relevant aspects of the material, to pay attention to the ways story components are sequenced and fit together, and to reconstruct the story after it has been read (Mandler, 1978; Mavrogenes, 1983; McConaughy, 1982).

Story grammars have been developed to describe the structure of a particular kind of narrative text. They are meant to reflect both the external structure of stories and the internal cognitive structures within readers (Mandler, 1987; McConaughy, 1982). Four major story grammars are typically discussed in the literature: Mandler and Johnson's (1977; Johnson & Mandler, 1980), Rumelhart's (1975, 1977), Stein and Glenn's (1979), and Thorndyke's (1977). These grammars were derived from oral folktale and fairy-tale traditions in western cultures. With some variation in structural elements, all of these grammars include a *setting,* a series of *episodes,* and a *resolution.* In the *setting,* the central character is introduced, and location and time may be described. Within each episode is an *initiating event* that causes the central character to have a *reaction* and to formulate a goal. The central character *attempts* to achieve the goal or solve the problem. (An attempt is sometimes referred to as the *action.*) For each attempt, there is either a successful or failed *outcome,* sometimes called a *consequence.* If there is more than one episode in the story, the consequence of each episode is the initiating event of the subsequent episode. Thus, the consequence acts as the consequence of the preceding episode and the initiating event of the next episode. *Resolution,* or *ending,* represents the final outcome or long-range consequence of the action. In Figure 3.1, the story structure of *The Three Bears* is represented.

The psychological reality of story grammar has been confirmed by a number of researchers. In studies in which readers were presented with stories that were well formed and stories that varied in differing degrees from well-formed stories, recall was found to be directly related to how closely the stories conformed to ideal story structure (Mandler, 1978; Stein & Nezworski, 1978). When asked to divide into parts

	Setting	Once upon a time, there was a family of bears—a papa, a mama, and a baby. They lived in the woods.
Episode 1	Initiating Event	Mama Bear made porridge for breakfast, but it was too hot to eat.
	Reaction	The bears decided to go for a walk in the woods while the porridge cooled off.
	Action	Goldilocks walked up to the Bears' house. Because no one was home, she walked in.
Episode 2	Consequence	Goldilocks saw three bowls of porridge.
	Reaction	Because she was hungry, she decided to eat some porridge.
	Action	The porridge in the big bowl was too hot. The porridge in the middle-sized bowl was too cold. The porridge in the small bowl was just right, and she ate it all up.
Episode 3	Consequence	She saw three chairs.
	Reaction	Because she was tired, she decided to sit down.
	Action	The big chair was too hard. The middle-sized chair was too soft. The small chair was just right. Suddenly, the chair broke.
Episode 4	Consequence	Goldilocks walked upstairs.
	Reaction	Because she was tired, she decided to lie down.
	Action	The big bed was too hard. The middle-sized bed was too soft. The small bed was just right, and she fell asleep.
	Consequence	The bears came home. They saw that someone had eaten their porridge, sat in their chairs, and slept in their beds. Baby Bear's porridge was all eaten up, his chair was broken, and someone was in his bed.
	Ending	Goldilocks woke up. When she saw the bears, she ran out of the house and never came back again.

FIGURE 3.1   Story Structure of *The Three Bears*

stories that systematically varied in structure, adult readers demonstrated sensitivity to story structure constituents regardless of the content (Mandler, 1987).

Children have also been found to expect stories to have a predictable structure, with their schemata becoming more differentiated as they become older (Buss, Yussen, Mathews, Miller, & Rembold, 1983; Fitzgerald, Spiegel, & Webb, 1985; Golden, 1984; McClure, Mason, & Barnitz, 1979; McConaughy, 1980; Pappas & Brown, 1987; Whaley, 1981). When presented with stories that followed the rules of story grammar and stories that deviated from ideal story structure, even children in second grade have been observed to have better comprehension and recall of the well-formed stories (Brennan, Bridge, & Winograd, 1986; Feldman, 1985; Glenn, 1978; Hartson, 1984).

Yet some children seem to develop a sense of story structure sooner, or with less difficulty, than other children. Several researchers have found a positive relationship between reading ability and story schema, with more able readers demonstrating more highly developed story schemata (Fitzgerald, 1984; Krein & Zaharias, 1986; Rahman & Bisanz, 1986; Weaver & Dickinson, 1982; Wilkinson & Bain, 1984).

Studies of textual schema have found that (a) story schemata enhance reading comprehension and can be taught to deaf students explicitly and nonexplicitly; (b) although deaf children use story schema to recall and create stories, their schemata are less well developed than those of hearing children, though deaf children with deaf parents have been found to perform as well as hearing children; (c) internalization of story structure is related to writing development; and (d) stories with structures that reflect less predictable story lines encourage higher level cognitive processing than stories with structures that reflect highly predictable story lines (Akamatsu, 1988; Donin, Doehring, & Browns, 1991; Griffith & Ripich, 1988; Luetke-Stahlman, Griffith, & Montgomery, 1998; Schirmer, 1993; Schirmer & Bond, 1990; Schirmer & Winter, 1993; Yoshinaga-Itano & Downey, 1986).

Schema for Expository Text. It is difficult to examine readers' schemata for expository text because there is no single structure for writing that, according to *The Literacy Dictionary* (Harris & Hodges, 1995), is used for the purpose of setting forth or explaining. Almost all expository writing includes a combination of structures.

Much of the research on expository text structure has focused on the five patterns identified by Meyer (Mulcahy & Samuels, 1987; Ohlhausen & Roller, 1988; Richgels, McGee, Lomax, & Sheard, 1987). Meyer (1975; Meyer & Freedle, 1984) found the following five basic expository text organizations, often referred to as *rhetorical predicates* in the literature. In each of these structures, information is organized hierarchically.

1. *Collection.* A collection structure is information grouped by association and by sequence, such as in a time sequence or a list. Richgels, McGee, Lomax, and Sheard (1987) illustrated this structure with the following graphic organizer:

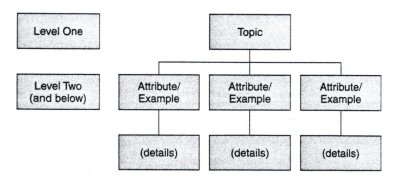

From Richgels, D. J., McGee, L. M., Lomax, R. G., & Sheard, C. (1987, Spring). Awareness of four text structures: Effects on recall of expository text. *Reading Research Quarterly, 22*(2), 177–196. Reprinted with permission of Donald J. Richgels and the International Reading Association. All rights reserved.

2. *Description.* A description structure is a specific type of grouping by association in which one element is subordinate to another. In a description, an attribute, specific, or setting is presented to support the topic.

3. *Causation.* In a causation structure, elements are not only grouped by association and sequenced, but they are causally related. Richgels and associates illustrated this structure with the following graphic organizer:

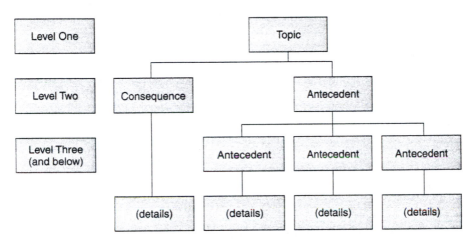

From Richgels, D. J., McGee, L. M., Lomax, R. G., & Sheard, C. (1987, Spring). Awareness of four text structures: Effects on recall of expository text. *Reading Research Quarterly,* 22(2), 177–196. Reprinted with permission of Donald J. Richgels and the International Reading Association. All rights reserved.

4. *Problem/solution.* A problem/solution structure contains all the elements of a causation structure with the addition that at least one aspect of the solution matches the content and blocks a cause of the problem. Richgels and associates used the following graphic organizer to illustrate this structure:

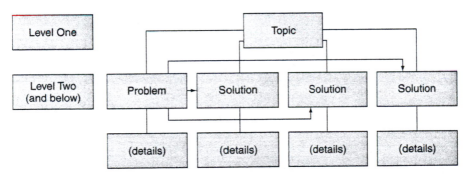

From Richgels, D. J., McGee, L. M., Lomax, R. G., & Sheard, C. (1987, Spring). Awareness of four text structures: Effects on recall of expository text. *Reading Research Quarterly,* 22(2), 177–196. Reprinted with permission of Donald J. Richgels and the International Reading Association. All rights reserved.

5. *Comparison.* A comparison structure is organized on the basis of similarities and differences. The following graphic organizer was developed by Richgels and associates to illustrate this structure:

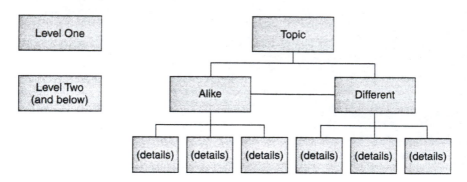

From Richgels, D. J., McGee, L. M., Lomax, R. G., & Sheard, C. (1987, Spring). Awareness of four text structures: Effects on recall of expository text. *Reading Research Quarterly, 22*(2), 177–196. Reprinted with permission of Donald J. Richgels and the International Reading Association. All rights reserved.

Research suggests that awareness of expository text structure increases with age and reading ability and that awareness of text structure is related to comprehension and recall of text information (Horowitz, 1985a, 1985b; Langer, 1985; McGee, 1982; Ohlhausen & Roller, 1988; Richgels, McGee, Lomax, & Sheard, 1987; Taylor & Samuels, 1983; Williams, Taylor, & deCani, 1984).

Surface Structure Schema.   *Surface structure* is a construct used in transformational–generative grammar to refer to the relationship among the syntactic and morphologic elements of a spoken, sign, or written sentence. Surface structure is contrasted with *deep structure,* or the meaning of a sentence. Sentences can have different surface structures but the same deep structure. (For example, John threw the ball. The ball was thrown by John.) Sentences can also have the same surface structure but different deep structures. (For example, Mary asked John to fix the bike. Mary promised John to fix the bike.)

Readers use content schema and textual schema for deep structure processing, but to get to the deep structure of a passage, they need to first process the surface structure efficiently. Schemata for surface structure include *word recognition, text cohesion, sentence transformations,* and *figurative language.*

Understanding at the word level involves *lexical cues, graphophonic cues, structural cues,* and *context cues.* The goal of word recognition strategies is to identify a word as being in the reader's vocabulary and therefore activate a content schema for the word. *Lexical cues* are cues that signal an immediate recognition of the word as a whole. All of the other word recognition cues are used to enable the reader to figure out the identity of individual words. *Graphophonic cues* are used by readers to analyze a word with predictable letter–sound relationships. When readers use *structural cues,* they are analyzing a word through roots, prefixes, suffixes, and compounds. *Context cues* include syntactic and semantic cues. Syntactic cues are the help that the order of known words offers readers, and semantic cues are the help that the meaning of known words offers readers when they are trying to identify an unknown word in the same context. (Detailed descriptions of word identification skills are provided in many current reading methodology textbooks such as Leu & Kinzer, 1999; Savage, 1998; and Vacca, Vacca, & Gove, 2000.)

When readers have highly developed schemata for word recognition, they are able to quickly and successfully identify words in written discourse. The more attention readers need to give to word recognition the less attention they can give to processing text at a deep structure level (Beck, 1989; Holdaway, 1979; Wood, 1985).

Research on word recognition has found that (a) some deaf students, oral and ASL, effectively use phonological-based codes to identify words in print; (b) some deaf students use fingerspelling and others use signs as nonphonological-based codes; (c) rapid identification of known words in print is an important factor in fluent reading and is no different for deaf and hearing readers; and (d) less skilled deaf readers may be slower and make more errors in word recognition than more highly skilled deaf readers (Bebko, 1998; Brown & Brewer, 1996; Fischler, 1985; Hanson, 1989; Hirsh-Pasek, 1987; Kelly, 1995; Leybaert, 1993; Paul, 1996; Schaper & Reitsma, 1993; Siedlecki, Votaw, Bonvillian, & Jordan, 1990).

To understand text at and beyond the sentence level, the reader must note the links, ties, order arrangements, or patterns that connect and integrate text elements and provide discourse with unity and clarity. The reader's subjective judgment regarding how well a text "hangs together" is referred to as *coherence of text* (Chapman, 1979; Harris & Hodges, 1995). When readers have well-developed schemata for text cohesiveness, they are able to identify anaphoric references (expressions, usually pronouns, that substitute for a preceding word or group of words), follow the sequence of action signalled by words such as *then* and *before,* understand the order of events through use of verb tenses, and recognize other cohesive ties in text. Although content and textual schemata are primary factors in reading comprehension, ability to process cohesive ties does have an effect on comprehension (Chapman, 1979; McClure, Mason, & Barnitz, 1979).

Some linguistic structures are clearly more difficult for youngsters to comprehend than others. The surface structure of simple active declarative sentences, such as "Mary painted the picture," provide a direct signal to the deep structure. *Transformations* of this sentence complicate the reader's road to the deep structure, however, as indicated by even simple questions, such as "What did Mary paint?", negatives, such as "Mary didn't paint the picture," and passives, such as "The picture was painted by Mary." Schemata for English grammatical constructions obviously have an influence on the reader's ability to process written text, since confusion at the sentence level can create misunderstanding at the discourse level.

The reader's ability to understand *figurative language* depends on content, textual, and surface structure schemata. When skilled readers encounter figurative language, their schemata for surface structure tell them that the expression makes no literal sense. They then must use their content and textual schemata to remind them that sometimes writers use nonliteral language, such as similes, metaphors, hyperbole, irony, and other figures of speech. Finally, they must use context cues available in the surface structure of the text as well as their prior understanding of the passage as a whole to deduce the possible meaning of the figurative language.

Investigations of sentence-level understanding have provided evidence that (a) while specific syntactic structures are particularly difficult for deaf children to comprehend, difficulties with syntax may be less of a factor in comprehension than ability to identify words in print through phonological or nonphonological recoding; (b) syntactic difficulties may depress the deaf child's ability to apply knowledge of vocabulary while reading; (c) deaf readers, like hearing readers, are sensitive to underlying morphophonological relationships among English words; (d) limited context inhibits the deaf child's comprehension whereas more extended context facilitates comprehension; and (e) text that is rewritten to control for syntactic complexity and sentence length may result in material that is more difficult for deaf students to understand because of the lack of text coherence (Hanson & Wilkenfeld, 1985; Israelite & Helfrich, 1988; Kelly, 1996; Lillo-Martin, Hanson, & Smith, 1992; McKnight, 1989; Stoefen-Fisher, 1987–1988; Wilbur & Goodhart, 1985; Wilbur, Goodhart, & Montandon, 1983).

Emergent Literacy

Emergent literacy, which has its roots in the work of Dewey and Piaget, replaced the concept of reading readiness in the mid-1980s (Christie, Enz, & Vukelich, 1997; Teale & Sulzby, 1986). According to emergent literacy theorists, the development of literacy in the young child is a continuous process, which occurs as the child is encouraged to notice and interact with written language (Hiebert & Raphael, 1998; Strickland & Morrow, 1989b).

The traditional concept of reading readiness considered early childhood and kindergarten as a period of preparation for learning to read. Hall (1987) observed that this view of literacy development was based on the following assumptions:

- Reading and writing are primarily visual–perceptual processes involving printed unit/sound relationships.
- Children are not ready to learn to read and write until they are five or six years old.
- Children have to be taught to be literate.
- The teaching of literacy must be systematic and sequential in operation.
- Proficiency in the "basic" skills has to be acquired before one can act in a literate way.
- Teaching the "basic" skills of literacy is a neutral value-free activity. (p. 2)

The scope of emergent literacy includes the kinds of literacy learning that take place prior to formal school instruction or prior to the time when children learn to read and write in what adults would interpret as conventional ways (Holdaway, 1979; Teale, 1987).

Teale (1987) considered the terminology *emergent literacy* to be extremely significant. *Literacy* emphasizes the developmental relationship between reading and writing. *Emergent* emphasizes the process and continuity of development and suggests the importance of home and community over formal teaching.

Hall (1987) observed that the emergent literacy view of literacy development is based on the following assumptions, which look quite different from the reading readiness assumptions:

- Reading and writing are cognitive and social abilities involving a whole range of meaning-gaining strategies.
- Most children begin to read and write long before they arrive at school. They do not wait until they are "taught."
- Literacy emerges not in a systematic, sequential manner, but as a response to the printed language and social environment experienced by the child.
- Children control and manipulate their literacy learning in much the same way as they control and manipulate all other aspects of their learning about the world.
- Literacy is a social phenomenon and as such is influenced by cultural factors. Therefore, the cultural group in which children grow up will be a significant influence on the emergence of literacy. (p. 8)

What Do Young Children Learn about Literacy?

The reading readiness view of reading was based on the notion that children arrived at school with little or no knowledge of literacy. Research with hearing and deaf students has shown that children learn a great deal about literacy before they are engaged in formal reading instruction (Adams, 1990; Andrews & Mason, 1986; Applebee, 1978; 1980; Bock & Brewer, 1985; Cox & Sulzby, 1982; Dyson, 1984; Garton & Pratt, 1998; Isom & Casteel, 1986; Mason & Allen, 1986; Mavrogenes, 1986; Morrow, 1989; Rottenberg & Searfoss, 1992; Snow, Burns, & Griffin, 1998; Sulzby, 1982; Teale, 1987; Williams, 1994).

Children learn that reading and writing have purposes, functions, and uses. They learn that print conveys a message and that people can communicate their ideas and feelings through reading and writing.

Children develop attitudes toward literacy during their early years. They learn whether reading and writing are valued by the adults around them.

Children learn the conventions of reading and writing; they learn that books are read from front to back, and print from left to right and top to bottom on a page (if they are reading English, that is). They also learn that print is followed word by word and, furthermore, that print consists of letters, words, spaces, and punctuation. They learn that print is different from pictures.

Children become aware of some decoding strategies. They learn to distinguish between words and between letters, notice repetitions and patterns among words, identify letters, and make the connection between written words and spoken and sign words. They also learn that words are composed of distinct sounds and that there is a correspondence between these sounds and the letters and letter clusters of words.

Children learn that the written language system has major differences from their oral or sign language system. Mason and Allen (1986) described these differences as physical, situational, functional, form, and structural.

1. *Physical differences* involve language in print versus language in voice or through-the-air. The authors use the example of speed. "Readers can vary their speed but listeners cannot. The same language sample, such as a paragraph from a speech, may take 6 minutes to write but as little as 1 minute to read aloud and half a minute to read silently" (p. 11).

2. *Situational differences* involve the face-to-face context of oral and sign language versus the decontextualized nature of reading. For example, speakers and signers can modify their information as they receive feedback from their communication partners.

3. *Functional differences* refer to the different purposes for which written language and spoken and sign language are used. For example, written language can be used to record a body of information for many readers to use over time.

4. *Form differences* relate to physical differences but include the restrictions in written language for expressing meaning. For example, spoken language can use intonation, pitch, and loudness, and spoken and sign language can use stress and rhythm.

5. *Structural differences* refer to the more formal, precise, and explicit nature of written language when compared to spoken and sign language.

Young children also develop knowledge about the world that builds their content schema, and they develop a sense of story that builds their story schema.

How Do Young Children Learn about Literacy?

Children use their environment to make sense of print; they pay close attention to restaurant signs, messages on tee shirts, advertisements in newspapers and magazines, labels on food products, and the many other kinds of environmental print they encounter. While researchers argue over the relationship between environmental print awareness and learning to read continuous text, it does appear that knowledge of environmental print plays a role in literacy development (Garton & Pratt, 1998; Mavrogenes, 1986; Teale, 1987). Research suggests that "experience with environmental print is an intrinsic part of becoming a literate language user, but that such experiences operate in conjunction with many other oral and written language experiences" (Hall, 1987, p. 28).

Children also learn about literacy through storybook reading. Researchers have studied parent–child interactions and teacher–child interactions during storybook reading, and they have studied how children function independently with storybooks. It has been found that when parents and teachers read to children, they rarely read word-for-word. Instead, they encourage much conversation, and this conversation changes as the same story is reread over time (Hall, 1987; Mason & Allen, 1986; Pappas & Brown, 1987). As Teale (1987) noted, "The words of the author are surrounded by the language and social interaction of the adult reader and the child(ren). In this interaction the participants cooperatively seek to negotiate meaning. Viewing storybook reading as social interaction has revealed that reading books aloud to children is fundamentally an act of construction" (p. 60).

Children use their emerging understanding of literacy in their pretend readings of storybooks, their imaginative play, and the stories they tell (Cox & Sulzby, 1982; Galda, 1984; Hiebert & Raphael, 1998; Isenberg & Jacob, 1983; Pappas & Brown, 1987; Purcell-Gates, 1989; Sachs, Goldman, & Chaille, 1984).

Why Do Young Children Want to Learn about Literacy?

From the moment they become aware of print, children seem strongly motivated to learn to read and write. Most cultures in the United States place a high value on literacy, and children seem to figure that out quickly. Children are surrounded by print. They see adults reading and writing, and they clearly like to emulate adult behavior. When adults read them a story, ask what they want for dinner while looking at a menu, or tell them about a birthday party after opening the mail, children are implicitly told that literacy is part of social interaction. They observe a purpose and need for reading and writing each time they see a parent cutting out a food coupon, reading the directions for assembling a new toy, following a recipe to prepare a special dessert, looking through the TV listing to decide on a television program, and doing the other myriad activities involving literacy. And they see that reading and writing are important when they see adults reading a book, newspaper, or magazine and writing a letter, shopping list, or e-mail message.

Research on the literacy acquisition of young children has shown that successful learners exhibit the literacy behaviors shown below during their preschool years (Snow, Burns, & Griffin, 1998, p. 61).

Birth to Three-Year-Old Accomplishments
- Recognizes specific books by cover.
- Pretends to read books.
- Understands that books are handled in particular ways.
- Enters into a book-sharing routine with primary caregivers.
- Vocalization play in crib gives way to enjoyment of rhyming language, nonsense word play, etc.
- Labels objects in books.
- Comments on characters in books.
- Looks at picture in book and realizes it is a symbol for real object.
- Listens to stories.
- Requests/commands adult to read or write.
- May begin attending to specific print such as letters in names.
- Uses increasingly purposive scribbling.
- Occasionally seems to distinguish between drawing and writing.
- Produces some letter-like forms and scribbles with some features of English writing.

Three- to Four-Year-Old Accomplishments

- Knows that alphabet letters are a special category of visual graphics that can be individually named.
- Recognizes local environmental print.
- Knows that it is the print that is read in stories.
- Understands that different text forms are used for different functions of print (e.g., list for groceries).
- Pays attention to separable and repeating sounds in language (e.g., Peter, Peter, Pumpkin Eater, Peter Eater).
- Uses new vocabulary and grammatical constructions in own speech.
- Understands and follows oral directions.
- Is sensitive to some sequences of events in stories.
- Shows an interest in books and reading.
- When being read a story, connects information and events to life experiences.
- Questions and comments demonstrate understanding of literal meaning of story being told.
- Displays reading and writing attempts, calling attention to self: "Look at my story."
- Can identify 10 alphabet letters, especially those from own name.
- "Writes" (scribbles) message as part of playful activity.
- May begin to attend to beginning or rhyming sounds in salient words.

Reprinted with permission from *Preventing Reading Difficulties in Young Children.* © 1998 by the National Academy of Sciences. Courtesy of the National Academy Press, Washington, DC.

Capability and Achievement of Deaf Students

Both hearing children and children who are deaf begin to develop as readers and writers from the point in early childhood when they become aware of print in their environment and the uses of print by significant individuals in their lives. Preschool children have been found to demonstrate developmentally appropriate knowledge and understanding of written language and uses of literacy even when language acquisition is delayed in comparison to hearing children (Rottenberg & Searfoss, 1992; Williams, 1994; Williams & McLean, 1997). However, as children who are deaf are engaged in formal reading and writing instruction in school, literacy development typically does not proceed at a pace considered average for hearing students (Holt, 1993; LaSasso & Mobley, 1997; Wolk & Allen, 1984). Wolk and Allen conducted their study with 1,664 students enrolled in special education programs and found that the average deaf student gained one-third of a grade equivalent change each school year. If it takes three years to progress one level in reading, this observation seems to explain mathematically why many deaf students graduate from high school with a fourth grade reading level.

Achievement of the average deaf student tells us very little though about the potential of any single child. There is considerable evidence to suggest that many children who are deaf achieve at levels commensurate with hearing children and that the reading process itself is not different for deaf children (Erickson, 1987; Ewoldt, 1978; Geers & Moog, 1989; Griffith & Ripich, 1988; Hayes & Arnold, 1992; Livingston,

1997; Paul, 1998). If the reading process itself is not different even though performance is often different, all of us need to analyze the literacy learning environment in which we immerse students who are deaf. Several researchers have suggested that the factors most critical to success in reading can be found in the quality of reading instruction provided to deaf children (Limbrick, 1991; Livingston, 1997; Truax, 1992). In Chapter 4, I will present the best teaching practices for helping deaf children to become competent and confident readers and writers.

Literature and Literacy Development

During the period when whole language first became popular among teachers in the United States, there was considerable debate surrounding the role of literature in literacy development (Goodman, Y., 1989; Sawyer, 1987). The lines of this debate were never drawn between the pros and cons of actually using literature to teach reading. Instead, the heat from this debate emanated from differing definitions of literature and differing views on how literature should be packaged for instruction. The debate subsided, but it is still crucial for teachers to consider the role of literature in the literacy development of deaf children. Literature is currently packaged in many forms for instruction, and all teachers must decide which forms will best enhance the literacy acquisition of the children they teach.

Basal Readers

A *basal reader* is a book in a basal reading series, which is "a collection of student texts and workbooks, teacher's manuals, and supplemental materials for developmental reading and sometimes writing instruction, used chiefly in the elementary and middle grades" (Harris & Hodges, 1995, p. 18). Basal reading series were traditionally characterized by controlled vocabulary, progressive difficulty, and detailed teaching instructions. However, current basal reading series look quite different from these traditional basals. Indeed, most contemporary publishers highlight the literature content of series by referring to them as *anthologies* rather than basals. Presently, the majority of teachers use basals as the foundation of their reading instruction, the percentage being 80–90 percent in some studies and over 90 percent in other studies, within classrooms of hearing and classrooms of deaf students (The Commission on Reading, 1989; LaSasso & Mobley, 1997; Reutzel & Larsen, 1995).

One of the major criticisms leveled against basals has been the contrived nature of text selections. To create texts in an easy to progressively more difficult sequence, authors traditionally developed stories and passages in which sentence length and complexity were monitored, vocabulary was controlled, and content selection was limited. In numerous studies, it has been found that contrived texts are actually more difficult for youngsters to read, regardless of whether the youngsters are deaf or hearing (Bouffler, 1984; Davison & Kantor, 1982; Ewoldt, 1984; Gourley, 1978; Hare, Rabinowitz, & Schieble, 1989; Israelite & Helfrich, 1988). Israelite and Helfrich concluded that "deaf students should be reading well-written stories created by skilled children's authors, instead of basal materials developed to meet a predetermined set of rules for syntax, sentence length, or vocabulary" (p. 271).

A number of other criticisms have also been brought against basals. The following ones were taken from the report on the state of reading instruction in the United States produced by The Commission on Reading of the National Council of Teachers of English (1989):

- Basal reading systems leave very little room for other kinds of reading activities in the schools where they have been adopted.
- Basal reading series typically reflect and promote the misconception that reading is necessarily learned from smaller to larger parts.
- The sequencing of skills in a basal reading series exists not because this is how children learn to read but simply because of the logistics of developing a series of lessons that can be taught sequentially, day after day, week after week, year after year.
- Students are typically tested for ability to master the bits and pieces of reading, such as phonics and other word-identification skills, and even comprehension skills. However, there is no evidence that mastering such skills in isolation guarantees the ability to comprehend connected text, or that students who cannot give evidence of such skills in isolation are necessarily unable to comprehend connected text.
- So much time is typically taken up by "instructional" activities (including activities with workbooks and skill sheets) that only a very slight amount of time is spent in actual reading—despite the overwhelming evidence that extensive reading and writing are crucial to the development of literacy.
- Basal reading series typically reflect and promote the widespread misconception that the ability to verbalize an answer, orally or in writing, is evidence of understanding and learning.
- Basal reading series typically tell teachers exactly what they should do and say while teaching a lesson, thus depriving teachers of the responsibility and authority to make informed professional judgements. (pp. 88–89)

Studies of teachers who use basals have found that they use these series for a number of reasons (Canney & Neuenfield, 1993; Greenlaw, 1990; Shannon, 1982). Primarily, they feel that these materials can be used successfully to teach reading. They also believe that basals embody scientific truth, they incorporate a variety of good children's literature, and they provide a well-organized plan for the teaching of reading. Many teachers also rely on basals because of state and district policies that favor the adoption and use of basals. In Shannon's study, teachers reported that their major reason for using published materials was to fulfill administrators' expectations while these same administrators thought that the teachers were using these materials because of belief in their effectiveness.

Trade Books

A *trade book* is defined as "a book published for sale to the general public" and "commercial books, other than basal readers, that are used for reading instruction," according to *The Literacy Dictionary* (Harris & Hodges, 1995, p. 258). When educators discuss literature-based programs for teaching reading, they usually mean that trade books, as well as other materials published for a wide audience such as newspapers and magazines, should be used for instruction. The difference between trade books and basal readers can be illustrated by imagining both kinds of books in a classroom library. Which books would youngsters spend time reading if they were given a choice?

Educators who advocate using literature in reading programs believe that there is a great difference between reading stories or excerpts from books and reading whole books. Huck (1987) called it *getting children hooked on books*. "Instead of reading 'bits and pieces' of a story, they have a chance to become engrossed in an entire book" (p. 376). Smith and Bowers (1989) made the point that "it takes more than ten pages for a student to understand and really fall in love with a book" (p. 345).

While most basals now include literature, many educators question whether the adaptations maintain the integrity of the original literature. Reutzel and Larsen (1995) examined five top-selling basal series and found that the publishers made significant changes including censorship, lost illustrations, and missing plot elements. They concluded that "the change in the current basal readers, though less dramatic than in previous years, may in fact have more insidious effects upon teachers and children than the alterations that were so obvious in the past. At least in the past, neither teacher nor student ever mistook a basal for a book" (p. 505).

Unlike the basal readers, the use of trade books requires the teacher to make decisions regarding pedagogy because instructional planning resides with the teacher and not the author of the basal reader. Hiebert and Colt (1989) identified three patterns of reading instruction that incorporate a blend of instructional format and literature selection:

Pattern 1. Teacher-selected literature in teacher-led groups.
Pattern 2. Teacher- and student-selected literature in teacher- and student-led small groups.
Pattern 3. Student-selected literature read independently.

Hiebert and Colt (1989) advocated the use of all three patterns within the same classroom. Smith and Bowers (1989) identified these same patterns but noted two other decisions that teachers need to make. The first decision is whether to integrate literature into content subject instruction, and the second decision is whether to use literature to replace or to supplement basal readers.

Huck (1987) presented five components she believed to be crucial to the success of a literature-based approach:

1. A read-aloud program for youngsters at all grade levels.
2. Daily opportunity to read self-selected books.
3. In-depth discussion groups.
4. The use of literature across the curriculum.
5. Time for children to respond in various ways to books.

When teachers decide to use trade books as the centerpiece of reading instruction, they must choose each book individually and develop all instructional ideas. Most publishers offer reading packages and theme collections, books that the editor has grouped together at different reading levels, as a compromise. Accompanying the books are supplementary materials and teaching suggestions.

Whether teachers use trade books, basal readers, or publishers' collections, they must carefully evaluate the materials, decide how appropriate they are for individual students who are deaf, and develop instructional strategies incorporating the materials.

Readability

One of the side issues in literature-based reading programs is *readability*. When teachers choose their own books or use books from a publisher's collection, they have to be able to determine if the texts will be comprehensible to the youngsters.

A number of factors, within texts and within readers, contribute to readability. Content, structure, cohesiveness, format, typography, literary form and style, vocabulary difficulty, sentence complexity, idea or proposition density, level of abstractness, and organization are *within-text* factors. *Within readers,* motivation, ability, interest, purpose for the reading, cultural background, knowledge of vocabulary, extent of background knowledge and experience with the topic, and knowledge of text structure contribute to the ease with which the text will be comprehended (Dreyer, 1984; Harris & Hodges, 1995; Irwin & Davis, 1980; Israelite, 1988; Koenke, 1987; Lange, 1982; Marshall, 1979; Zakaluk & Samuels, 1988).

The most frequently used tool for determining readability is a readability formula. Most formulas rely on two factors, average sentence length and vocabulary difficulty. Clearly, these two factors do not exhaust all of the possible variables that influence text readability. When used as probability statements or estimates though, formulas can provide predictive information regarding how easily a text will be understood by the average reader (Dreyer, 1984; Fry, 1989; Koenke, 1987). But they will not predict precisely whether a given reader will interact successfully with a particular text (Lange, 1982). Interestingly, when they updated the Dale-Chall readability formula, Chall and Dale (1995) noted that classic readability formulas are a valuable tool for assessing the difficulty level of reading material and continue to be widely used.

The use of readability formulas has been actively discouraged by a number of educators. I think there are two reasons for this phenomenon. The first is that whole language advocates found it anathema to use only two characteristics of a text for evaluating the potential interactions between reader and text. The problem with this criticism is that readability formulas are not meant to be the only measure of text comprehensibility. The use of formulas should be augmented with other methods for estimating the readability of text. As Lange (1982) wrote, "In the final analysis, it is not the use of readability formulas that presents problems, but the use of the formulas either as the only evaluation of a text or as the starting point for adapting a text to 'fit' a particular reading level" (p. 861).

Lange's last point leads to the second criticism of readability formulas, that readability formulas have been used to create texts written at specific difficulty levels. The problem with this criticism is that readability formulas were never meant to be writeability formulas. Fry, developer of the Fry Readability Graph, argued that "readability formulas are not and never were intended to be writer's guides. . . . The most common misuse of formulas is for writers to take the two simple inputs of most formulas and manipulate them irrationally" (1989, p. 293).

The use of readability formulas is simple and straightforward, and computer technology can make the process relatively quick. Virtually all word-processing programs incorporate readability measures. For example, Microsoft Word uses the Flesch Readability Ease Score and Flesch-Kincaid Grade Level Score, which can be viewed through the spell- and grammar-check command. However, formulas cannot be used without other methods of determining readability, although it might be very tempting to rely solely on computer software, with its aura of scientific validity. Some of the other readability approaches suggested in the literature are useful for determining readability.

One suggestion is for teachers to read the target texts themselves, using their own knowledge and understanding of their students to compare against the demands of the text (Dreyer, 1984; Israelite, 1988; Rush, 1985). A second suggestion is to give a selection of the text to the youngsters for a trial reading (Rush, 1985). A third suggestion is to use a cloze procedure, in which the youngsters are given a reproduced portion of the text from which words have been systematically deleted (Rush, 1985). In the second and third suggestions, the teacher needs to predetermine a criterion level of comprehension that the students can demonstrate through answering questions, retelling the passage, or filling in syntactically and semantically appropriate words in the cloze passage.

A fourth suggestion is to use a checklist for evaluating the comprehensibility of text. Teachers could create their own checklists using within-reader and within-text characteristics discussed previously in this section, or use one published in the literature, such as the Irwin and Davis readability checklist (1980). In Figure 3.2, I have presented my own readability checklist.

The checklist is designed to help the teacher figure out how close a match there is between the deaf child and the material before instruction. In other words, if the deaf child read the material independently, would he or she encounter several new words or only a few, would the concepts be unfamiliar or not, and would the level of abstraction be appropriate? In Chapter 4, I will discuss how to choose instructional models and strategies based on these readability factors.

Chall and associates (1996) developed another kind of readability measure that they termed *qualitative assessment of text difficulty*. They created six sets of exemplars, one each for literature, popular fiction, life sciences, physical sciences, narrative social studies, and expository social studies. Each set consists of passages at different reading levels, from easiest to hardest. To use this measurement tool, the teacher compares the text being assessed to one set of exemplars and determines readability by choosing the passage that seems to represent the closest match.

The true test of readability ultimately resides within the interaction of reader and text. I agree with Israelite's suggestion regarding the evaluation of readability by teachers of children who are deaf that "teachers reserve evaluation until they have observed their students interacting with texts, for in the final analysis, the most informed judgments are those of the readers, themselves" (1988, p. 17).

FIGURE 3.2   Readability Checklist

Book Title: _____

Author(s): _____

Other Readability Data: _____

Evaluation: (Circle your ratings along the 5 point scale)

Readability Factors within Texts

Word Frequency	(few new words)	1 2 3 4 5	(many new words)
Concept Density	(few new concepts)	1 2 3 4 5	(many new concepts)
Level of Abstraction	(low level of abstraction)	1 2 3 4 5	(high level of abstraction)
Organization	(clearly organized)	1 2 3 4 5	(not clearly organized)
Cohesiveness	(highly cohesive)	1 2 3 4 5	(not cohesive)
Clarity in Presentation of Ideas	(very clear)	1 2 3 4 5	(not clear)
Format/Design/Typography (e.g., print size, length of line of print, length of paragraph, color, typeface, punctuation)	(well designed)	1 2 3 4 5	(poorly designed)
Use of Illustrations	(many, good illustrations)	1 2 3 4 5	(few and/or poor illustrations)
Sentence Complexity	(simple sentence structures)	1 2 3 4 5	(complex sentence structures)
Vocabulary Difficulty	(simple vocabulary)	1 2 3 4 5	(difficult vocabulary)

		1 2 3 4 5	
Literary Form and Style	(familiar form and style)	1 2 3 4 5	(unfamiliar form and style)
Textual Structure	(familiar and consistent)	1 2 3 4 5	(unfamiliar and/or inconsistent)

Readability Factors within Readers

Interest	(high interest)	1 2 3 4 5	(low interest)
Motivation	(high motivation)	1 2 3 4 5	(low motivation)
Extent of Background Knowledge	(considerable)	1 2 3 4 5	(limited)
Vocabulary Knowledge	(extensive)	1 2 3 4 5	(narrow)
Knowledge of Text Structure	(thorough)	1 2 3 4 5	(incomplete)
Purpose for the Reading	(clear)	1 2 3 4 5	(not clear)

Additional Comments:

Recommendation:

— Appropriate as independent reading material

— Appropriate as instructional reading material

— Appropriate as reading material for story reading (read-aloud/in sign)

— Not appropriate

Metacognition and Literacy

Metacognition refers to thinking about thinking, reflecting on one's own cognitive processes, or monitoring one's own thinking (Babbs & Moe, 1983; Guthrie, 1982). When applied to the reading process, *metacognition* (sometimes labeled *metacomprehension* in the context of reading) includes readers' awareness and control over their own comprehension (Raphael, Myers, Tirre, Fritz, & Freebody, 1981).

A. Brown (1980) identified four elements of metacognition. The first element is *knowing when you know* (and knowing when you do not know). For readers, it means knowing when they understand and knowing when they do not. The second element is *knowing what you know.* In schema theory, knowing what you know means being able to activate relevant schemata while reading. The third element is *knowing what you need to know.* For readers, it means being able to benefit from knowing the purposes for reading. The fourth factor is *knowing the utility of active intervention.* In reading, this element involves the ability to invoke strategies to improve comprehension.

Strassman (1997) conducted a review of the research on the linkages between metacognition and reading in children who are deaf. Three issues emerged from this body of research. First, instructional practices that emphasize skills and school-related activities such as completing worksheets, answering teacher questions, and memorizing vocabulary words may hinder metacognitive knowledge and control in deaf students. Second, reading material that is typically given to deaf students because it matches their assessed reading levels may actually be low level and, therefore, may not provide opportunity for deaf students to develop and practice metacognitive strategies. Third, deaf learners benefit from metacognitive strategy instruction.

It is our goal as teachers to help youngsters who are deaf become conscious of their own reading and writing processes and use their self-awareness for monitoring and directing their own learning. Metacognition lies within the core of an autonomous and empowered learner. In the next two chapters, I will discuss instructional strategies in reading and writing that can enable children who are deaf to reach this goal.

Development of Writing

In the past, this section would not have been titled "development of writing." It would perhaps have been called "stages of writing," and the models of writing would have been discussed, models that conceptualized composing as proceeding in linearly sequenced and discrete stages, such as prewriting to writing to rewriting. Or, perhaps, it would have been called "types of writing" in which modes of discourse that conceptualized composing as mastering aspects of narration, description, exposition, and argumentation would have been discussed. Traditional writing paradigms resulted in teaching strategies designed to provide instruction in skills and rules, practice in mastering techniques, and evaluation based on how error-free finished products were (Hull, 1989; Laine & Schultz, 1985; Shah, 1986). The emphasis on teachers' comments, corrections, and grades on children's completed compositions led researchers to label this view of writing instruction as a writing-as-product approach. "Writing was a skill that one either possessed or did not, a process students experienced through native genius or discovered through trial and error" (Hull, 1989, p. 106).

In the early 1970s, researchers began to ask different questions about writing. Instead of only asking questions about the teaching, evaluation, and development of writing skills, they started to ask questions about what individuals think about when they write. Findings from this body of research caused a shift in the ways that writing, writers, and teaching writing were understood.

Current writing-as-process approaches conceptualize writing as a problem-solving process. Prewriting-writing-rewriting are no longer seen as linear and discrete stages. When writers engage in prewriting, their planning, rehearsing, and organizing are interrelated with their writing and revising. Movement between rehearsing, writing, rereading, and revising is ongoing and dynamic. Writers are in a continuous discovery state.

We used to think that writers had only one problem to solve: How can I communicate my ideas? In other words, what words and what grammatical constructions should I use? We now know that writers have many problems to solve. Who is my audience? What style do I want to use? Have I expressed my intent? Will the reader understand my meaning? And so on. The questions are internally generated and help writers to monitor their own progress. Through self-questioning while rehearsing, writing, and revising, writers come to understand and clarify their ideas. In a writing-as-process paradigm, editing is viewed as a final step in the composing process. In this view, editing is not equated with revision but rather is a part of revision, when the writer makes adjustments in spelling, punctuation, and other surface mechanics (Britton, Burgess, Martin, McLeod, & Rosen, 1975; Calkins, 1994; Emig, 1971; Graves, 1983).

Hull (1989) captured the essence of this conceptualization of writing when she wrote that "literacy researchers are learning of late to broaden their notions of writing as a complex cognitive process, of students as possessing immature or incomplete or perhaps flawed representations of that process, of research as the description of process, and of pedagogy as providing instruction on the process as well as occasions to experience it" (p. 113).

Writing Process

In the discussion of language development, syntax, semantics, and use were examined separately to emphasize that these language processes work interdependently within the individual. Literacy development was examined in the same way by pulling apart spoken language, sign language, writing, and reading while recognizing their interrelationships. To examine the writing process, each aspect will also be discussed separately. But for the writer, whether emergent or experienced, highly skilled or novice, the process is recursive. It seems as if each researcher has developed his or her own set of terminology to describe the subprocesses. The following terminology will be used here: planning, writing, and revising. Support for these processes can be found in the research literature beginning in the 1970s (Birnbaum, 1982; Calkins, 1994; Dyson, 1983, 1986; Emig, 1971; Flower & Hayes, 1980; Graves, 1975; Humes, 1983; Newkirk, 1987).

Planning

Planning includes generating ideas for topic and content, organizing, and setting goals. Planning for some writers involves prewriting, such as in the form of outlines, notes, or even a rough draft, and can also include rehearsal activities, such as drawing and conversing with others. And planning often means quiet thinking. Planning takes place before, during, and after writing.

Writing

Writing has been called drafting, translating, and articulating as well as many other terms. It has been observed that skilled writers recognize that what they put on paper (or computer) is tentative, whether it is a word, sentence, paragraph, or complete piece.

Revising

Revising includes rereading (or reviewing) and rewriting. Revising can mean rereading a word, thinking about several other choices, using a dictionary or thesaurus, crossing a word out, trying a new word in its place, rereading the new word, and so on. Revising can mean rereading a phrase or sentence and then trying out several structures. Revising can mean going back to a paragraph several pages ago, rereading it, and moving it several pages ahead. Revising can mean feeling satisfied with the meaning and style, but going back over the last few sentences to change punctuation or check spelling.

The research on the writing process has been conducted with hearing children, and the assumption has been that teaching approaches based on this paradigm are equally valuable for deaf children. Most of the literature describes how these approaches have been implemented in classrooms of deaf students (Johnson, 1992; Kluwin & Kelly, 1992; Pogoda-Ciccone, 1994; Truax, 1987). Indeed, the research on the writing process has focused largely on instructional implications of the theory. In Chapters 4 and 5, I will describe teaching approaches that reflect understanding and respect for the role of the writing process in children's writing development.

Emergent Writing

Children write long before they begin to use conventional print symbols. Their writing development is linked to their spoken and sign language development and to their reading development.

Harste, Woodward, and Burke (1984) identified eight concepts that served to organize the patterns they found in the writing of children between the ages of three and six: (a) organization, (b) intentionality, (c) generativeness, (d) risk-taking, (e) social action, (f) context, (g) text, and (h) demonstrations.

Organization

The first concept is *organization*. Children as young as three years old have been found to distinguish between scribbles and drawing and to invest their scribbles with written language meaning (Dyson, 1986). Organizational patterns have also been observed in young children's attention to syntactic, semantic, and pragmatic features in their own early writing (Harste, Woodward, & Burke, 1984; Hoffman & McCully, 1984).

Children's attempts at using graphophonic cues also reflect their efforts at figuring out the organizational principles of writing. Harste, Woodward, and Burke (1984) found that young children use three spelling strategies: the phonemic (spelling the way it sounds), the graphemic (spelling the way it looks), and the morphemic (spelling the way it means).

Bear and Templeton (1998) reported that the developmental spelling research suggests six stages of spelling knowledge through which children pass.

- Prephonemic—using pictures, squiggles, and letters to represent words.
- Semiphonemic/early letter name—using letters to represent sounds in words but only providing a partial mapping of all the sounds in a word.
- Letter name—using letters to map all the sounds in a word.
- Within-word pattern—moving from reliance on one letter–one sound to manipulating more complex letter patterns.
- Syllable juncture—attending to the morphologic features of polysyllabic words.
- Derivational constancy—spelling almost all words correctly and appreciating spelling–meaning connections.

Intentionality

According to Harste, Woodward, and Burke (1984), the second concept is *intentionality*. From the time children begin to use scribbles, they appear to invest their written symbols with meaning. In other words, they intend for their scribbles to be viewed as writing.

Generativeness

The third concept is *generativeness*. Young children have been found to arrange and rearrange their written language to create varieties of meanings and forms, and to serve changing needs within the child both to think about meaning and to communicate meaning. Generativeness in language means the ability to create an infinite variety of meanings from a finite set of words and a finite set of rules for combining these words. Generativeness in emergent writing means that the child is able to take a finite set of written symbols and create an infinite variety of meanings.

Risk-Taking

The fourth concept is *risk-taking*. By the time children are four years old, they seem more aware of the constraints of real literacy and less willing to try something new in their written language. By five and six, they often prefer to produce text with which they feel safe. However, Harste, Woodward, and Burke (1984) called this attitude a "learned vulnerability, not something inherent in the literacy process" (p. 140).

Social Action

The fifth concept is *social action*. Harste, Woodward, and Burke (1984) observed that children as young as three years of age recognized that written language, along with other forms of language, is social as well as personal in nature. "Not only do writers assume there are readers and speakers assume there are listeners, but interaction with real or supposed social others involving all of the expressions of language is an integral part of any instance of the language and language learning process" (p. 145).

Context

The sixth concept is *context*. The young children studied by Harste, Woodward, and Burke (1984) demonstrated sensitivity to the importance of the linguistic, situational, and cultural contexts of their written language. For example, they typically used more formal language registers in their written language than in their spoken language.

Text

The seventh concept is *text*. Early in their writing development, children were found to seek unity in their written language and to recognize that the text in their heads, what is called *text potential,* is not identical to the text they create.

Demonstrations

The eighth concept is *demonstrations*. Harste, Woodward, and Burke (1984) found that young children are keen observers of the literacy behaviors of others. The children's writings often contained features they had observed in environmental print, storybooks, the creations of other children, and the writing of parents and teachers.

Sulzby (1989, 1992) identified seven categories of emergent writing. She found that children move back and forth between these categories and sometimes combine several categories within the same composition.

- Drawing as writing—The child uses pictures to represent writing.
- Scribble writing—The child uses continuous lines to represent writing.
- Letter-like units—The child makes separate marks, often in a series, that have some characteristics of letters.
- Nonphonetic letter strings—The child writes strings of letters that do not reflect letter–sound relationships.
- Copying from environmental print—The child copies print from the environment.
- Invented spelling—The child writes words based on letter–sound relationships.
- Conventional writing—The child writes most words based on correct spelling.

Williams (1994) examined the literacy environments and activities of three profoundly deaf preschool children, one oral and two who signed, and found that despite the children's language delays, they demonstrated knowledge and understanding of written language that were developmentally appropriate. Her observations of the children at home showed that their "delayed language acquisition did not prevent them from experiencing, participating in, and using written language in their homes in ways that are similar to the ways hearing children experience, participate in, and use written language at home" (p. 145). Likewise, she found the same parallel with written language used at school. She concluded that "despite the differences between the deaf and hearing children's experiences with verbal language, their experiences with literacy were remarkably similar. Written language practice and use crossed the boundaries of language acquisition" (p. 149). Johnson, Padak, and Barton (1994) examined the developmental spelling strategies of eighty-six children with hearing loss, who primarily used oral/aural modes of communication, and found that the strategies they used to invent spellings were developmentally and phonologically similar to those used by hearing children.

The research in emergent writing has shown that children begin to explore writing long before they enter school. When we look at the young child engaged in imaginative play, drawing, writing, reading, communicating with others, talking and signing to him- or herself, we are witnessing the child's ability to represent reality in thought. As teachers, we need to recognize our students' cognitive potentials and language abilities, whether they are preschoolers or high schoolers.

Writing Development through the School Years

We do not have a very neat and clear picture of how writing develops during the school years against which we can compare the writing of youngsters who are deaf. What the literature provides is a theory about the writing process and implications for instruction. Unlike the literature in language acquisition, no models of writing acquisition are available that could be used to analyze the writing of children who are deaf. The reader might very well ask, "Is that all? Can't you tell me when I can expect my students to use traditional spelling? When will their paragraphs look like paragraphs? When will their stories be one paragraph long? two paragraphs? ten? When will they stop using illustrations? When will their stories conform to story structure? When will 'The End' no longer signal the end? When will they be able to write reports, diaries, letters, essays, thank-you notes, directions, recipes, and all of the other kinds of writing?"

The answer is, at least for now, it depends on the child and the learning environment. Do children who are deaf learn to write differently than children who are hearing? Do they have greater difficulties? Is the process more difficult? Is it less fun? No. At least, it does not have to be. The literature is replete with studies and observations of deaf youngsters becoming successful writers (Bensinger, Santomen, & Volpe, 1987; Cambra 1994; Ciocci & Morrell-Schumann, 1987; Conway, 1985; Nower, 1985; Olson, 1987; Schirmer, Bailey, & Fitzgerald, 1999; Staton, 1985; Truax, 1985).

In the next two chapters, I will discuss strategies and activities that have been used successfully with children who are deaf to enable them to develop as writers and readers. In Chapter 6, I will discuss techniques for monitoring their progress.

Relationships between Reading and Writing Development

Reading and writing both involve the construction of meaning through text (Schewe & Froese, 1987; Squire, 1984). Tierney and Pearson (1983) took this view even further by demonstrating how the composing process in writing can be used to understand the reading process. They found that both writers and readers engage in *planning* (goal-setting and knowledge mobilization), *drafting* (refinement of meaning as readers and writers deal with print), *aligning* (assuming of stances and roles in relation to the author or audience), *revising* (interpreting, changing hypotheses, analyzing, modifying purposes), and *monitoring* (conversing with oneself to decide how well one's goals have been met).

Fitzgerald (1989) found that revision specifically draws on similar thought processes during reading and writing because readers and writers are both actively involved in comparing the text (the actual text for readers and the evolving text for writers) to their goals and expectations. When readers and writers experience consonance, they continue reading and writing. When writers experience dissonance, they revise their text. When readers experience dissonance, they revise their understanding, goals, beliefs, or expectations.

Another parallel between reading and writing observed by some researchers is that achievement levels in reading and writing seem to be related. In other words, better readers tend to be better writers, although this pattern does not hold true for all children (Shanahan, 1980; Stotsky, 1983; Tierney & Leys, 1986). It has been suggested by some investigators that reading and writing are reciprocal processes that are mutually reinforcing. Others claim that reading influences writing development, while yet others believe writing influences reading development (however, the movement of influence does not work in reverse according to these two viewpoints). Smith (1983) argued that everyone who becomes a competent writer "must read like a writer in order to learn how to write like a writer. There is no other way in which the intricate complexity of a writer's knowledge can be acquired" (p. 562).

In their study of three theoretical models of the reading–writing relationship, Shanahan and Lomax (1986) found that second and fifth grade children used both their reading knowledge in writing and their writing knowledge in reading, and that in general the children used more reading information in writing than vice versa. However, they noted that the children in their study may not have had much opportunity to write and that in an instructional program that emphasized writing, writing knowledge might exert more influence on reading than they found.

Dobson (1989) studied the emergent literacy of kindergarten and first grade children and found that they transferred strategies learned in writing to reading, and reading to writing. He concluded that "reading and writing are mutually supportive and connected at each step to learners' knowledge of the system of written language and how it works" (p. 100). Mason, Peterman, Powell, and Kerr (1989) found support for the conclusion that at early reading levels, writing activity affects reading while at higher reading levels, reading affects writing.

By focusing on the parallels between reading and writing, it is tempting to ignore the differences. Yet as a number of authors have pointed out, although reading development and writing development are closely related, they are individual processes; and important differences exist between them (Langer & Applebee, 1986; Noyce & Christie, 1989). Rosenblatt (1989) observed that the "transaction that starts with a text produced by someone else is not the same as a transaction that starts with the individual facing a blank page" (p. 171). She viewed cross-fertilization as possible but not automatic without instruction that encouraged youngsters to gain metalinguistic insights into their own reading and writing processes.

Final Comments

Literacy development involves reading development and writing development. The relationship between the development of face-to-face language and the development of literacy in children who are deaf is not completely clear, but we do know a great deal more today than we did even a decade ago. Most significant, we know that deaf children have the cognitive ability to become proficient readers and expressive writers, and that we do not have to wait for some arbitrary level of language development prior to initiating reading and writing instruction. Indeed, we know that literacy and language are interrelated and that learning environments that encourage the development of literacy also encourage the development of face-to-face language, and vice versa. We also know that children do not wait for us to teach them to read and write; they start to understand and use written symbols long before they come to school.

This chapter discussed what is currently known about the reading process and the writing process in children who are deaf. The next chapter will contain models, methods, and strategies for encouraging and enhancing the development of reading and writing in deaf children.

Suggested Readings

Dahl, K. L., & Farnan, N. (1998). *Children's writing: Perspectives from research.* Newark, DE: International Reading Association.

Hiebert, E. H., & Raphael, T. E. (1998). *Early literacy instruction.* Fort Worth, TX: Harcourt Brace.

Paul, P. V. (1998). *Literacy and deafness.* Boston: Allyn and Bacon.

Pressley, M. (1998). *Reading instruction that works: The case for balanced teaching.* New York: Guilford.

Snow, C. E., Burns, M. S., & Griffin, P. (Eds.). (1998). *Preventing reading difficulties in young children.* Washington, DC: National Academy Press.

4

Approaches to Promote Reading and Writing Development

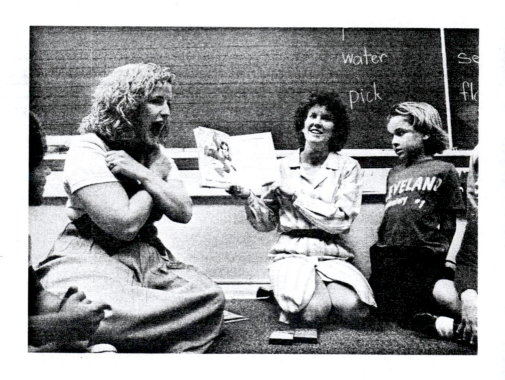

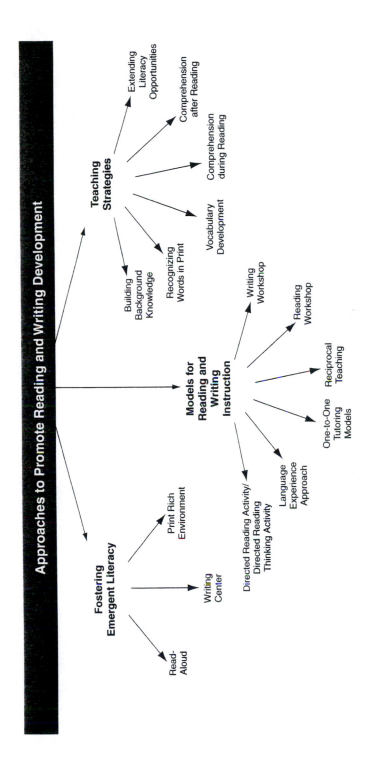

Approaches to Promote Reading and Writing Development

Fostering Emergent Literacy
- Read-Aloud
- Writing Center
- Print Rich Environment

Models for Reading and Writing Instruction
- Directed Reading Activity/Directed Reading Thinking Activity
- Language Experience Approach
- One-to-One Tutoring Models
- Reciprocal Teaching
- Reading Workshop
- Writing Workshop

Teaching Strategies
- Building Background Knowledge
- Recognizing Words in Print
- Vocabulary Development
- Comprehension during Reading
- Comprehension after Reading
- Extending Literacy Opportunities

133

Chapter 3 provided a theoretical framework of literacy development. This chapter will link theory with practice. I encourage readers to scrutinize critically these ideas and to ask at least three questions about each suggestion. Is this strategy grounded on sound theoretical principles? Has this strategy ever been used successfully with children similar to the ones I teach? Will I be willing to work through the problems if this strategy does not work smoothly at first?

Fostering Emergent Literacy

Several components of an early childhood curriculum seem to be central for supporting children's explorations into reading and writing. Parents and teachers have always known that these particular activities are valuable to young children. The last several years, however, have given us empirical evidence that when young children are provided daily opportunities to interact with print, they develop complex notions of reading and writing well before they are engaged in formal instruction.

Read-Aloud

If parents and teachers of deaf children were only able to consistently carry out one activity every day, I would strongly suggest that it be read-aloud. Read-aloud helps to develop children's story schema, background knowledge, and awareness of written language conventions. Read-aloud provides opportunities for meaningful conversations between teachers and children, and parents and children. Children who are read to regularly are likely to develop an interest in reading and a love of stories (Morrow & Weinstein, 1982; Wells, 1982).

Teachers of children who are deaf are sometimes reluctant to read aloud because they believe their students' language development levels are not advanced enough to enable them to understand the stories being read. This concern is not very different from that of parents of hearing infants and toddlers. Trelease (1995) responded to the question, "How old must the child be before you start reading to him?" by asking one of his own:

> "When did you start talking to your child? Did you wait until he was six months old?" "We started talking to him the day he was born," parents respond. "And what language did your child speak the day he was born? English? Japanese? Italian?" They're about to say English when it dawns on them the child didn't speak any language yet. (p. 27)

If we view reading and read-aloud as a milieu for creating readers, then we can begin read-aloud with children who are deaf long before they can understand every word and concept in the stories we read. We all can envision a classroom in which children are conversed with and read to because that is precisely the language-rich environment they need.

Some research has been conducted on the "how-to's" of read-aloud. One of the best sources on the subject is Trelease's *The Read-Aloud Handbook* (1995), although a number of authors have written about read-aloud. It has been suggested that teachers and parents make read-aloud part of a routine and carefully consider the children's attention spans. For most young children who are deaf, five minutes of watching or listening is a *long* time. It has also been suggested that well-written, enjoyable stories with a variety of themes be chosen. Teachers and parents are also encouraged to converse with children about the stories being read, before and after reading them (Butler, 1980; Rasinski & Fredericks, 1990). And reading the same story again and again over time is a time-honored and now research-proven activity (Martinez & Roser, 1985; Yaden, 1988).

Prescribing a set of behaviors for read-aloud is probably not necessary. Long before researchers decided that it was a great idea, parents read aloud to their children. Some evidence suggests that teachers and parents already know how to read to children effectively. Altwerger, Diehl-Faxon, and Dockstader-Anderson (1985) found that mothers match their read-aloud to the experiential, linguistic, and literacy background of their children by adapting, extending, clarifying, and sometimes disregarding the print. The researchers observed that "the mother begins to relinquish her role as text constructor for her child, and moves to a closer reading of the print as she perceives the child better able to bear the responsibility alone" (p. 483).

One of the few studies on read-aloud with deaf children was conducted by Rogers (1989). The five- to nine-year-old children in this study were read to four nights each week in their dormitory rooms at bedtime, with several parents continuing the read-aloud during weekends and vacations. Rogers reported positive results in the children's language development, ability to converse about stories, and comprehension.

Based on observations of deaf adults reading stories to children, Schleper (1995) recommended that teachers who read aloud in ASL keep the written words visible so that the child can move back and forth between the ASL rendition and the English words. He also suggested that teachers progress from telling to reading with successive readings of the same story, elaborating more when a story is new to the child and maintaining the integrity of the text as the story becomes more familiar. Read-aloud should be an enjoyable and mutually rewarding activity for children and adults.

Shared Book Experience

Read-aloud traditionally has taken two forms. The school form has been *one teacher-group of children*. The home form is *one parent-one child*. By combining features of school and home, two new forms of read-aloud are currently being suggested to augment the traditional school form.

The first form, *one-to-one* story reading in school between the teacher and one child, can provide the child with an enriching experience. However, demands on the teacher's time may make this an impractical suggestion in many classrooms of children who are deaf. The research to support this activity has been accomplished with a team of research assistants individually assigned to one child each (Morrow, 1987, 1988).

The second form is story reading with *big books*. This form is modeled on lap reading between parent and child in which the open book is viewed by both parent and child simultaneously, with the parent sometimes tracking the actual words with his or her finger. By using enlarged texts called big books (or using the regular book with a group of no more than three children sitting close enough to the teacher to see the print), the teacher can provide a lap reading experience to a group of children (Brown, Cromer, & Weinberg, 1986; Holdaway, 1979, 1982; Trachtenburg & Ferruggia, 1989). For the teacher who is signing, the book can be placed on an easel, or one of the children can hold the book.

Big books are currently available commercially, and many of them are accompanied by regular-sized copies for classroom libraries. Children can look through the same story over and over again during free play or book time, share it with another child, or ask an adult to reread the story during lap reading.

The shared book experience is sometimes used as a model for early reading instruction (Eldredge, Reutzel, & Hollingsworth, 1996; Reutzel, Hollingsworth, & Eldredge, 1994). In this model, the teacher sits in front of the children with a big book, introduces the story, and leads a discussion about the cover, title, and illustrations. The children are encouraged to predict the story line, after which the teacher reads the story aloud/in sign. The teacher engages the children in a discussion of the story, and then the children are asked to retell the story; either one child retells it to the group, or they take turns retelling it to a peer. The teacher rereads the book several times throughout the year, and each time increases the students' attention to the written language by inviting them to read and point out print and language patterns.

Writing Center

Writing centers are a new idea in preschool and kindergarten classrooms. In a writing center, the teacher creates a special table at which children can sit and select paper in an array of sizes and colors, pens, pencils, felt-tipped markers, and crayons. Most important, the writing center is a place at which children can choose what to do with these materials. It has been observed that most young children start by doing a great deal of drawing at these centers but gradually and spontaneously combine scribbling and then writing with their drawings (Crowell, Kawakami, & Wong, 1986; Heald-Taylor, 1984; Noyce & Christie, 1989; Strickland & Morrow, 1988).

Ewoldt (1987) found significant growth in the writing of three- to seven-year-old deaf children who were given opportunities to engage in self-selected reading and writing over a three-year period. Manson (1982), a teacher in the Ewoldt study, observed that "one of the advantages that became apparent as the project continued was that freedom of expression in drawing and/or writing allowed proficiencies to emerge individually while simultaneously exposing the students to additional print concepts as they emerged for classmates" (p. 36).

Print Rich Environment

A classroom environment that implicitly communicates the message that *literacy is valued here* can exert a powerful influence on early literacy development. Strickland and Morrow (1989) have observed that "purposefully arranging the physical setting to develop literacy can wield an active and pervasive influence on the activities and attitudes of teachers as well as on those of the children in their classrooms" (p. 178).

One way to create a print rich environment is through the use of *environmental print.* Labeling objects in the classroom, creating charts of classroom routines and rules, and using print in bulletin boards are just a few ways that teachers can meaningfully display print in the classroom. Some educators recommend that environmental print for deaf children be written in phrases and sentences to provide a full English model.

A *library center* is another essential part of a print rich classroom environment. It has been suggested that the library center be comfortable, obvious, and inviting. It should afford privacy and display books attractively. If possible, the library center should contain variety in terms of reading levels, topics, and genres. And children should be given time to use the library center (Morrow & Weinstein, 1982; Strickland & Morrow, 1988).

Preschool and kindergarten classrooms with children who are deaf should provide a setting in which the children are encouraged to engage in reading and writing activities. The classroom layout developed by Leu and Kinzer (1999) includes a reading center with bookshelves, writing center table, Author's Corner easel and sign, author's chair, and flip chart. This classroom also includes flip charts and signs at each activity center—dramatic play center, science area, art area, math center, and computer stations—and the room has a special table for constructing signs. In addition, there should be comfortable chairs in which children can read alone or with others, bulletin boards, and lots of books.

By the time deaf children complete kindergarten, if we have provided them with extensive opportunities to engage in literacy activities, they should demonstrate the same accomplishments as hearing children who become successful readers (Snow, Burns, & Griffin, 1998). Keep in mind, some of the milestones are dependent on audition and should be modified for children who cannot access the sounds within words. For example, deaf children who do not hear the differential sounds within word parts, such as *dak, pat,* and *zen,* can, with help, learn to identify them visually in print and through fingerspelling.

Kindergarten Accomplishments
- Knows the parts of a book and their functions.
- Begins to track print when listening to a familiar text being read or when rereading own writing.
- "Reads" familiar texts emergently, i.e., not necessarily verbatim from the print alone.
- Recognizes and can name all uppercase and lowercase letters.
- Understands that the sequence of letters in a written word represents the sequence of sounds (phonemes) in a spoken word (alphabetic principle).

- Learns many, though not all, one-to-one letter sound correspondences.
- Recognizes some words by sight, including a few very common ones (a, the, I, my, you, is, are).
- Uses new vocabulary and grammatical constructions in own speech.
- Makes appropriate switches from oral to written language situations.
- Notices when simple sentences fail to make sense.
- Connects information and events in texts to life and life to text experiences.
- Retells, reenacts, or dramatizes stories or parts of stories.
- Listens attentively to books teacher reads to class.
- Can name some book titles and authors.
- Demonstrates familiarity with a number of types or genres of text (e.g., storybooks, expository texts, poems, newspapers, and everyday print such as signs, notices, labels).
- Correctly answers questions about stories read aloud.
- Makes predictions based on illustrations or portions of stories.
- Demonstrates understanding that spoken words consist of a sequence of phonemes.
- Given spoken sets like "dan, dan, den" can identify the first two as being the same and the third as different.
- Given spoken sets like "dak, pat, zen" can identify the first two as sharing a same sound.
- Given spoken segments can merge them into a meaningful target word.
- Given a spoken word can produce another word that rhymes with it.
- Independently writes many uppercase and lowercase letters.
- Uses phonemic awareness and letter knowledge to spell independently (invented or creative spelling).
- Writes (unconventionally) to express own meaning.
- Builds a repertoire of some conventionally spelled words.
- Shows awareness of distinction between "kid writing" and conventional orthography.
- Writes own name (first and last) and the first names of some friends or classmates.
- Can write most letters and some words when they are dictated.

Reprinted with permission from *Preventing Reading Difficulties in Young Children.* © 1998 by the National Academy of Sciences. Courtesy of the National Academy Press, Washington, DC.

Models for Reading and Writing Instruction

The approaches discussed in this section and the strategies section are important when helping the deaf child move from being an emergent to a proficient and fluent reader. In the past, researchers thought that children learned to read at the early grade levels and read to learn at the later grade levels; however, we now know that learning to read and reading to learn occur simultaneously and continue virtually throughout our lifetimes. Some of the models and strategies discussed in this section, though traditional, have endured because they help hearing and deaf children become motivated and autonomous readers and writers. And some of the models and strategies represent relatively new ideas and reflect emerging theories about the processes of reading and writing.

No one model, set of materials, or collection of strategies is right for every deaf child, and no method of instruction that is effective in classrooms of deaf children is ineffective in classrooms of hearing children. The models and strategies presented here make sense for all children, but they make particular sense for children who are deaf. Teachers of deaf children must wear a metaphoric fishing vest with multiple pockets to hold their knowledge of different models, strategies, techniques, tactics, and approaches. From this vest, the teacher can choose the appropriate teaching idea for a given child at a specific time. In this section as well as the following section, the best teaching ideas will be presented, along with a framework for making good instructional decisions.

A *model* is a structure for approaching the teaching of reading and writing. Even though far fewer models than strategies are discussed in the literature, models maintain their relevance much longer than strategies. A model provides the teacher with a set of instructional steps; within each step, the teacher may employ a variety of strategies while the steps remain relatively constant over time. They provide the support a child needs to progress as a reader and writer.

The models I present here meet two criteria. First, they have been successfully used with hearing and deaf children. Second, they represent models along a continuum of support. The models at one end of the continuum provide substantial support for deaf children because they are designed to assist children at the earlier stages of reading development and children struggling with reading. The models along the rest of the continuum offer fading and differential levels of support because they are designed to meet the literacy learning needs of children who are becoming increasingly proficient readers and writers.

Directed Reading Activity/ Directed Reading Thinking Activity

The *Directed Reading Activity (DRA)* was first suggested by Betts (1946). It was adapted as the basic lesson format by most basal reading series in preference to the older and questionable round-robin format. With half a century of changes and adjustments, the DRA is still widely recommended as a format for daily reading instruction. The DRA includes the following steps:

1. *Concept Development.* This step is sometimes called prereading activities, preparation, and background building. In this step, the teacher is trying to activate and build the deaf child's content schema so that new information in the text will connect to the child's prior information. This step also includes the presentation and teaching of new vocabulary.

2. *Sight Vocabulary.* In this step, the teacher introduces words for the youngsters to learn to recognize immediately as a whole. Sight vocabulary involves learning to recognize, in print, words one already knows in speech or sign. Building a child's sight vocabulary with six to eight words daily that the child immediately encounters in text is considered to be a particularly critical activity for youngsters who are deaf because other word identification strategies, such as phonic analysis, may not prove to be particularly useful.

3. *Guided Reading.* In this step, the teacher divides the story or chapter into segments for silent reading. For young children who are deaf, a segment might be one sentence or one paragraph. For older children, a segment is usually one or two pages, and sometimes several pages. If the youngsters can read the whole story or chapter with no guidance from the teacher, the DRA is probably not the most appropriate model to be using. For each segment, the teacher sets a purpose, asks the children to read the segment silently, encourages the children to discuss the purpose-setting question and several other comprehension questions, and asks each child to orally or in sign reread relevant sentences or paragraphs to clarify answers.

   a. *Purpose Setting.* In this part of the guided reading step, the teacher sets a purpose, either through a question (such as "What will happen to Jennifer when she meets the old woman?") or through a statement (such as "Find out why the old woman has been hiding.").

   b. *Silent Reading.* At this time, the children are asked to silently read the segment. Some children will subvocalize or sign to themselves. Silent reading and reading aloud, in voice or sign, serve different purposes. For most children, comprehension is best achieved through silent reading (Holmes, 1985; Taylor & Connor, 1982). Indeed, because adult fluent readers rarely read aloud, it should make us wonder why silent reading in school should seem so strange. Furthermore, in classrooms of severely or profoundly deaf children, it is not possible to both read and watch at the same time, so we find children reading aloud to an audience of one, the teacher, or perhaps worse, children reading very little because most of their time is spent watching the reader. There is a place for purposeful oral or sign rereading of a passage, which will be discussed shortly.

   c. *Questions.* When the children have completed reading the segment silently, their attention is drawn back to the purpose previously set by the teacher. The teacher then asks several additional questions. The children's answers often lead to purposeful oral or sign rereading.

   d. *Purposeful Oral or Sign Rereading.* When the child has answered a question correctly or incorrectly, the teacher can ask, "What part of the story made you think of that answer? Please read it to all of us." Thus, the rereading has a purpose. For the child, the purpose is to share more information about an answer. For the teacher, the purpose can be to identify problems related to the child's silent reading, to help the child develop fluency, or to encourage the child's voice or sign expression.

   The questions and purposeful rereading in voice or sign can provide the teacher with diagnostic information regarding the children's reading abilities. This information can then be used to design strategy lessons that can be taught as minilessons during the DRA or at another time during the day. Strategy lessons will be discussed in greater depth later in this chapter.

4. *Discussion.* When the cycle of purpose setting, silent reading, questions, and purposeful rereading is complete, global questions are asked to stimulate discussion about the central story line and to engage the children in higher-order thinking.

5. *Skills Development.* Traditionally, skill-building activities have involved worksheets on sight vocabulary, word meaning, phonic analysis, structural analysis, and other skills considered to be essential for fluent reading. One purpose is for the student to practice a skill that was needed in the story or segment of the story that he or she just finished reading with the teacher. The other purpose is to provide seatwork for one group of children while the teacher works with another group.

6. *Enrichment.* In this step, the teacher creates opportunities for the children to extend their comprehension through activities such as field trips, dramatizations, art projects, writing, and other reading.

The *Directed Reading Thinking Activity (DRTA)* was developed by Stauffer (1969). The difference between the DRA and DRTA is that in a DRTA, the teacher helps students set their own purposes for reading by encouraging them to make predictions. After silent reading, the teacher uses questions to direct the youngsters back to their predictions for confirmation, modification, and creation of new predictions for the upcoming passage.

Two types of questions are typically asked in a DRTA. The first are questions requiring speculation and prediction, such as "What do you think?", "Why do you think so?", and "Can you prove it?" The second are questions requiring support for conclusions, such as "What makes you think that?", "Why?", and "How do you know that?" (Haggard, 1988; Widomski, 1983). Some evidence suggests that the DRTA results in better comprehension and recall of stories than the DRA (Marshall, 1984). The kinds of questions asked in a DRTA encourage higher-order thinking in children who are deaf.

The DRTA is a time-intensive instructional model that provides support in many areas for students who are deaf. Kurt Schaefer is a resource room teacher of deaf children in a public elementary school. When Kurt considered the models he might use with his students, he recognized that the DRTA offers the kinds of support that many of his students need. In Step 1, Concept Development, this model provides a place for him to build background knowledge of topics of which his students have little or incomplete information or experience. He can also use this step as an opportunity to focus on vocabulary development, another area of weakness for many of his students. In Step 2, Sight Vocabulary, this model provides a place for building the children's sight vocabulary a few words every day, which all of his children need. While he teaches these sight words, he often points out letter–sound relationships and structural features that he hopes they will apply when they encounter new words. During the Guided Reading, Step 3, he can closely monitor their comprehension and provide direct instruction when they are confused or even when they are unaware that they have misunderstood an important event or character description. One of the key features of this step is silent reading, which has cognitive benefits and fosters greater student engagement (Wilkinson & Anderson, 1995). In Step 4, Discussion, this model provides a place for him to encourage his students to analyze, synthesize, evaluate, and critique what they have read. For the Skills Development, Step 5, he provides the students with activities that they can carry out independently, such as creating a personal dictionary for new vocabulary words, or with a peer, practicing new sight words. The

Enrichment activities that he develops for Step 6 typically involve writing. For example, he asks the students to react in a journal to what they have read, and he responds to their written comments at least once each week. Other examples of writing activities are provided later in this chapter.

Language Experience Approach

In the *language experience approach,* frequently referred to as the LEA, youngsters dictate ideas or experiences to the teacher, the teacher records their dictation into the form of an experience story, and the story becomes the youngsters' reading material. It is used as an adjunct strategy for beginning reading instruction or as a remedial instruction model.

Through the language experience approach, children become aware of the relationship between spoken or sign language and written language, and they experience success in reading and understanding text precisely because they created the text. The language experience approach also capitalizes on deaf children's motivation to discuss and read about their own personal experiences (Ewoldt & Hammermeister, 1986; Hammermeister & Israelite, 1983).

The language experience approach also has some drawbacks. It can leave children with the impression that the relationship between spoken or sign language and written language is a direct one and that writing is a one-step process in which one's first thoughts are recorded into a final draft. Furthermore, most experience stories follow no common narrative or expository text structure. As Heller (1988) noted, "Group dictated stories that are recorded verbatim often lack the continuity that distinguishes a story from lists of sentences" (p. 130).

Experience stories can be individually dictated or group-dictated. The steps usually include the following when used with deaf students (Ewoldt & Hammermeister, 1986; Johnson & Roberson, 1988):

1. The teacher introduces a stimulus. It can be an object, animal, field trip, movie or videotape, art project, celebration, or anything else that is likely to stimulate a discussion.
2. The children dictate their thoughts or impressions about the experience. The teacher transfers the children's words onto a large sheet of paper, overhead transparency, chalkboard, or the computer.
3. The children read the story aloud, in voice or sign, while the teacher points to each word. Known words can be underlined and later written on word cards for each child's word bank.
4. The children copy the experience story, or the teacher makes a copy for each child's notebook, which the children can illustrate.
5. The children use the experience story and word bank over time. For example, stories are usually reread periodically to the teacher, peers, and parents. Also, words are continuously added to the word bank.

One of the challenges in using the language experience approach arises when the deaf child's dictated story differs noticeably from standard written English. If the teacher writes the story as dictated, the text may be a poor model of written English. If the teacher modifies the story, the implicit message is that the child's language is inferior or flawed. Also, one of the benefits of the language experience approach may be lost if the child has difficulty with patterns that do not match his or her own expressive language. One suggestion has been offered to solve this problem.

Gillet and Gentry (1983) proposed that teachers create at least two written stories for every language experience activity. The first should be a transcription of the child's language exactly as dictated. The second story should be the same story translated into standard written English. The second story is introduced as another story about the same topic, and both stories are then used in the conventional language experience activities.

Another challenge in using the language experience approach involves making it clear that the first draft and the final draft of a story are not the same. Karnowski (1989) advised teachers to write "sloppy copy" at the top of the experience chart and then engage the children in discussion that encouraged ongoing revision of the dictated story. The same process-oriented approach to creating a language experience story can also solve another problem of language experience activities, the fact that the "stories" the children produce tend to be strings of sentences with no cohesion and no text structure. Heller (1988) recommended that teachers ask questions designed to promote thinking of the text as a whole and to encourage the children to actively monitor their dictation. Both Karnowski and Heller suggested that dictated stories be read, reread, and rewritten by the children and teacher before a final draft is created.

The language experience approach is most typically thought of as appropriate for young deaf children. However, teachers of adolescent and adult deaf students often use language experience as a strategy to help these students gain confidence in themselves as readers. LEA seems to be particularly valuable in helping those students who have been unsuccessful with traditional reading approaches to realize that they can be successful readers. Once these students have developed some confidence with experience stories, other types of reading materials can be introduced.

Mr. Schaefer knows that several of the deaf children in the kindergarten class are engaged in LEA instruction, and he feels that this approach is helping to build early literacy skills and vocabulary. Kurt is also finding that the LEA is the best approach for Louis, a fourteen-year-old young man who reads at the late first-grade level. He has an extremely negative attitude toward reading and books, which is not surprising given how frustrating it is for him and how much failure he has experienced. With the LEA, Louis feels successful at reading his own stories while gradually building a core of sight words. Soon, Kurt is planning to introduce sophisticated picture books to Louis by asking him to read aloud/sign to younger deaf children. This activity will provide a fun transition to books as well as a reason to reread for fluency.

One-to-One Tutoring Models

The most time-intensive models involve one-to-one tutoring. Several models have targeted children who are at risk of school failure at the early stages of reading development. These models are designed to provide instruction that will prevent reading failure. To describe preventive one-to-one tutoring models, Slavin, Karweit, and Wasik (1994) use the analogy of a town with a playground located on the edge of a cliff. Occasionally, a child would fall off this cliff and be badly hurt. Although the town council discussed the matter, they could not decide whether to put a fence at the top of the cliff or an ambulance at the bottom. Sadly, education has often been more interested in putting an ambulance at the bottom of the cliff to help children who are failing academically than in putting a fence at the top of the cliff to prevent academic failure. Remedial reading programs, such as Chapter 1/Title I pullout programs, are the ambulance at the bottom of the cliff whereas one-to-one tutoring programs, such as Reading Recovery and Success for All, are the fence at the top of the cliff. These programs involve a major commitment by schools or school districts because of the investment in training and the ongoing costs of tutoring.

Reading Recovery
Reading Recovery is a preventive tutoring program originally developed by Marie Clay (1985) in New Zealand that was brought to the United States in the mid-1980s by Gay Su Pinnell and other researchers at Ohio State University. As designed by Clay, the children chosen to receive Reading Recovery instruction are those in the lowest 20 percent reading achievement group in their first-grade classrooms. The tutors are certified teachers who have received intensive training for a full academic year. Each day, the children are tutored for thirty minutes until they either reach the level of performance of their classmates in the middle reading group or until they receive sixty lessons without achieving this level of performance. The children who do not achieve performance equivalent to the average reader in their classrooms are often referred for special education services.

Reading Recovery lessons include four major steps. First, the child rereads familiar books with the goal of reading for fluency and focusing on comprehension. Second, the child reads aloud a book that was new the previous day as the teacher takes a running record by marking errors and substitutions and notating behaviors. Third, the child writes a message or story; the teacher rewrites it onto sentence strips, cuts the strips, and asks the child to reassemble and read the text. During this step, the teacher may also use magnetic letters to work on letters and sounds. Fourth, the teacher introduces a new book by talking about it and looking at the pictures; then the child reads the book.

Substantial research on the instructional effectiveness and cost effectiveness of Reading Recovery has been done, and although later results are not as positive as those of earlier studies, this model has helped many children at the early stages of reading development (Barnes, 1997; Center, Wheldall, Freeman, Outhred, & McNaught, 1995; Hiebert, 1994; Pinnell, Lyons, DeFord, Bryk, & Seltzer, 1994; Rasinski, 1995; Shanahan & Barr, 1995; Wasik & Slavin, 1993). Although Reading Recovery has been used with deaf children, no research results have yet been published.

Mr. Schaefer does not use the Reading Recovery model, but he does incorporate one of the steps in his literacy instruction. At least twice each week, he brings two deaf students together, and they take turns reading a familiar chapter or short story to each other. He has also discussed this activity with several of the regular classroom teachers because he believes that it could work well with teams of deaf and hearing students.

Success for All

Success for All is a comprehensive schoolwide program designed for schools with large numbers of disadvantaged students (Slavin, Madden, Karweit, Livermon, & Dolan, 1990). In one part of the program, students in grades one through three who exhibit difficulties in learning to read receive one-to-one tutoring by certified teachers. Initially, first graders are identified for tutoring through individually administered reading inventories and are reassessed every eight weeks. Unlike the Reading Recovery model, students in Success for All can receive individual tutoring for a year or longer. Each day, the student is tutored for twenty minutes by teachers who have received six days of training. In addition to this daily, one-on-one interaction, teachers integrate this tutoring program with the schoolwide reading program, and tutors teach one, ninety-minute reading class and tutor three children per hour each day.

Success for All tutoring sessions typically follow three steps. First, the student reads aloud a story he or she has previously read in tutoring and in the reading class. Second, the teacher conducts a one-minute drill of the letter sounds taught in class. Third, the student and teacher read aloud a shared story, described as "interesting, predictable stories that have phonemically controlled vocabulary in large type and other elements of the story in small type. The teacher reads aloud the small-type sections to provide a context for the large-type portions read by the students. The tutor works with the student to sound out the phonemically regular words, asks comprehension questions about the whole story, and has the student reread passages out loud to gain fluency. Writing activities are also incorporated into the reading activities" (Wasik & Slavin, 1993, p. 189).

The school at which Mr. Schaefer teaches does not use Success for All, so many of the features of this integrated program are not available to individual teachers, even though some of the aspects are clearly beneficial to deaf children learning to read. Success for All emphasizes the direct teaching of metacognitive strategies for comprehension. For example, Kurt often asks his students to go back to the text and reread a section to clarify information they did not understand. Other metacognitive strategies will be discussed later in this chapter.

Pikulski (1994) found that the research on one-to-one tutoring programs and early reading intervention programs indicates that several factors appear central to effectiveness:

- Coordination between the tutoring program and in-class program and excellent instruction in both programs.
- Small-group or individual instruction for students experiencing difficulty with reading and a greater amount of time in reading instruction compared to children not experiencing difficulty.
- Special reading instruction focused at the first-grade level.

- Literature that uses natural, simple language patterns and reflects predictable plot structures and characters.
- Rereading texts for fluency and comprehension.
- Strategies for phonemic awareness, phonic analysis, and word patterns.
- Writing activities.
- Ongoing assessment, particularly of oral reading fluency.
- Communication between home and school.
- Continuous professional development and support for teachers.

Reciprocal Teaching

Reciprocal teaching is a model developed by Palincsar and Brown (1986, 1988) for enhancing reading comprehension through dialogue that encourages collaborative problem solving between teachers and students. In reciprocal teaching, four activities form the basis of the dialogue: (a) *summarizing* involves identifying the main idea, (b) *question generating* involves creating appropriate questions about the passage, (c) *clarifying* involves monitoring comprehension and using repair strategies when comprehension has broken down, and (d) *predicting* involves making and testing hypotheses. Palincsar and Brown reported that these four activities were chosen because successful readers routinely employed them; they represent activities that readers engage in before, during, and after reading; and students are forced to monitor their understanding by focusing on information presented in the text itself

Palincsar (1986) described a typical reciprocal teaching lesson as beginning with a review of the four activities. The students are then encouraged to make predictions, after which they read the passage. The "teacher," who can be the classroom teacher or one of the students, asks questions, and the students respond. The teacher summarizes and asks for modifications to the summary, or the teacher asks for a summary. The summary leads to a discussion of any clarifications that are needed by any of the students. In the last part of the daily dialogue, the students make predictions for the next passage, and a new teacher is chosen.

The transition from teacher-directed to student-directed reciprocal teaching lessons occurs gradually. "During the initial days of instruction, the adult teacher is principally responsible for initiating and sustaining the dialogue. He or she models and provides instruction regarding the four strategies. However, with each day of instruction, the teacher attempts to transfer increased responsibility to the students while providing feedback and coaching them through the dialogue" (Palincsar, 1986, p. 119).

Andrews (1988) found that using the reciprocal teaching procedure for teaching prereading skills to kindergarten and first-grade students with severe-to-profound and profound hearing losses resulted in significant gains in their letter, word, and story knowledge. Reciprocal teaching has been found to be an effective instructional approach for teaching comprehension to students who have both good decoding and comprehension skills as well as students who have poor comprehension skills (Moore, 1988; Rosenshine & Meister, 1994).

Mr. Schaefer uses reciprocal teaching with two of his deaf students, one in fourth and the other in fifth grade. These students do not need the degree of support that DRTA provides, but they do need to develop comprehension–fostering and comprehension–monitoring strategies. In the reciprocal teaching model, Kurt does not simply ask comprehension questions; rather, he teaches his students a few key comprehension strategies within the context of reading actual text.

Reading Workshop

Reading Workshop is built on the belief that three basic principles underlie a supportive literacy program—time, ownership, and response. In Reading Workshop, only the first five to ten minutes of class time are spent in direct teacher instruction (i.e., strategy lessons or minilessons). The greatest proportion of the reading instruction period is devoted to independent reading. Atwell (1998) developed the following rules for Reading Workshop with her classes of middle school students:

1. You must read a book. Magazines, newspapers, and comic books don't have the chunks of text you need to develop fluency, and they won't help you discover who you are as a reader of literature.
2. Don't read a book you don't like. Don't waste time with a book you don't love when there are so many great ones out there waiting for you.
3. If you don't like your book, find another one. Browse, ask me or a friend for a recommendation, or check the "Favorite Books" list or display.
4. It's all right to reread a book you love. This is what readers do.
5. It's okay to skim or skip parts if you get bored or stuck; readers do this, too.
6. Record every book you finish or abandon on the form in your reading folder. Collect data about yourself as a reader, look for patterns, and take satisfaction in your accomplishments over time.
7. Understand that reading is thinking. Do nothing to distract me or other readers. Don't put your words into our brains as we're trying to escape into the worlds created by the authors of our books.
8. When you confer with me, use as soft a voice as I use when I talk to you: whisper.
9. Read (and write in your reading journal) the whole time.
10. Read as well and as much as you can. (pp. 116–117)

Reading Workshop is a model for students who are relatively autonomous readers. None of the deaf students that Kurt teaches are ready for this level of instructional support. However, he has found that the classroom rules developed by Atwell work very well with his Sustained Silent Reading program, which will be discussed later in the chapter.

Writing Workshop

Writing Workshop is a teaching model that evolved from the research on process writing that was conducted in the early- and mid-1970s. In Writing Workshop, the process of prewriting-writing-rewriting that was observed in skilled writers was applied as planning-writing-revising stages in the teaching model. These stages are not seen as linear or discrete in the Writing Workshop model because the research on the writing process showed that skilled writers move back and forth between these operations. However, the concept of stages gives the teacher a framework for the kinds of activities the child engages in at each step in the writing process. The overeaching environment is one that provides each child with choice, time, and a real audience to his or her writing.

Stages in the Writing Process

Planning.   Planning can include choosing a topic, identifying a purpose, considering the audience, and choosing the form for the writing. Choosing a topic can be particularly difficult for some children. Graves (1983) noted that "children who are fed topics, story starters, lead sentences, even opening paragraphs as a steady diet for three or four years, rightfully panic when topics have to come from them" (p. 21).

It has been suggested that each child should keep a writing folder or author's folder. One page in this folder can be a list of topic ideas that the child is encouraged to generate from personal experiences and interests, from topics he or she has read about, and from other students' ideas. The list of topics is meant to be a growing and changing list.

Planning also includes rehearsal activities. For some children, drawing serves an important rehearsal function. For others, discussion is vital. Sometimes a young author needs to gather information through an experience or through reading.

Writing.   Writing is the stage of getting one's ideas on paper (or the computer screen). Calkins (1994) preferred the term *drafting* to writing because drafting more clearly demonstrates the tentativeness of the writer's early efforts.

The author's folder continues to be valuable to youngsters during the writing stage. By having an author's folder in which to keep writing-in-progress, the child has choice over whether to keep working on one piece of writing or to switch to another piece that may be at a different point toward completion.

It is at the writing stage that children's concerns over spelling need to be addressed. If children believe that every word in a draft must be correctly spelled using standard orthography, they may be unwilling to do any writing at all. A number of educators have recommended that children should be encouraged to use letters or written symbols that make sense to them (Calkins, 1994; Graves, 1983; Harste, Short, & Burke, 1988). It is assumed that using invented spelling allows the child's writing to flow more freely. When Clarke (1988) studied the effects of invented versus traditional spelling on the writing of first graders, she found that children who used invented spelling wrote longer texts at the beginning of the study and showed greater increase in text length after five months.

However, not all children are comfortable with invented spelling. Wood (1989) proposed that teachers present children with invented spelling strategies, such as drawing, scribbling, using strings of letters, and phonetic spelling, and model how these strategies can be used to write and read back what has been written. Contrary to these views, Atwell (1998) tells her students to "get into the habit of punctuating and spelling as conventionally as you can while you're composing; this is what writers do" (p. 116).

Revising.   Revising has been defined as seeing again, a re-vision (Calkins, 1994; Tompkins, 2000). Calkins believed that writers ask the same basic questions of themselves over and over again:

- What have I said so far? What am I trying to say?
- How do I like it? What is good here that I can build on? What is not so good that I can fix?
- How does it sound? How does it look?
- How else could I have done this?
- What will my readers think as they read this? What questions will they ask? What will they notice? Feel? Think?
- What am I going to do next? (pp. 222–223)

Movement between planning, writing, and revision can happen at the word level, sentence level, paragraph level, and text level. At one point, the writer may change a single word a dozen times and at another point write several paragraphs without stopping to reread and revise. Editing is usually thought of as a final cleanup for the written conventions of spelling, capitalization, grammatical structure, and writing style, yet many writers cannot move forward if a word is spelled incorrectly, the punctuation confuses the meaning, a sentence seems awkward, or the copy is messy.

Teachers typically report that youngsters do not like to revise and are reluctant to do much more than peripheral revision. In her review of the literature on revision, Fitzgerald (1987) found that researchers had made the identical observation. It appeared that without extensive support from teachers or peers, beginning writers do little independent revision and that even older and more experienced writers tend to make editing revisions only. Yet the research also supports the positive effects of revision on the writer's thought processes and on the quality of the final written composition.

Fitzgerald (1988) found some support in the literature for three kinds of instructional strategies that encouraged children to revise their writing. The first is *naturalistic classroom support*. In this strategy, natural opportunities to think about and experiment with revision are provided. Naturalistic classroom support is provided whenever children are given lots of time to write and lots of time to talk with others about their writing. The second strategy is *direct instruction in the problem-solving process of revision*. In this strategy, the teacher demonstrates the revision process, provides guided practice, and gives the youngsters written suggestions about revision. The third strategy is *procedural facilitation of revision*. In this strategy, the teacher provides the youngsters with a set of evaluative statements that they can use to assess their writing and guide their revisions. Some examples are, "People won't see why this is important," "This is good," "I'm getting away from the main point," "I'd better give an example," "I'd better change the wording" (p. 128). Teachers can develop evaluative statements that are appropriate for individual children.

Many teachers include revision checklists or editing/proofreading lists inside the author's folder. Ultimately, the author's folder contains a rich history of the child's writing: topic ideas, drafts, completed pieces, self-evaluations and teacher evaluations, and writing suggestions.

Publishing.   Not every piece that children write leads to publishing, but the opportunity to publish provides youngsters with the sense that they are writing for a real audience. Graves (1983) contended that "publishing serves as a specific anchor for the future during the composing. Even more important, when the child is composing a new piece, publishing is a hardcover record of past accomplishments" (p. 54).

Many schools have taken on publishing as a schoolwide project that has included the purchasing of book-binding equipment, the involvement of parent volunteers, and the establishment of a school publishing house. Regardless of how simple or elaborate the publishing process is, most children seem to enjoy seeing some of their work placed and catalogued into a well-used classroom or school library. As Hubbard (1985) noted, "If the goals of an effective writing program include helping writers go beyond themselves, taking pride in their work and their classroom community, then publishing books should be an integral part of that program" (p. 662).

Conferencing

Calkins (1994) observed that conferences fell into five categories: content, design, process, evaluation, and editorial. In *content conferences,* the focus is on the subject of the writing, and the conference partner asks questions that help the writer figure out what he or she knows about the topic, needs to learn about it, and what he or she wants to convey to the reader. In *design conferences,* the focus is on the form of the writing, and the conference partner asks questions that help the writer make decisions about mode, style, amount of detail, focus, and balance.

Process conferences focus on the writing process, and the conference partner asks questions that help the writer reflect on the strategies—planning, self-questions during revising, and editing checklists—he or she is using that work well and those that are not working well. *Evaluation conferences* focus on evaluating the writing, and the conference partner asks questions that encourage the writer to be a critical reader of his or her own writing. In *editorial conferences,* the focus is on mechanics, and the conference partner draws the writer's attention to correct usage of spelling, punctuation, capitalization, and sentence structure.

There are not only different categories of conferences but different forms of conferences as well. One-to-one conferences can be between the teacher and one student or between two peers. When they are between peers, the teacher has to make sure that the youngsters are taught how to interact with one another in conferences, often the topic of several minilessons.

Group conferences can be conducted for the purpose of seeking advice or for sharing. Harste, Short, and Burke (1988) make this distinction with the terms *Author's Circle* and *Author's Chair.* In *Author's Circle,* the author reads his or her piece to the group and gives the group direction regarding the kind of feedback being solicited.

"Author's Circle is under the direction of whichever author is presenting a piece. The presenting author shares the piece of writing, tells what he or she particularly likes about it, asks if it is clear, and identifies sections that are weak and that require the group's suggestions for improvement" (p. 69). In *Author's Chair,* the child reads to the group a composition that he or she likes just the way it is.

Minilessons

Minilessons are five- to ten-minute lessons that are often used to open writing workshop class periods. Minilessons offer a whole-group forum for the teacher to provide direct instruction in a skill or concept with which the youngsters have been grappling in their writing. Atwell (1998) organized minilessons around three broad categories:

- *Procedural*—the rules and routines of the workshop.
- *Literary Craft*—techniques, styles, genres, authors, and works of literature.
- *Conventions*—spelling, punctuation, sentence structures, paragraphing, capitalization.

In a whole language approach, a Writing Workshop model provides little direct instruction or intervention. Even the five- to ten-minute minilesson that opens the class period is increasingly being replaced by longer, interactive discussions with students about writing (Atwell, 1998). This limited support can be problematic for students who are struggling with writing and with English, such as children who are deaf, children with learning disabilities, and children learning English as a second language (Reid, 1994; Schirmer, Bailey, & Fitzgerald, 1999; Stoddard & MacArthur, 1993).

Mr. Schaefer uses a writing process approach, but not a Writing Workshop model with his deaf students. He spends considerable time teaching the qualities of good writing as well as the stages of the writing process itself. In addition to creating many opportunities for his students to write on self-selected topics, he assigns writing projects that are related to instruction in the content areas, such as science and social studies. Indeed, he helps many of his students work on reports that are assigned by their regular classroom teachers. Kurt believes that his feedback to the students is crucial for helping them understand how well they are succeeding, so he uses a variety of criteria for evaluating each piece of writing. However, he also requires them to evaluate their own writing using the same criteria. Some of the students' classroom teachers use a Writing Workshop model, and their major difficulty is peer conferencing because using an interpreter is cumbersome and feels intrusive. Most of the time, the students bring their writing to the resource room and conference with Kurt.

Teaching Strategies

Most teachers own crates of files or index boxes full of teaching strategies gathered from preservice and inservice coursework, education journals and magazines, web sites, workshops, books, and other teachers. The goal of this section is not to randomly add to this array of ideas. Rather, the goal here is to connect pertinent and proven strategies to the instructional models that you are using with the deaf students you teach.

Building Background Knowledge

For teachers using the DRA or DRTA model with their deaf students, building background knowledge is the first step for each new piece of reading, and with other models, such as reciprocal teaching, it can be an added step that activates prior knowledge or provides new information helpful to comprehension. It can also be an important step in the planning stage of the writing process. Which strategy the teacher chooses and the amount of time allotted to the activity depend largely on the extent to which the students are already familiar with the topic.

When students are relatively knowledgeable about the topic and the goal is to activate their knowledge, engaging the students in a brief discussion is generally adequate. This type of discussion is probably the easiest and most efficient way to activate background knowledge with students who are deaf; however, it is simply too brief for building new knowledge. The following activities have been effectively used with both deaf and hearing students.

Reconciled Reading Lesson

Reutzel (1985a) noticed that some of the best ideas for prereading activities were those suggested for enrichment in the teacher's manuals of basal reading series. He proposed that an enrichment activity should be the first step instead of the last step in a DRA or DRTA. In a *reconciled reading lesson,* activities such as performing a play, writing a recipe, and viewing a film are conducted before rather than after reading the story. Furthermore, the youngsters are engaged in a full discussion of the story prior to reading. For example, if the students were getting ready to read *The Diary of Anne Frank,* the teacher doing a typical background building activity for the DRTA model might engage the class in a discussion of the events involved in World War II and the Holocaust. If the teacher used a reconciled reading lesson format, instead of simply having a discussion and drawing on the students' knowledge of these historical events, the teacher might show the movie of *The Diary of Anne Frank* or *Schindler's List* and then engage the class in a discussion of the book they would be reading.

In their study of forty-five children in grades one through five, Prince and Mancus (1987) found strong support for the finding that reconciled reading lessons improved story comprehension. Because of the amount of time needed for a reconciled reading lesson, it would seem to be most appropriately used when the youngsters are getting ready to read material, such as a novel, which will take at least two weeks to complete.

Previews

A *preview* is a summary of text material that is read in advance of the full text. Most of the research on previews has specifically related to previews of expository text, which will be discussed in Chapter 5. However, there is some support for the use of previews with narrative text. Graves, Cooke, and Laberge (1983) found that previews significantly improved the comprehension and recall of the seventh and eighth graders in their study, and that the students reported they liked the previews and found them useful. It should be noted that the previews used in this study did not take the form of brief, introductory statements. Rather they were designed to seriously engage the students in the upcoming passages and to tell the students a great deal about the stories. Previews began with a series of short questions and statements that were followed first by a story synopsis, then by an identification of each character, and finally by a definition of several difficult words.

Previews would seem to be a particularly valuable strategy for deaf children preparing to read material with a possibly unfamiliar text structure. For example, one teacher developed a preview for *The Diary of Anne Frank,* which one of the deaf students in her high school resource room was getting ready to read in his regular classroom. He had not previously read a book written as a diary and, furthermore, was not completely familiar with the historical context of the book. In the preview, the teacher included information about the author, the other key individuals in the book, and background information on the period during which Anne Frank kept her diary. This preview enabled the youngster to participate more fully in the class discussions and to gain greater appreciation of the book.

Semantic Mapping

Semantic mapping is "a categorical structuring of information in graphic form" (Heimlich & Pittelman, 1986, p. 1). Semantic mapping has most commonly been used for vocabulary development, prereading, postreading, and as a study skill technique. As a prereading activity, the teacher writes a central story concept on the board and circles it. Lines are drawn to radiate from the circle. These lines are sometimes called *web strands.* From each line, a new circle is drawn within which the teacher writes a question about the story. The youngsters are encouraged to make predictions that are written, circled, and connected by lines to the questions (Freedman & Reynolds, 1980; Sinatra, Stahl-Gemake, & Berg, 1984; Spiegel, 1981).

Semantic mapping is a relatively quick way to activate interest in an upcoming story and to encourage thinking that goes beyond the literal level. Teachers using this strategy with children who are deaf have noted that the predictions help the children become interactive readers, and the semantic map itself becomes a focal point throughout the reading for seeing how the story components fit together.

ReQuest

In the *ReQuest* procedure (Manzo, 1969), the students read the title and first sentence of a story and look at the picture. They then ask the teacher anything they want to know about the title, sentence, and picture. When the teacher finishes answering all of their questions, the procedure is repeated for the second sentence. If the students run out of questions to ask, the teacher can suggest questions. Teacher questions not only add to the students' understanding of the upcoming passage, but they also serve as a model for good questions. After all the questions are answered, the teacher asks the students what they think will happen in the passage. At that point, the youngsters read the passage silently.

Larking (1984) found that after two months of using this Reciprocal Questioning procedure, the seventh-grade students in his study asked significantly more inferential and evaluative questions, and their reading comprehension scores improved significantly. Larking further found a positive relationship between reading comprehension scores and the number of higher-order questions the youngsters asked.

For youngsters who are deaf, an added benefit of the ReQuest procedure is that it encourages language development in the area of asking questions, including all types of wh- questions and *yes/no* questions.

Mr. Schaefer has found that his deaf students recall new information better when they have had a personal experience related to it. Because experiential activities are so time consuming, he tends to involve his students in these activities when they are beginning a new novel rather than a new short story. Indeed, he has included a greater number of novels in his reading program because he does not have to conduct background-building activities as often as when the students read short stories that are unrelated in topic. The fact that many classroom teachers are theming their instruction has also been advantageous; in fact, much of the background building and activating that used to be part of Kurt's instruction is now essentially a part of science and social studies units.

Kurt varies the activities he uses for background building. For his students who use ASL, he has sometimes modified a procedure developed by Andrews, Winograd, and DeVille (1996) called the *ASL summary technique*. In this technique, the teacher first tells the students a story in ASL, and then they read the story silently. After reading, the students retell the story and discuss it. The teacher can use student retellings as an opportunity to note the differences between English and ASL syntactic forms, the relationship between these forms, and the meanings they express. In the technique developed by Andrews and her associates, at this point, the teacher is supposed to fill in gaps in understanding. Instead, Kurt uses the reciprocal teaching technique of having the students go back to the written text to clarify information. He also uses the DRTA technique of having the students read aloud/sign sections of the text in response to a question or point of discussion.

Recognizing Words in Print

Models that provide significant teacher support, such as the DRTA and one-to-one tutoring, incorporate steps for teaching children to recognize words in print. The debate about the role of phonemic awareness and phonic analysis in reading development notwithstanding, it is obvious that fluency and comprehension depend on the relatively rapid and effortless identification of words in print. Readers have basically four approaches for word identification—automatic word recognition, phonic analysis of letter–sound relationships, structural analysis of meaningful units within words, and context cues.

Word identification strategies must be taught early, which is why the DRA, DRTA, and the one-to-one tutoring models incorporate steps for teaching sight vocabulary, phonic analysis, structural analysis, and context cues. In a balanced reading program, strategies are taught and practiced in isolation and reinforced within the context of text reading. Dozens of learning activities have been developed and published in magazines for teachers, curriculum packages and workbooks, textbooks, and web pages. Minilessons and strategy lessons are two of the best strategies for teaching word recognition to deaf readers, and they fit well into the DRTA lesson format as well as other instructional models.

Minilessons and Strategy Lessons

Minilessons and strategy lessons involve children in brief, clear, and concise discussions of specific aspects of the reading and writing process. Minilessons occur before reading whereas strategy lessons occur during and after reading. As discussed in the sections on Reading and Writing Workshops, minilessons can encompass a broad range of topics from genre to understanding anaphoric references, revision strategies to conferencing skills.

Minilessons for word recognition should focus primarily, if not exclusively, on words that the children will immediately encounter in text. As part of a DRTA, minilessons can combine the teaching of sight vocabulary with instruction on phonic or structural analysis. In this strategy, each word is presented in isolation on a flashcard or within a brief phrase for contextual support on a sentence strip. The teacher shows the word to the students, says it, signs it, fingerspells it, and discusses the meaning. The teacher then points out letter–sound relationships, onset and rimes, and roots and affixes within each word. It is more useful to concentrate on a few of these, particularly when a pattern is present in more than one sight word. For example, when Mr. Schaefer is teaching a sight word with the past tense -*ed,* he might point out only the verb inflections in other sight words. The students then practice reading all the sight words and signing, saying, and fingerspelling them.

During reading, strategy lessons occur as needed when the child has difficulty identifying a word. The teacher takes a few minutes to teach the letter–sound relationships, the root and affixes, or the semantic or syntactic cues available in the context of the word. Kurt often focuses strategy lessons on the word identification features he taught during the minilesson.

After reading, strategy lessons should reinforce a skill that the students have just applied and can be followed by activities designed to provide practice in applying the skill to new words in additional contexts. These strategy lessons are part of the skills development step of the DRTA.

Strategy lessons serve three important goals. They enable the teacher to focus on specific reading skills on an as-needed basis, when the skill is relevant to the deaf child's current reading needs. Strategy lessons also explicitly let the child know that individual skills are important because they are applicable to the reading process and not because they are an end in themselves. Furthermore, strategy lessons implicitly communicate the message that the most important part of the reading class period is reading, as the strategy lessons involve considerably less time than actual reading of text material.

Vocabulary Development

A direct relationship has been found between vocabulary knowledge and reading comprehension. However, the relationship between vocabulary instruction and reading comprehension is tenuous (M. Graves, 1986; Mezynski, 1983; Roser & Juel, 1982; Stahl & Fairbanks, 1986). The implication seems to be that although vocabulary knowledge is critical to reading comprehension, we do not always teach new vocabulary in ways that enable children to develop or use deep-level word concepts.

One of the problems faced in discussing vocabulary development is defining what is meant by "new" words. M. Graves (1986) identified six word-learning tasks to distinguish between levels of the child's current word knowledge. One task is learning to read known words (referred to as sight vocabulary in a previous section). The other tasks are learning new meanings for known words, clarifying and enriching the meanings of known words, learning new labels for known concepts, learning words that represent new and difficult concepts, and moving words from the youngster's receptive vocabulary to productive vocabulary.

Three qualities of effective vocabulary instruction have been identified: *integration, repetition,* and *meaningful use* (McKeown, Beck, Omanson, & Pople, 1985; Roser & Juel, 1982; Stahl, 1986; Stahl & Fairbanks, 1986). Integration involves relating new words to the child's background knowledge. Repetition involves providing the child more than one encounter with the meanings and uses of new words. Meaningful use involves developing rich conceptual frameworks for new words and providing opportunities for the youngster to encounter new words in real text.

Kibby (1995) suggested three approaches to increasing vocabulary knowledge:

Promote natural growth in meaning vocabulary by
- stimulating interest in words and things through activities such as word games, quizzes, puns, malapropisms, derivations, cartoons, oxymorons, and spoonerisms.
- developing word consciousness through activities that encourage students to note words they come across that they don't know.
- teaching and reinforcing words and things continually.
- stimulating wide reading.

Promote lifelong vocabulary learning through indirect vocabulary instruction that includes
- using context clues.
- developing dictionary skills and the motivation to use dictionaries.
- identifying meaning through roots and affixes.

Promote the learning of specific words through direct vocabulary instruction that includes
- teaching words in advance of reading.
- planning which words to teach and how to teach them.
- moving from the known to the unknown when teaching vocabulary.
- using a variety of methods.

Studies of deaf children have shown that (a) vocabulary knowledge is positively related to reading comprehension, (b) deaf students demonstrate better understanding of the semantic properties and relationships of words than word definitions, (c) students with hearing loss do not have greater difficulty learning novel words than hearing children, (d) didactic vocabulary instruction has not been shown to be effective in improving comprehension, and (e) deaf students are able to derive some word meanings through context within authentic text (Conway, 1990; Davey & King, 1990; deVilliers & Pomerantz, 1992; Garrison, Long, & Dowaliby, 1997; Gilbertson & Kamhi, 1995; Kelly, 1996; LaSasso & Davey, 1987; Nolen & Wilbur, 1985; Paul, 1996).

Definition-Based Approaches

Definition-based approaches commonly take two forms. In one form, the youngsters are asked to look up the definitions of a list of words in the dictionary, copy them, and write a sentence for each word. In the other form, the teacher briefly discusses the meaning of the new words in an upcoming reading selection. Often, these two approaches are followed by worksheets in which words and definitions are manipulated through crossword puzzles, columns to be matched by drawing a line from the word to its definition, or cloze sentences. Studies have shown that definition-based approaches can be effective when ample time is spent in teacher–student discussion about the new vocabulary (Eeds & Cockrum, 1985; McKeown, 1993; Vaughan, Castle, Gilbert, & Love, 1982) because simply learning a dictionary definition does not lead to vocabulary development.

For youngsters who are deaf, opportunities to discuss word meanings provide a milieu for language development not only in the area of vocabulary but also in the areas of conversation and pragmatics. Deaf children using ASL can compare and contrast the ASL equivalents of English vocabulary words, which helps to build their vocabulary in both languages.

However, looking up lists and lists of words in a dictionary, writing their definitions, and creating isolated sentences for each word is usually tedious for the child and is not likely to result in significant word learning. Furthermore, dictionary definitions are often written in complicated sentence structures that children who are deaf have difficulty understanding, and the definitions themselves often include words that are unfamiliar to the children.

Context-Based Approaches

A number of issues surround the power of *context-based approaches* for teaching vocabulary. One issue is the connection between direct instruction and context-based learning. It has been found that direct instruction, whether through a definition-based approach or concept-based approach, is more effective when combined with context. In other words, youngsters ultimately need to encounter a word in context to develop a full sense of its meaning (Gipe, 1980; Gipe & Arnold, 1979). This issue may help explain why youngsters who are deaf often have difficulty remembering the meaning of words they have been taught. Teaching the meaning is important, but not sufficient.

A second issue is the probability that new words can be learned through context. Obviously, when context is explicit, it is more likely that youngsters will be able to derive the meaning of a new word. Nevertheless, even when context is not particularly supportive, it has been found that youngsters will acquire some aspects of a word's meaning but often not complete enough to write a definition or choose a synonym. With further exposures to the word in various contexts, more complete understanding of the word's meaning usually takes place (Jenkins, Stein, & Wysocki, 1984; Moore, 1987; Nagy, Herman, & Anderson, 1985; Schatz & Baldwin, 1986). This issue serves to remind us that one or two encounters with a word is simply not enough to build full understanding.

Based on their own study of eighth graders' ability to develop word knowledge from context as well as their review of the literature, Nagy, Herman, and Anderson (1985) concluded that "incidental learning from context accounts for a substantial proportion of the vocabulary growth that occurs during the school years" (p. 233).

A third issue is what I call the reality issue. In reality, the teacher cannot teach all of the new words the students will encounter in every reading selection. By necessity, deaf students will need to figure out the meanings of many words through context. Blachowicz and Fisher (1996) suggest that students be taught to:

- Look. Before, at, and after the word.
- Reason. Connect what they know to what the author has written.
- Predict a possible meaning.
- Resolve or re-do. Decide if they know enough, should try again, or consult an expert or reference. (p. 24)

This strategy can be used effectively within the lesson format of models, such as the DRTA and one-to-one tutoring, when the students encounter a word they do not know. And practice in using these skills can be carried out with cloze paragraphs in which words are deleted. Another approach is the use of captioned video, which appears to provide a motivating medium for vocabulary development (Koskinen, Wilson, Gambrell, & Neuman, 1993).

Concept-Based Approaches
Concept-based approaches are grounded on the assumption that new knowledge is gained from finding new relationships in old knowledge and from relating new information to old knowledge.

Semantic Mapping.   In *semantic mapping* for vocabulary development, the teacher starts by writing a word that represents a key concept. The youngsters are asked to think of words that relate to the key word. These words are grouped around the key word in categories, either preset by the teacher or created by the youngsters. The teacher then suggests new words and encourages a discussion about where these words might fit into the map (Duffelmeyer & Banwart, 1993; Heimlich & Pittelman, 1986; Johnson, Pittelman, & Heimlich, 1986). Figures 4.1 and 4.2 repre-

sent two different vocabulary semantic maps developed in classrooms of children who are deaf.

Two aspects of semantic mapping seem to account for much of its power as a teaching strategy. The first aspect is that the map provides a visual display of the relationships between concepts in a key word. The second aspect is that it involves intense discussion, which in turn encourages active thinking. As Stahl and Vancil (1986) noted, "It is this active thinking that leads to effective vocabulary learning" (p. 66).

In one variation of the semantic map approach, definitions are combined with mapping. In this approach, called a *word map,* the map becomes a visual display of the definition. The word is placed in the center of the map, and three questions form the three categories surrounding the word: What is it? What is it like? What are some examples? (Schwartz & Raphael, 1985).

Semantic Feature Analysis.   In a *semantic feature analysis,* the teacher chooses a word or phrase that represents a major topic or category about which the students will

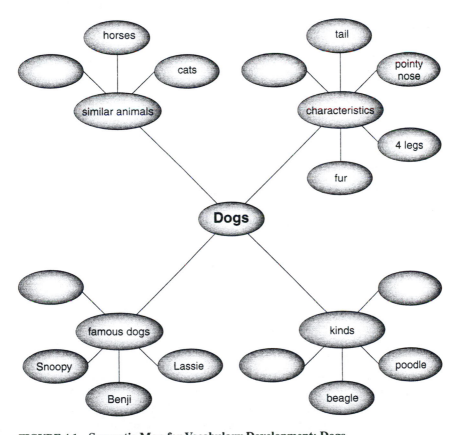

FIGURE 4.1   Semantic Map for Vocabulary Development: Dogs

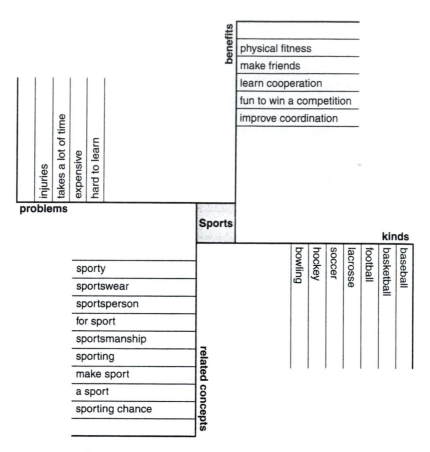

FIGURE 4.2   Semantic Map for Vocabulary Development

read. In a column, the teacher lists some words related to the topic. In a row, the teacher lists some features shared by some of the words already listed in the column. At the intersection of row and column, the teacher asks the students to put a plus (+) if the word possesses the feature and a minus (–) if the word does not possess the feature (or a Likert-type scale from 0 to 5 can be used). The students are also asked to add words to the column and features to the row. Student discussion is as critical to the semantic feature analysis as it is to the semantic mapping strategy, particularly discussion that focuses on the students' reasoning (Anders & Bos, 1986). An example of a semantic feature analysis is provided in Figure 4.3. This semantic feature analysis was developed by an upper elementary reading group. One of the students in the group was deaf. The group had been reading a story in which the characters were playing in a school orchestra. The semantic feature analysis helped the children get a clearer idea of musical instruments, which the teacher felt was an important concept in the story.

	strings	blow into	hit	pluck	press
harp	+	−	−	+	−
violin	+	−	−	+	+
piano	+	−	−	−	+
clarinet	−	+	−	−	+
drum	−	−	+	−	−
flute	−	+	−	−	+
tamborine	−	−	+	−	−

FIGURE 4.3   Semantic Feature Analysis: Musical Instruments

In semantic mapping, the discussion is generally quite congenial because all ideas can be accommodated in the map. But in semantic feature analysis, the youngsters have to come to a consensus, so the discussion tends to involve pragmatic skills, such as persuading, disagreeing, expressing opinions, and suggesting.

Concept Attainment.   When using the *concept attainment model,* the teacher begins by presenting examples and nonexamples of a key word. The teacher then encourages the youngsters to identify critical or relevant attributes of the concept, in other words the attributes or characteristics important to the meaning of the word. The youngsters are encouraged to separate the relevant attributes from the irrelevant attributes. The teacher can then ask the youngsters for subordinate terms (examples of the concept), superordinate terms (more general concepts), and coordinate terms (concepts that share some of the same attributes as the targeted concept). Or the teacher can ask for further examples and nonexamples of the key word (McNeil, 1992; Wixson, 1986).

The concept attainment model is unique in that it encourages the child who is deaf to think about how aspects of a word's meaning relate to other concepts. One teacher who used this model periodically with a group of middle school students reported to me that although the model wasn't appropriate for all vocabulary instruction, it provided a nice divergence from his typical vocabulary lessons. He also found that the comparing and contrasting encouraged by the model carried over into other discussions of concepts in reading as well as other subject areas.

Concept Wheel.   When using a *concept wheel,* the teacher starts by asking the students to brainstorm all the things that come to mind about a given word. The teacher writes all their ideas on the board and then directs the children to a page in their books where the word is written and also to the glossary that provides a definition. The teacher asks the students to decide on three words from their list that will help them remember the target word. The words are written inside a circle that has been divided into quarters. Because each child may have a different list of three words, their concept wheels are individualized. According to Rupley, Logan, and Nichols (1999), the steps can be reversed, with the children given the concept wheel first and asked to supply the name of the wheel.

ASL Handshape Games.   In *ASL handshape games,* the students must think of as many words as possible in ASL. In one form of the game, each successive person adds to a sequential story by using a sign that incorporates the next letter of the alphabet. In another form, one handshape is chosen, and each successive person or team must think of a sign that reflects the handshape.

Comprehension during Reading

Instruction during reading can be particularly powerful in teaching deaf children to be strategic readers. Models such as reciprocal teaching and Reading Workshop have built-in strategies, such as predicting, self-questioning, retelling, conferencing, and journaling, that can be used within other instructional models. Most of the strategies presented here are designed to encourage deaf children to be metacognitive—to reflect on their own comprehension, recognize when they do not understand, and strategically carry out activities to enhance comprehension.

Comprehension Questions

Comprehension questions can be used to assess children's comprehension, or they can be used to extend comprehension. Assessment will be discussed in Chapter 6. In this section, we will examine the kinds of questions that help children who are deaf understand text more deeply and that provide models of self-questions.

Levels of Questions.   Comprehension taxonomies have been widely used by teachers for constructing varying types of comprehension questions. The most frequently used taxonomy is Bloom's classification of the intellectual objectives of education into six lower to higher levels: knowledge, comprehension, application, analysis, synthesis, and evaluation (Bloom, Engelhart, Furst, Hill, & Krathwohl, 1956). Another popular taxonomy is Barrett's (1976), which was specifically designed to distinguish among the cognitive and affective dimensions of reading comprehension through four major levels: literal, inferential, evaluation, and appreciation. Both taxonomies are further divided into multiple subcategories that teachers can use in creating comprehension questions.

Tatham (1978) cautioned that taxonomies should be viewed as classification systems and not as developmental frameworks of comprehension skills. "These taxonomies are nothing more than efficient systems for organizing types of reading behavior under clearly defined labels. The labels can be very useful when teachers want categories in which to place comprehension questions from instructional materials in order to analyze the types of thinking these questions promote" (p. 193).

In 1978, Pearson and Johnson proposed what they referred to as a simple taxonomy of questions that was designed "to capture the relationship between information presented in a text and information that has to come from a reader's store of prior knowledge" (p. 157). Their taxonomy included three types of questions: textually explicit, textually implicit, and scriptally implicit. *Textually explicit questions* have answers that are obvious in the text. *Textually implicit questions* have answers in the text, but the answers are not obvious. To answer a textually implicit question, the reader must use inference. *Scriptally implicit questions* have answers that come from the reader's prior knowledge; the answers are not in the text, but the question is related to the text. "It is similar to textually implicit comprehension in that an inference is involved; however, it is different in that the data base for the inference is in the reader's head, not on the page" (p. 162).

The *Question–Answer Relationship* (QAR) program was developed by Raphael (Raphael, 1982, 1984, 1986; Raphael & McKinney, 1983; Raphael & Pearson, 1985; Raphael & Wonnacott, 1985) and based on the Pearson and Johnson question taxonomy.

Raphael (1986) divided question–answer relationships into two primary categories: (a) In the Book and (b) In My Head. The *In the Book* category includes two types of QARS. The first is called *Right There* and is the appropriate strategy to use when the answer can be found explicitly stated within a single sentence of the text. The second is called *Think and Search* or *Putting It Together* and is the appropriate strategy to use when the answer can be found in the text but requires the reader to synthesize information from different parts of the text.

The *In My Head* category also includes two types of QARS. The first is called *Author and You* and is the appropriate strategy when the reader needs to combine background knowledge with text information. The second is called *On My Own* and is the appropriate strategy when the answer cannot be found in the story and could even be answered if the story was not read. *On My Own* questions require the reader to rely completely on background knowledge.

Regardless of the taxonomy used, teachers are strongly encouraged to ask some questions that promote higher-order thinking along with the questions they ask that require recall of factual information (Daines, 1986; Hansen & Pearson, 1983). It seems self-evident that the difficulties experienced by many youngsters who are deaf in thinking critically, creatively, and abstractly are due in large part to their lack of experience in this kind of thinking. When children have not been asked questions that encourage higher-order thinking, it is very hard for them at first to think at levels beyond the literal. Instead of giving up and assuming that deaf children cannot answer inferential, evaluative, and other higher-level questions, these are precisely the kinds of questions they need to be asked. But teachers need to realize that promoting higher-order thinking takes time.

Schirmer and Woolsey (1997) found that upper elementary-level deaf students could answer comprehension questions that required analysis, synthesis, and evaluation without having answered literal questions, but to do so, they needed support in identifying salient story details, building accurate and pertinent background knowledge, applying background knowledge appropriately, and communicating effectively.

Comprehension questions can enhance another dimension of thinking, that of thinking about text structure.

Questions That Highlight Text Structure.   It may be possible to teach children to identify the parts of a story, but there is no strong evidence that learning to analyze the grammar of stories and other texts will improve children's reading comprehension (Dreher & Singer, 1980; Johnson & Bliesmer, 1983; Schmitt & O'Brien, 1986). If this finding seems familiar, it is because more than a decade ago educators learned that being able to analyze sentences into their grammatical components was not found to be related to the children's spoken, reading, or writing abilities.

Research into text structure does, however, have implications for instruction. Instead of teaching children the labels for text components, it has been suggested that teachers use questions to bring significant text components and the causal relationships between components to the children's attention. Through questions that highlight the information that reflects the basic structure of narrative or expository text, the teacher in essence can "show" children what it means to understand written discourse. Ultimately, such questions over time help deaf and hearing children to internalize the structure of text into their textual schemata (Carnine & Kinder, 1985; Mavrogenes, 1983; McConaughy, 1980; Schirmer & Bond, 1990).

Teachers can create questions that emphasize text structure by first analyzing the structure of the texts themselves and then creating questions based on key components. Figure 4.4 shows questions that were developed for *The Three Bears*. (The reader might want to look back at the story structure of *The Three Bears* presented in Figure 3.1).

Text structure questions can serve two objectives. They not only can guide children who are deaf in recognizing the underlying structure of typical narrative and expository text, but they can also be developed to encourage different levels of thinking.

Think Time.   One characteristic of comprehension questions that many of us tend to forget is that wonderful questions will not enhance comprehension if children are not given time to think about their answers. It has been observed that teachers give children an average of one second to answer a question. After one second, teachers ordinarily repeat or rephrase the question, answer it themselves, call on another student, or ask another question (Gambrell, 1983; Rowe, 1974; Tobin, 1986).

What happens when teachers wait three seconds, five seconds, or longer before soliciting an answer? In Tobin's (1986) study of students in grades six and seven, he found that waiting between three and five seconds resulted in significantly fewer failures of students to respond, greater length of student responses, and better comprehension. In a review of studies involving wait time, Tobin (1987) found that a wait time of between three and five seconds seemed to be optimal for improving the quality of teacher and student discourse and for affecting higher cognitive-level achievement. In Gambrell's review of the literature (1980), she found evidence that a wait

FIGURE 4.4   Comprehension Questions Based on Story Structure

	The Three Bears
Setting	1. Where did the three bears live?
Initiating Event/Reaction	2. Why did the three bears go for a walk?
Action	3. Who showed up at the Bears' house?
Consequence	4. What did Goldilocks do when she entered the house?
Reaction/Action	5. What happened when Goldilocks tasted the porridge, sat in the chairs, and walked upstairs?
Consequence	6. What happened when the three bears came home?
Ending	7. What did Goldilocks do when she woke up?

time of five seconds or more resulted in student responses that were longer, more appropriate, and demonstrated higher-order thinking. She also found that when teachers increased their wait time, they tended to ask more varied questions and to stimulate greater student involvement.

In reviewing her own series of studies on wait time in elementary and high school classrooms along with a review of the studies conducted by other researchers, Rowe (1986) found that wait time influenced students and teachers in a number of ways. When the interval between the end of a teacher question and the start of a student response was three to five seconds as compared to only one second:

1. the length of student response increased 300 percent to 700 percent.
2. students were much more likely to use evidence and logical argument to support their inferences.
3. students engaged more often in speculative thinking.
4. students asked considerably more questions.
5. students paid more attention to each other.
6. "I don't know" responses decreased dramatically.
7. off-task behavior decreased.
8. greater percentages of students participated, particularly from groups rated as poor performers.
9. student confidence increased.
10. test performance improved on cognitively more complex test items.
11. classroom discourse more closely resembled discussion than question–answer routines.
12. teachers asked fewer questions, and those they asked tended to invite clarification and elaboration.
13. teacher expectation for student performance rose, particularly with students for whom they had previously held low expectations.

Wait time is particularly pertinent to deaf children who are in regular education classes and receive information from the teacher through an interpreter. Because interpreting is not simultaneous with the teacher's utterances, unless the teacher waits between asking a question and soliciting answers, the child who is deaf may have no opportunity to answer and certainly no opportunity to think.

Predicting

It is believed that good readers are constantly predicting, testing their hypotheses to confirm or disconfirm them, and integrating information by separating important ideas from less important ideas and interpreting the important ideas (A. Brown, 1980; McNeil, 1992). Hansen (1981) found that teaching children to use their prior knowledge to predict upcoming story events improved their comprehension.

Several instructional models, including the DRTA and reciprocal teaching, ask students to predict what will happen next and discuss their predictions after reading the segment or chapter. Teaching students how to make predictions can be a minilesson, and discussing the accuracy of their predictions can be a strategy lesson. When Mr. Schaefer introduces the concept of prediction to his deaf students, he accepts any prediction they provide. As they become comfortable with this strategy, he asks them to justify their predictions with evidence from the text and their own background knowledge. And as they continue reading, he urges them to determine when their predictions are correct, when they are not, and why.

Self-Questioning

Self-questioning is a strategy that has emerged from three bodies of research—active processing, metacognitive theory, and schema theory (Wong, 1985). According to the active processing perspective, self-questioning is critical to the reader's active engagement in comprehension because the act of generating questions creates an interaction between the reader and the text. According to metacognitive theory, self-questioning is crucial to the reader's ability to focus on important information and to monitor his or her own comprehension. In schema theory, self-questioning grows out of the connection between background knowledge and the learning of new information. According to schema theory, self-questioning is seen as a fundamental strategy for the reader to use in activating relevant background knowledge.

In her review of the literature, Wong (1985) found that self-questioning is effective in enhancing comprehension when children are given explicit instruction in how to generate questions and ample time to think while reading. Bergman (1992) suggested that students be taught to ask the following questions:

- To get the gist—What is the story about? What is the problem? What is the solution? What makes me think so?
- To predict–verify–decide—What's going to happen next? Is my prediction still good? Do I need to change my prediction? What makes me think so?

- To visualize–verify–decide—What does this person, place, or thing look like? Is the picture in my mind still good? Do I need to change my picture? What makes me think so?
- To summarize—What's happened so far? What makes me think so?
- To think aloud—What am I thinking? Why?
- To solve problems or help when I don't understand—Shall I guess, ignore and read on, re-read or look back? Why? (p. 599)

The Reading/Language in Secondary Schools Subcommittee of the International Reading Association (1989) wrote that effective learners talk to themselves; they have an inner voice that guides and monitors their cognitive activities.

This view of the role of an inner voice is an extension of Vygotsky's concept of inner speech, which was discussed in Chapter 1. Vygotsky viewed inner speech as speech turned into inward thought. Some researchers believe that inner speech is used by individuals to consciously clarify and guide their thoughts. Many reading researchers believe that this same inner voice is used by good readers to clarify and guide their thoughts during reading. It seems logical that inner speech does not have to be in voice but that for some individuals who are deaf, inner speech is in sign.

Based on his study of the comprehension monitoring strategies used by second-, fourth-, sixth-, and eighth-grade readers and adult readers, Winser (1988) proposed that young readers and poor readers would benefit from instruction that helps them gain conscious control of reading strategies. He found that good readers use the following alternative strategies when comprehension difficulties arise and that they are able to consciously choose the appropriate strategy:

1. Read on—moving further on into the text.
2. Sound out—referring to phonemes/graphemes. [For some deaf students, this strategy might be fingerspelling.]
3. Inference—using prior knowledge.
4. Reread—repeating the reading. [This strategy might involve signing the segment.]
5. Resume task—continuing to read.
6. Suspend judgment—being prepared to wait for more information.
7. Aware—indicating knowledge of comprehension problem. (p. 259)

Mr. Schaefer has found that encouraging children who are deaf to use their inner voice or sign and to generate their own questions requires that he spend a substantial amount of time modeling appropriate questions and self-talk. Within all of the instructional models he uses he encourages these thinking behaviors during and after reading.

Mental Imagery

Mental imagery is generally thought of as the formation of visual or spatial representations in one's mind, although all sensory modalities can be represented in imagery. It has been suggested that mental imagery can serve two metacognitive functions.

First, mental imagery can be a means for activating background knowledge prior to reading (Gambrell, 1982; Johnson, 1987; Long, Winograd, & Bridge, 1989). Second, mental imagery can serve a comprehension monitoring function (Gambrell & Bales, 1986; Gambrell & Jawitz, 1993; Sadoski, 1983, 1985).

Because sign language is a visual–spatial language, it might be argued that mental imagery could be a particularly powerful strategy for many deaf youngsters to use in comprehending text. Fusaro and Slike (1979) found that imagery influenced the ease with which nine- to twelve-year-old deaf children learned to identify words.

In a study of elementary-level deaf students, Schirmer (1993) found that when they were encouraged to engage in mental imagery, they exhibited qualities of thinking that revealed how they were processing narrative text. Their responses reflected their efforts to make sense of each story. They expressed ideas about the characters and plot that went beyond the authors' words, but their ideas were consistent with story line, character development, and their own prior knowledge and experiences.

Mental imagery instruction fits easily into the DRTA lesson format as well as other models. Before reading, the children are told, "Make pictures in your mind to help you understand and remember." After reading, the children are asked, "Do you have any pictures or scenes in your mind that you remember from this part of the story?" As with the other metacognitive strategies, the teacher of deaf children must model his or her own mental images when this strategy is first introduced. It is very valuable for the children to share and discuss their imagery with peers.

Scaffolded Conversations

In a balanced reading program, sometimes the teacher sustains the dialogue with students through questions, yet at other times, the dialogue is conversational in nature. Conversations about what children are reading or writing are called *scaffolded conversations* when the teacher is consciously providing a support structure for ways to think about the text. Scaffolding is a relatively new term to education that uses the metaphor of the scaffold, which in construction parlance is a temporary platform for supporting workers building a structure. In current learning theory, a scaffold is a temporary supportive structure that enables learners to complete a task they would not be able to complete without support. These supports are removed or faded in stages until the learner is able to complete the task independently.

In the scaffolded conversations model, the teacher engages the children in a discussion of the material, which can be a paragraph, page, chapter, or complete text. Within this discussion, the teacher contributes his or her ideas in ways that act as a scaffold for children to think about and respond to the material (Beed, Hawkins, & Roller, 1991; Echevarria, 1995; Goldenberg, 1993).

For Mr. Schaefer, using scaffolded conversations means turning his questions into statements. For example, one day a couple of students in third grade were reading an *Amelia Bedelia* story. When he had developed his lesson plan, Kurt had incorporated questions such as, "Why does Amelia Bedelia make so many mistakes?" and "What mistakes did she make?" In his scaffolded conversation lesson, instead of asking questions, he comments, "I thought this book was very funny. Tell me what you thought." If the children do not discuss the mistakes Amelia Bedelia made, he says, "I was surprised the first time Amelia Bedelia followed Mrs. Rogers' directions and cut the bathroom towels because she was supposed to change them. She thought 'change' meant to make them different. But Mrs. Rogers meant 'change' to put the old ones in the hamper and put clean ones on the shelf. Tell me what surprised you."

Comprehension after Reading

Opportunity to respond is a key element of all learning; for young readers, it may be essential. Strategies that teachers of deaf children employ after they have read a story, novel, text chapter, newspaper or magazine article, and other material can provide the opportunity for the children to share their responses with others who can support and extend their ideas. These strategies fit into virtually all of the instructional models for teaching literacy.

Literature Discussions

Literature discussions enable children to discuss their thoughts and impressions with the teacher and peers who can provide other perspectives, share information, help solve problems, explore ideas, provide immediate feedback, and clarify thinking. Many educators believe that peer-led literature discussions are best able to accomplish these outcomes, and there is some research to indicate that peer-led discussions are richer and more complex than teacher-led discussions (Almasi, 1995; Kletzien & Baloche, 1994; Koskinen & O'Flahavan, 1995; Langer, 1994; Leal, 1993). On the other hand, less able readers have been found to experience greater difficulty participating in literature discussions, displaying their knowledge, and constructing meaning collaboratively (Wollman-Bonilla, 1994). Literature discussions can occur within the context of one-to-one reading conferences, reader's chair, and book club.

Reading Conferences.   *One-to-one conferences* between teachers and students can be scheduled for as little as five minutes and as long as fifteen minutes. These conferences can be used to teach children how to respond to literature through supporting their ideas about what they are reading, through questions with no "known" answers, and through real conversations about mutually interesting stories and characters (Hansen, 1987; Strickland, Dillon, Funkhouser, Glick, & Rogers, 1989).

Once the children know the kinds of open-ended questions that should be asked during conferences and they have learned how to be an interested listener/partner, peer conferences can be used to proportionally increase the students' opportunities to engage in literature discussion.

Reader's Chair.   During reader's chair, one student shares what he or she has read or is currently reading with a group of fellow students and then "chairs" the subsequent discussion. I use the term *reader's chair* because the functions of this type of literature response group are quite similar to author's chair in writing workshop.

In their study of four elementary classrooms (one first/second grade, one second grade, one gifted/talented third grade, and one sixth grade), Strickland and her associates (1989) found that student-led literature discussion groups were a valuable resource for learning language, learning through language, and learning about language. They observed that:

> one of the most significant features of these discussion groups is that it puts the student in the role of expert or resource. The presenter makes the decisions about what is important to reveal about the book and what is to be read aloud. Not only do students have a greater sense of control over the talk, they have more opportunities to talk in an interactional pattern that is likely to criss-cross among the group members rather than remain dyadic. (p. 199)

Book Club.   During book club, youngsters who are reading the same book come together periodically to discuss what they are reading. I use the term *book club* because the purpose and function of this type of literature response group are similar to book clubs for adults. In an adult book club, a small group of enthusiastic readers decides on a book they are all interested in reading and then get together for a discussion after the members have had time to read the book. This activity is also sometimes referred to as *literature circles* (Simpson, 1995).

Raphael and her associates use the term *Book Club Program* for the reading instruction model they developed (Goatley, Brock, & Raphael, 1995; McMahon & Raphael, 1997; Raphael & McMahon, 1994). This model includes four components—reading, writing, community share, and book club. During the reading component, students read daily for at least fifteen minutes either aloud or silently, with a partner or alone, or the teacher or peer reads aloud to the class. During the writing component, the students make entries into their reading logs. Community share is a teacher-led whole-class discussion. Books clubs are small, student-led discussion groups in which the students control the content and flow of the discussion. One of the students in the Book Club Program wrote the following:

> When we talk with our peers, we find out about other people's ideas, have a chance to say something really important, get to tell what the author should do better or different, ask questions about the book, and express our feelings and ideas. Also, sometimes books were hard for me to understand. In Book club, other students, or the teacher, helped one another to understand the story. So, a big advantage of Book club was talking with friends. (McMahon & Raphael, 1997, p. 24)

In group discussions, particularly when there is one deaf child and several hearing children, it is challenging for the deaf child to track the movement of the discussion from child to child. And the larger the group, the less opportunity each child has to contribute ideas. Mr. Schaefer teaches his deaf students how to participate in these types of discussions by role-playing literature discussions in the resource room.

Reading Response Journals

In addition to literature discussions, *reading response journals* can provide youngsters who are deaf with a meaningful way to respond actively to the literature they are reading. Harste, Short, and Burke (1988) called this kind of journal a *literature log*. They considered it to be one type of learning log. In a learning log, children are asked to write about their reaction to something new they learned that day or their response to how they went about learning it. In a literature log, children are asked to write their responses and reactions to what they are reading.

Reading logs are a component of the Book Club Program. Raphael and her associates found that it was helpful to provide the students with think sheets as a scaffold for writing in logs. For example, think sheets might include spaces for the children to write unusual vocabulary, questions for the author, a comparison of a current and previous book, and the quality of book club discussions.

Berger (1996) suggested that students be given a guide for writing a reader response journal. She asked her students to write a response after every two chapters and to answer at least four questions. What do you notice? What do you question? What do you feel? What do you relate to? Hancock (1993b) developed the following guidelines for her students:

- Feel free to write your innermost feelings, opinions, thoughts, likes, and dislikes.
- Take time to write down anything that you are thinking while you read.
- Don't worry about the accuracy of spelling and mechanics in the journal.
- Record the page number on which you were reading when you wrote your response.
- Relate the book to your own experiences and share similar moments from your life or from books you have read in the past.
- Ask questions while reading to help you make sense of the characters and the unraveling plot.
- Make predictions about what you think will happen as the plot unfolds.
- Talk to the characters as you begin to know them.
- Praise or criticize the book, the author, or the literary style.
- There is no limit to the types of responses you may write. (p. 472)

One type of focused reading response journal is a character journal, which is a diary written by the child as if he or she were a character in the story. The child writes in the first person and responds to the events occurring in the character's life. When Hancock (1993a) used character journals with her eighth graders, she found that they preferred to write two types of entries, one as the character and the other as a spectator, so that they could respond as themselves and share their own thoughts.

Retelling

Retelling stories after reading provides children who are deaf with the chance to make sense of the text as a whole. In the past, retellings have been used predominantly to assess reading comprehension (Gambrell, Pfeiffer, & Wilson, 1985). However, viewing retellings as reconstructions and using them to monitor comprehension may be considerably less valuable than viewing retellings as constructions and using them as a strategy to enhance comprehension.

Verbal Retelling. Retelling significantly improves reading comprehension and recall (Gambrell, Pfeiffer, & Wilson, 1985; Koskinen, Gambrell, Kapinus, & Heathington, 1988). Gambrell and her associates observed that "practice in verbal rehearsal of what has been read results in significant learning with respect to the comprehension and recall of discourse, and that what has been learned, as a result of practice in retelling, transfers to the reading of subsequent text" (Gambrell, Pfeiffer, & Wilson, 1985, p. 220).

Practice in retelling has been found to improve both the richness of children's retellings as well as their reading comprehension (Kapinus, Gambrell, & Koskinen, 1987; Morrow, 1985). Story retelling has also been found to help develop children's story schema (French, 1988; Morrow, 1985, 1986). French (1988) observed that deaf elementary students who retold stories as a group activity were able to learn from each other which components of a story carried the most meaning.

Several guidelines have been suggested for using retellings in the classroom. Y. Goodman (1982) encouraged teachers to use unaided retellings followed by open-ended questions that serve to prompt the child. Koskinen, Gambrell, Kapinus, and Heathington (1988) advised teachers to model retelling for students with no retelling experience, guide students' practice of retelling through prompts, and provide students with opportunities for repeated practice with partners. They further suggested that students be given guidance in how to provide positive feedback when someone else is retelling a story. French (1988) reported that in the language arts program at the Kendall Demonstration Elementary School, retelling with deaf students was conducted as a group activity that the teacher recorded on the board, chart paper, or overhead transparency.

Story Maps and Story Frames. *Story maps* are a type of semantic map. In a story map, the key elements of a story and the relationships between elements are displayed graphically. Story maps are typically used after children have finished reading a story, chapter, or book. The story map is created as a group activity through in-depth discussion (Davis & McPherson, 1989; Idol, 1987; Keeler, 1993; Reutzel, 1985b).

The most common type of story map is the main idea–sequential detail map. Reutzel (1985b) presented the following steps for constructing this type of map:

1. Construct, in sequence, a summary list of the main idea, major events, and major characters in the story.
2. Locate the main idea in the center of the map.

3. Draw enough ties projecting out symmetrically from the center circle to accommodate the major events/characters on the summary list.
4. Enter the major concepts or events in circles attached to these ties, including them in
sequence clockwise around the center circle.
5. Enter subevents and subconcepts in clockwise sequence around the circles containing major events or concepts in the story map. (pp. 400–401)

Other types of story maps are character perspective and comparison maps, inferential story maps, cause–effect relationships, comparison/contrast maps, and drawing conclusions story maps (Davis & McPherson, 1989; Emery, 1996; Reutzel, 1985b;
Richards & Gipe, 1993). Story maps can be used by youngsters after reading to write
a summary of the story, write a book report, or as a conceptual model to create an original composition (Olson, 1984; Pehrsson & Denner, 1988; Sinatra, Stahl-Gemake, &
Morgan, 1986).

Story frames are summaries with information left out for the youngsters to
fill in. Some authors view them as story-level cloze (Cairney, 1987; Cudd & Roberts,
1987). Story frames are usually based on story structure components, but they have
also been used to guide children in analyses of characters, setting, and other aspects
of the text. The teacher can include a great deal of information in the frame and expect
just a small amount of writing from the children, or the teacher can provide minimum
guidance in the frame and expect the children to write quite a lot. Figure 4.5 illustrates
a story frame developed for *The Three Bears.*

When using semantic maps or story frames, there is a tendency for all ideas
to be seen as equally important. It is, therefore, important for teachers to use these
activities in ways that help children clearly differentiate between central story ideas or
central story problems and supporting details (Au & Scheu, 1989; Moldofsky, 1983).

Drama. *Drama* can provide youngsters who are deaf with an experiential mode for
responding to literature. It is believed that drama can have a positive influence on reading comprehension, student motivation to read, and oral and sign language development (Bidwell, 1990; Wagner, 1988).

It has been suggested that children in preschool and kindergarten be provided
with structured and free-play opportunities to recreate stories that are read aloud to
them (Christie, 1990; Galda, 1982). Pellegrini and Galda (1982) compared the effects
of dramatic play, discussion, and drawing as story reconstruction activities used to follow up read-aloud to 108 kindergarten, first- and second-grade children. They found
that dramatic play was the most effective facilitator of comprehension.

At the elementary and middle school levels, it has been suggested that youngsters be provided with opportunities to create dramatic presentations of novels, parts
of novels, or stories. Performances can be improvisational, or the students can write
a script based on the actual story, which is a technique sometimes referred to as *Readers Theatre* (Bidwell, 1990; Shepard, 1994; Wolf, 1993, 1994). In her investigation
comparing drama with discussion, Gray (1986) found that the sixth-grade students

Title _The Three Bears_

This story takes place _in the house of the three bears._
They live in the woods .

In this story, the problem starts when _Mama bear makes_
porridge, but it is too hot to eat. So the Bears
go for a walk in the forest .

After that, _Goldilocks visits the house._

_____ .

Next, _She eats some porridge. The porridge in the_
big bowl is too hot. The porridge in the middle size
bowl is too cold. The porridge in the small bowl
is just right, and she eats it all up .

Then, _she sits down. The big chair is too hard._
The middle chair is too soft. The small
chair is just right, but it breaks .

After that, _she goes upstairs. She lays down on_
the big bed, but it is too hard. The middle
size bed is too soft. The small bed is just
right, and she falls asleep .

Finally, _the bears come home. They see that_
someone ate their porridge, sat in their
chairs and slept in their beds .

The problem is solved when _they see Goldilocks._

_____ .

The problem ends when _Goldilocks wakes up, sees_
the bears and runs out of the house .

FIGURE 4.5   Story Frame for _The Three Bears_

in her study who participated in creative dramatic presentation demonstrated better ability to answer inferential questions than the matched group of students who took part in a story discussion with the teacher.

Drama is a strategy that has been used for many years by teachers of children who are deaf. It can take a relatively brief amount of time if the presentation is impromptu, or it can become a class project that takes several weeks if the presentation is performed for parents and other youngsters in the school.

Extending Literacy Opportunities

Several other strategies are integral to creating a core literacy program for children who are deaf. These strategies extend the daily opportunities for children to be engaged in the meaningful use of reading and writing.

Sustained Silent Reading

It is a long-held belief that time spent in silent reading is vitally important to children's reading development. In their study of fifth- and sixth-grade children's reading growth over a four month period, Taylor, Frye, and Maruyama (1990) found a significant relationship between time spent reading in the classroom and reading achievement. Their results provided empirical support for "the conventional wisdom that it is valuable for students to actually read during reading class" (p. 359). Yet when researchers have examined how much time youngsters actually spend engaged in silent reading, it has been found that the average is eight minutes daily for students at the elementary level (Thurlow, Graden, Ysseldyke, & Algozzine, 1984; Ysseldyke & Algozzine, 1983).

The amount of time engaged by deaf students in classroom reading may be even less than hearing students experience. Limbrick, McNaughton, and Clay (1992) found that the amount of time deaf students engaged in reading was almost half as much as hearing students in the classrooms they studied. However, reading time could have increased substantially in recent years because of the emphasis placed on whole language approaches. But, time spent reading does not mean completing workbook pages or reading brief selections for the purpose of answering questions. When educators talk about the importance of providing children with ample time to read, they mean that the time should enable children to become immersed in the text.

Sustained silent reading has earned many acronyms over the years including DEAR (Drop Everything And Read), HIP (High Intensity Practice), SQUIRT (Sustained Quiet Uninterrupted Reading Time), and the original acronym, USSR (Uninterrupted Sustained Silent Reading).

Sustained silent reading has been found to positively affect reading achievement and improve attitudes toward reading among deaf and hearing youngsters from first grade through high school (Collins, 1980; Dry & Earle, 1988; Holt & O'Tuel, 1989; Kaisen, 1987; Minton, 1980; Sadoski, 1980; Summers & McClelland, 1982; Wiesendanger & Bader, 1989). Yet, to be successful, the research has shown that a sustained silent reading program should follow these guidelines:

1. Everyone in the room should read during the entire sustained silent reading time including every child, the teacher, aide, volunteer, and whoever else is in the classroom.
2. Each child should have a self-selected book that he or she is able to read independently. Many children will need guidance in choosing appropriate books, and younger children may need to have several books next to them.

3. The time period should be appropriate for the developmental levels of the children. It is advisable to begin the program at five minutes per day and gradually increase to no more than thirty- to forty-minute periods.
4. The children should be given frequent opportunities to choose new books from the classroom and school libraries.
5. Sustained silent reading periods should be designed to reflect careful scheduling, adherence to time limits, and protection from outside interruptions.

Read-Aloud and Storytelling

I want to discuss again the topic of read-aloud to reiterate my belief that read-aloud should be a core activity for youngsters of *all* ages and to emphasize again the value I place on this activity for school-aged children who are deaf. In addition to my support of this activity, Gillespie and Twardosz (1997) involved deaf residential children between four and eleven years of age in group storybook reading sessions in their group cottages and found that the children became more independent as readers and showed greater interest in books.

Teachers usually read aloud, in voice or sign, between five and fifteen minutes daily from a novel slightly beyond the instructional reading levels of most of the youngsters in the class. It has been suggested that teachers choose books they like themselves and that reflect a variety of interests and genres. They should preread any books they plan to read aloud, set aside time every day for reading aloud, allow time for discussion, tell the youngsters something about the author, and end the day's reading at the conclusion of a chapter or at a suspenseful moment (Butler, 1980; Lindberg, 1988; Trelease, 1995).

Storytelling is an ancient art and a tradition in deaf culture, but only recently have educators begun to realize the power of storytelling in literacy development. It has been observed that storytelling can promote reading comprehension, writing development, listening or receptive sign skills, and spoken or expressive sign skills. Children who observe storytelling are often highly motivated to read the same story, to write the story or a similar story, to write their reactions in a journal, and to pay attention to stories in their reading that would be appropriate ones for their own storytelling.

As observers of the storyteller, they learn to give helpful feedback, to critically evaluate the storyteller's expressive skills, and to observe and listen carefully. As the storyteller, they learn to use meaningful expression, to notice and use audience feedback, and to develop poise. Storytelling also provides youngsters with opportunities to develop awareness of the structure of stories through listening, watching, and telling folktales, mysteries, biographies, and other types of stories (Nelson, 1989; Peck, 1989; Roney, 1989).

Dialogue Journals

In a *dialogue journal,* the child and the teacher carry on a private, written conversation, which can last a month, a term, or a year. Staton (1988) considered dialogue journal writing to be a unique kind of classroom writing for deaf students. "Unlike much school-assigned writing, which is often only for purposes of evaluation, dialogue journals are functional, interactive, mostly about self-generated topics, and deeply embedded in the continuing life of the classroom" (p. 198).

The special characteristics of dialogue journal writing offer benefits that other kinds of writing cannot. I will discuss four of these benefits that I consider to be especially important to children who are deaf, though many other benefits have been reported in the literature.

One benefit is the conversational voice used in this type of writing. As Shuy (1987) pointed out, "Children already know how to talk, so conversational writing does what education has always claimed to do but, in reality, seldom manages to do—it starts with what the learner already knows and then tries to build on this knowledge" (p. 892).

Another benefit to dialogue journal writing is that it provides a forum for using language to accomplish goals. In other words, this kind of writing is functional. Conway and his associates (1988) reported that the deaf youngsters they observed expressed a variety of language functions in their dialogue journals including explaining, persuading, requesting help, reporting, apologizing, asking questions, and expressing feelings. Bode (1989) found that the function used most frequently by the first-grade students in her study of dialogue journal writing was complaining, and the second most frequently used function was asking questions that challenged the teacher. Bode believed that the use of these functions made it obvious how empowering dialogue journal writing can be for the child.

A third benefit to dialogue journal writing is that it enables the teacher to facilitate the deaf child's language development through mutual collaboration and support. As the teacher questions, expands, and restates in response to the child's written comments, the teacher is in essence providing a scaffold of language learning for the deaf child (Conway et al., 1988; Satterfield & Powers, 1996; Staton, 1988). For children using ASL, dialogue journal writing can help them understand the translation process from ASL to English. When they write in the journal, their sentences are likely to include ASL structures. When the teacher responds, he or she can rephrase the child's sentences into English. This written conversation can help the child understand how ASL is translated into written English.

A further benefit to dialogue journal writing is that it provides youngsters with an immediate and obvious connection between reading and writing. The written conversation is perpetuated when the child reads the teacher's comments and responds in writing, and the child knows that the teacher must read the child's comments to respond in writing.

Several guidelines have been suggested for maximizing the positive outcomes of dialogue journal writing. In terms of materials, bound composition books are generally recommended. In terms of time, most educators urge classroom teachers to set aside a specific time daily for reading and writing in the journals, with five to ten minutes being appropriate for younger children or children new to the activity and twenty minutes for older children (Gambrell, 1985; Strackbein & Tillman, 1987). Bode

(1989) noted, however, that children can be given the choice of responding immediately to the teacher's comments or keeping the journal with them throughout the school day and writing in it whenever they choose.

In terms of responding, the teacher is strongly encouraged to keep in mind that writing in the child's journal is like writing a letter to the child. In letters between pen pals, for example, one pen pal does not correct the spelling or punctuation of the other pen pal, and one pen pal does not give the other pen pal instructions and directions. Instead, pen pals generally share experiences and insights, react to each other's written thoughts, ask for clarification or more information, and respond to one another's questions. And pen pals respect the confidentiality of their communication.

Dialogue journals do not have to be written between teachers and students. In a study by Kluwin and Kelly (1991), deaf and hearing students in ten public school districts exchanged correspondence, and the researchers found that exchanging dialogue journals with hearing peers helped improve the writing skills of many of the deaf students. Kluwin (1996) offered several helpful hints to teachers. Students should be encouraged to take a conversational approach to resolving misunderstandings between journal partners, hearing students should not be told about typical problems of deaf writers, teachers should start by suggesting topics such as describing themselves and listing their likes or dislikes, teachers should be prepared to respond to the kinds of problems that children face and about which they may write, and hearing and deaf students should be matched by age, gender, and interests.

Technology offers another avenue for journal writing between peers or between deaf adults and deaf children. Cyber partners can be established without regard to physical location. They can engage in dialogue via e-mail, listservs, web chat rooms, or other types of interactive Internet programs.

Final Comments

The teaching models and strategies presented in this chapter are designed to form a core literacy program for children who are deaf. Teachers of deaf children must be knowledgeable about the best practices in literacy instruction because it is through literacy that deaf children will be able to fulfill their own educational and career goals. Teachers increasingly must be able to share their knowledge of literacy practices with parents and the array of professionals who are responsible for the educational programs of our children. Not only do teachers of deaf children need to reflect exemplary practice, but they must also be able to communicate effectively with general education teachers who are often the individuals teaching reading and writing to deaf students.

Deaf children can become proficient readers and skilled writers who use literacy to communicate and learn. They need teachers who deliver quality literacy instruction throughout their school years.

Suggested Readings

Atwell, N. (1998). *In the middle: New understandings about writing, reading, and learning* (2nd ed.). Portsmouth, NH: Heinemann.

Bear, D. R., Invernizzi, M., Templeton, S., & Johnston, F. (1996). *Words their way: Word study for phonics, vocabulary, and spelling.* Englewood Cliffs, NJ: Merrill/Prentice Hall.

Blachowicz, C., & Fisher, P. (1996). *Teaching vocabulary in all classrooms.* Englewood Cliffs, NJ: Merrill/Prentice Hall.

Tierney, R. J., Readence, J. E., & Dishner, E. K. (2000). *Reading strategies and practices* (5th ed.). Boston: Allyn and Bacon.

Vacca, J., Vacca, R. T., & Gove, M. K. (2000). *Reading and learning to read* (4th ed.). New York: Longman.

Willis, J. W., Stephens, E. C., & Matthew, M. I. (1996). *Technology, reading, and language arts.* Boston: Allyn and Bacon.

5 Learning through Reading and Writing in the Content Areas

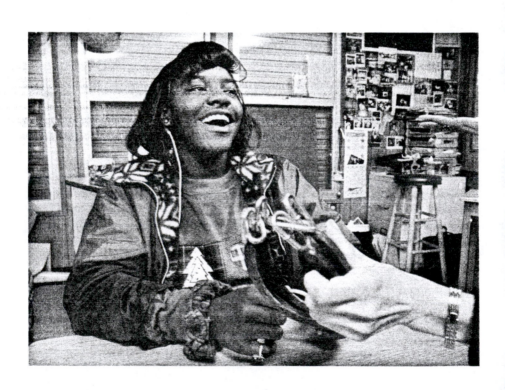

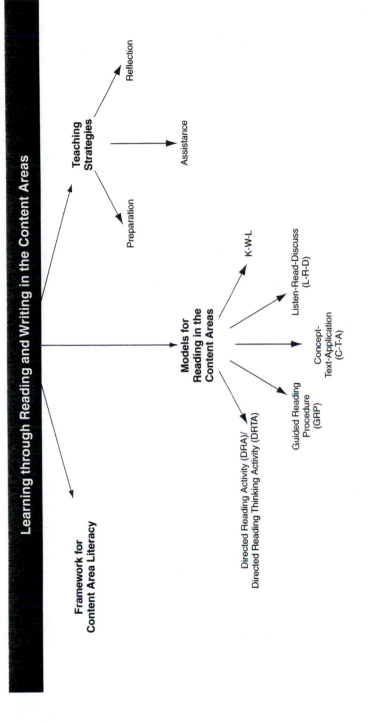

Learning through Reading and Writing in the Content Areas

Framework for
Content Area Literacy

Teaching
Strategies

Preparation

Assistance

Reflection

Models for
Reading in the
Content Areas

Directed Reading Activity (DRA)/
Directed Reading Thinking Activity (DRTA)

Guided Reading
Procedure
(GRP)

Concept-
Text-Application
(C-T-A)

Listen-Read-Discuss
(L-R-D)

K-W-L

Much of what has been written about reading and writing in the content areas centers on the secondary level, perhaps because at the primary and elementary levels, the curriculum tends to be more integrated, reading and writing play a particularly important role in the curriculum, and teachers of deaf children are more likely to view themselves as responsible for teaching all areas of the curriculum. Yet, clearly, teachers at all levels are confronted with the challenge of helping their students who are deaf read subject area material and gain skill in the style of expository writing.

In this section, I will present strategies for helping deaf children read and write in the content areas. I will not be presenting current theories of content area teaching. Content area material, specifically textbooks, present particular difficulties for youngsters who are deaf. Indeed, they present so much difficulty that many teachers use textbooks for reference only or rewrite portions for their students to read. Both of these strategies may be appropriate at times, but neither strategy enables the child who is deaf to become an independent reader of expository material, which they will need for success in college and in the workplace, as well as to be informed citizens throughout their lives.

Teachers of subject areas are always struggling with a double agenda; they are responsible for teaching the content curriculum of science, social studies, math, health, and other courses, but they are also responsible for teaching the skills that will give their students access to the body of written information on these subjects, written information that is as likely to be in the form of newspaper and magazine articles as in the form of textbooks, biographies, self-help books, reference materials, and Internet web sites.

Framework for Content Area Literacy

The theory and practice of literacy instruction discussed in Chapters 3 and 4 are applicable to content area literacy instruction. Virtually all of the models and strategies that teachers use to help deaf children become better readers and writers are just as effective with content area material. The teacher of deaf children can reach into his or her metaphoric "fishing vest" of models and strategies when children are reading expository text and accomplish goals related to literacy development and content learning.

The models and strategies that a teacher chooses for approaching the reading of particular text material should fit within an instructional framework that will enable the deaf child to read the material effectively and apply it to the learning of new content information. The framework developed by Richardson and Morgan (1997) views the reading and writing of content material as encompassing three steps—preparation, assistance, and reflection.

The preparation step involves preparing the learner to read the material by considering readability factors that ensure a reasonable match between the deaf reader and the text. Once these factors are taken into account, the teacher can determine what kind of learning scaffold the child needs to be able to interact meaningfully with the material. The prereading activities discussed in Chapter 4, such as background building, vocabulary development, and understanding the text structure, are the same types of preparation activities that teachers should use when they focus on content material.

The assistance step involves guiding the child through the material to ensure good comprehension. Again, these activities should be used with narrative text when the teacher's goal is developmental reading. In this step, the teacher encourages comprehension through questioning, metacognitive strategies, discussion, and summarization techniques.

The reflection step involves reviewing what was learned and expanding on the new knowledge. When the goal is content reading, this step includes activities that encourage synthesis of information, critical thinking, and extending the child's knowledge beyond the material in the text itself.

Models for Reading in the Content Areas

Models for reading in the content areas provide the same type of structure as models for teaching developmental reading. Each model provides the teacher with a set of instructional steps within which the teacher inserts appropriate strategies. As with the developmental reading models provided in Chapter 4, the models presented here meet two criteria. They have been successfully used with hearing and deaf children, and they represent models along a continuum of support. When choosing a model, consider the framework above. Does the model provide preparation for the child to read the material, assistance in reading it with good comprehension, and opportunities to reflect on new knowledge gained through the material?

Directed Reading Activity (DRA)/
Directed Reading Thinking Activity (DRTA)

Two models that seem to work as effectively with expository text as they do with narrative text are the DRA and DRTA (Alvermann & Swafford, 1989; Moorman & Blanton, 1990; Ryder, 1991), which were discussed in detail in Chapter 4. When used with subject area text, the steps in these approaches can enable students to read the material with good comprehension. However, they require that the teacher make a commitment of classroom time toward the actual reading of the text.

Most teachers of deaf children who use either approach include the first three steps (concept development, sight vocabulary, and guided reading) and eliminate the last two steps (skills development and enrichment). The concept development step tends to be used for presenting new terminology the student will encounter in the text. Instead of skills development and enrichment, teachers typically use the time that would be spent on those steps for presenting information on the topic that has not been covered by the text, for helping the students see relationships in the material that the text has not drawn, and for engaging the youngsters in activities, such as experiments, which help make the information more tangible.

Guided Reading Procedure (GRP)

In the *Guided Reading Procedure,* the assumption is made that the students are able to read the text independently but need guidance in comprehending it fully. The steps include the following: (a) a purpose is set, and the students read the text, being told to remember all they can, (b) as a group, the students tell everything they can remember, and the teacher records it on the board in no particular order, (c) the students are instructed to go back to the text to check on inconsistencies apparent from the differing information recorded on the board, (d) the students organize the information in the form of an outline, semantic map, or diagram. The remainder of the steps in the procedure are intended to be used for testing the students' recall of the information (Manzo, 1975).

Ankney and McClurg (1981) conducted a study in which they used the Guided Reading Procedure with fifth and sixth graders reading science and social studies textbooks and found that it took up a considerable amount of class time, was appropriate with highly factual material, was motivating to the students, and was best used with passages of 500 words or one and one-half pages of text at a time.

Because this strategy is built on the assumption that the students can read the text independently, it is not appropriate for many deaf students whose textbooks are written well above their reading levels. However, this strategy can be combined with the use of organizers, overviews, and other strategies, which will be discussed later in this chapter. This combination of strategies can enable many youngsters to read material that may otherwise appear to be too difficult for them.

Concept-Text-Application (C-T-A)

As developed by Wong and Au (1985), the *Concept-Text-Application* approach is quite similar to the DRTA. In the first phase, *concept,* the teacher assesses the students' background knowledge and introduces those concepts and vocabulary that are new to the students. In the second phase, *text,* the teacher sets a purpose, the students read the section silently, and the teacher asks literal-level questions. When the entire section is completed, the teacher engages the students in a discussion during which the information is organized into some type of visual structure. In the third phase, *application,* the teacher encourages the students to evaluate the material and to think divergently about the information.

The Concept-Text-Application approach requires both a fair amount of teacher planning time and class time. The visual structure may be a particularly worthwhile part of the strategy for deaf youngsters who may otherwise miss some of the information contributed during the class discussion.

Listen-Read-Discuss (L-R-D)

Listen-Read-Discuss was developed by Manzo and Casale (1985) as a basic lesson design from which content area teachers could create personal elaborations. In the

L-R-D approach, the teacher begins by presenting information from a portion of the text in the teacher's preferred style, such as lecture. The students are then directed to read the specific pages of the text covered in the lecture. The last step is discussion. An example of a teacher elaboration is for the students to be told that they need to locate some important details in the text that were omitted from the lecture.

Listen-Read-Discuss is actually just a reversal of the typical lecture approach used by many high school teachers and college/university instructors. Instead of lecturing on material the students have already read, in the L-R-D approach, the students read the material after the lecture. Thus, the material in the text and the terminology used are already familiar to the students, so they are more likely to be able to read the text independently.

K-W-L

The *K-W-L* approach developed by Ogle (1986) emphasizes the reader's prior knowledge. The first step in this approach is Step K, which Ogle defines as accessing *what I know.* In the first part of this step, the teacher writes the topic on the board, and the students brainstorm what they know about it. In the second part of this step, the students are encouraged to develop categories for the ideas they brainstormed. The second step is Step W—determining *what I want to learn.* In this step, the students are encouraged to create questions and are asked to write down the ones that interest them the most. The final step is Step L—recalling *what I did learn* as a result of reading. In this step, the students write or discuss what they have learned with specific attention to their original questions.

Teachers applying this approach with deaf students often use Step W to offer questions of their own that they know are likely to draw the children's attention to the most important information in the text. What is particularly attractive about using the K-W-L approach with students who are deaf is that it encourages them to become actively engaged in thinking about the relevance of the material before and after reading.

Teaching Strategies

Preparation

All of the models include a step designed to prepare the students for reading the material by building background knowledge, activating prior knowledge, and/or predicting content. However, none of the models include a step for guiding the teacher's choice of reading materials. For this step, teachers need to use the same strategies they used to choose developmental reading material, which were presented in Chapter 3.

The DRA and DRTA models include a step for building background knowledge and teaching new vocabulary. The DRA includes a step for the teacher to set a purpose, and in the DRTA, the teacher asks the students to predict what will happen. In the Guided Reading Procedure, preparation involves setting a purpose for the reading and asking the students to remember all they can. In Concept-Text-Application, the teacher introduces new concepts and vocabulary. The Listen-Read-Discuss model asks the students to read the material after the teacher presents the new information in the text they will be reading. K-W-L engages students in a discussion of what they already know about the topic and about what they want to learn.

Some of these planning activities are defined by the model, such as the first two steps in the K-W-L model. But there is typically little or no guidance provided for how the teacher should activate and build background knowledge, teach new vocabulary, or develop the child's knowledge of expository text structures. The teacher of deaf children can use the following strategies.

Expository Text Structure

Researchers have found that instruction in expository text structure has a positive effect on recall and comprehension (Armbruster, Anderson, & Ostertag, 1987; Roller & Schreiner, 1985; Taylor & Beach, 1984). This seems a logical finding given the difficulty many youngsters have in identifying the important information in their textbooks, their personal lack of experience with expository text when compared to the amount of experience they have with narrative text, and the mix of structures used in most expository materials.

The following two strategies represent contrasting approaches to teaching expository text structure. One promotes deductive learning and the other inductive learning. Expository text structures tend to incorporate several structures within the same passage, unlike narrative text, which typically maintains a consistent structure within one piece of writing. Using both learning approaches with different material across the variety of content areas over time will enable the deaf reader to internalize the set of expository text structures and use this emerging schema for comprehending future text material.

Seven-Step Approach. In the *seven-step approach* (my name for it because the authors did not give it one), the teacher uses well-structured textbook passages and graphic organizers to teach youngsters expository text structure (McGee & Richgels, 1985; Richgels, McGee, & Slaton, 1989).

Step 1. The teacher locates an actual passage from the students' textbooks that is a few paragraphs long, is well organized, clearly demonstrates one text structure (collection, description, causation, problem/solution, or compare/contrast), and contains clue words. A clue word gives the reader information about relationships between ideas. For example, the words *first, second,* and *next* are clues that the structure is based on collection. The words *therefore* and *because* are clues to a causation structure. *However* and *but* are clue words to a compare/contrast structure.

Step 2. The teacher creates a graphic organizer, which is a kind of outline with superordinate ideas at the top connected to subordinate ideas at lower and lower levels. Related ideas are connected with lines. Steps 1 and 2 are completed by the teacher in advance.

Step 3. The teacher explains the notion of text structure.

Step 4. The teacher explains the graphic organizer.

Step 5. The students write their own passages based on the graphic organizer.

Step 6. They read the actual text passage and compare it to their own compositions. The teacher then identifies the type of text structure they have just read and lists clue words that typically signal this type of structure. Steps 1 through 6 are repeated over time for each of the five expository text structures. At that point, Step 7 is added.

Step 7. The students read longer passages containing more than one structure and are encouraged to look at overall text structure.

Questioning Strategy. The *questioning strategy* developed by Muth (1987) is based on the assumption that teacher questions can focus students' attention on important relationships between ideas in expository text. In her view, good questions foster both internal connections (how text ideas relate to one another) and external connections (how text ideas relate to the reader's background knowledge). In the questioning strategy, teachers are encouraged to develop questions that build both internal and external connections while at the same time are aimed at the particular text structure the students are reading.

For the compare/contrast text structure, Muth (1987, p. 256) gave the following as examples of good questions in a passage about two breeds of horses. "What is the author comparing and contrasting?" and "What are the advantages of the Quarter horse for pleasure riding?" are two questions designed to build internal connections. "Which of the two horses would you pick and why?" is a question meant to build external connections.

For a passage on rust written in a causation structure, Muth (p. 257) used the example, "What is the cause–effect process that the author is describing?" as a question that helps build internal connections, and "When do you think things might rust in your house?" as the kind of question designed to build external connections.

Organizers and Overviews

Organizers and overviews consist of written information presented to the student prior to reading the actual text. In general, the information contained in an organizer or overview is intended to activate the reader's background knowledge and highlight key concepts in the material to be read.

The effectiveness of organizers and overviews with youngsters who are deaf is contingent on how independent the youngsters are in reading them and in thinking about how to apply the information. Thus, teachers need to spend time explaining the kinds of information contained in organizers and overviews, and providing their students with direction in how to use this information while they are reading the actual text.

Thematic Organizers. *Thematic organizers* and *advance organizers* are terms that are used almost interchangeably in the literature. The earliest reference to this strategy is the advance organizer, which was developed by Ausubel (1960). An *advance organizer* is written material that is (a) presented in advance of the actual text and

(b) designed to provide the reader with concepts that are more general, abstract, and inclusive than the actual text. According to Lenz, Alley, and Schumaker (1987), advance organizers generally include topics and subtopics, background information, new concepts, examples, new or relevant vocabulary, the organization or sequence of the new information, and an explanation of why the material should be read.

Alvarez (1983) modified the advance organizer strategy so that the organizer was written at the student's reading ability level, and it included information specifically related to the topic. He called this kind of organizer a *thematic organizer.* According to Risko and Alvarez (1983), the following elements characterize a thematic organizer:

1. Each organizer has three paragraphs that define the implied thematic concept of the passage and relate this concept to prior knowledge and/or experiences of the reader.
2. The concept is defined by presenting its various attributes and nonattributes.
3. Examples of how the concept relates to real-life experiences and the ideas in the text are given to further illustrate the meaning of the concept.
4. Following the three paragraphs are a set of statements written on the interpretive level. The students are instructed to indicate whether they agree with these statements during and/or after their reading. (p. 85)

The research suggests that organizers are particularly beneficial when students have weak background knowledge, they are taught to use the techniques, and the concepts in the text are abstract or poorly defined (Lenz, Alley, & Schumaker, 1987; Risko & Alvarez, 1986; Townsend & Clarihew, 1989).

The finding that children need to be taught to use thematic organizers was confirmed by Schirmer who found that thematic organizers did not activate the background knowledge of upper elementary and junior high school deaf students prior to reading text material when they were not given instruction on how to use them (Schirmer, 1993; Schirmer & Winter, 1993).

Structured Overviews.   Structured overviews have been called graphic organizers, graphic overviews, and conceptual maps, but the original term comes from Barron and Earle (Barron, 1969; Earle, 1969; Earle & Barron, 1973). A *structured overview* is a graphic representation of key concepts from the text presented in a hierarchical structure that shows the relationships among superordinate, coordinate, and subordinate concepts. The flow of the structured overview is not meant to reflect the sequence of ideas presented in the text. An example is presented in Figure 5.1.

Brown (1981) recommended that the following steps be used in preparing a structured overview:

1. Read the text assignment analytically to identify and write down major concepts.
2. Add to the list any terms relative to the concepts that the students might already know.
3. Arrange them in a schema to represent hierarchical and parallel relationships among terms. (p. 200)

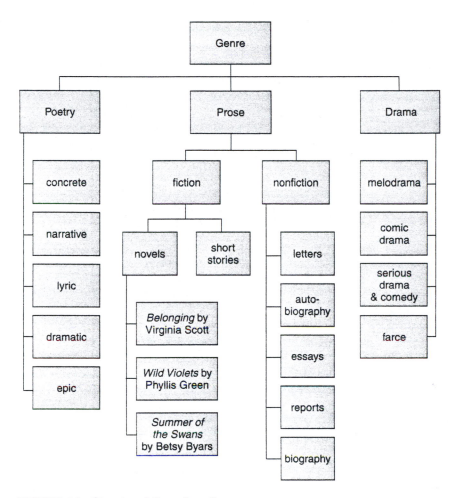

FIGURE 5.1   Structured Overview: Genre

The research on structured overviews indicates that they are more effective in improving comprehension when used along with other strategies, such as self-questioning or a study strategy, and when they are used both before and after reading (Alvermann & Boothby, 1986; Billingsley & Wildman, 1988; Darch, Carnine, & Kameenui, 1986).

Anticipation Guides.   An *anticipation guide* is a set of statements about a topic to which students must respond before reading about the topic. The responses are generally written as agree-disagree, likely-unlikely, or similar dichotomous formats.

According to Duffelmeyer (1994), constructing an anticipation guide "entails four tasks: identifying the major ideas presented in the text; considering what beliefs your students are likely to have; creating statements to elicit those beliefs; and arranging the statements in a form that requires students to respond to each one either positively or negatively" (p. 453). Effective statements relate to the main ideas in the text, draw on the students' prior knowledge, are general rather than highly specific, challenge students' beliefs, motivate students to read the material, and stimulate their thinking.

Vocabulary

Teaching the vocabulary of new concepts is important for all students but crucial for deaf students who may not always see others use complex and diverse vocabulary in their sign conversations. All of the vocabulary development strategies in Chapter 4 are effective for teaching the new vocabulary within content area material, but one strategy was developed specifically for teaching content area vocabulary.

Possible Sentences.   *Possible sentences* involves teaching new concepts so that they are related to each other and to the overall topic of a text chapter (Moore & Moore, 1986; Stahl & Kapinus, 1991). First, the teacher chooses six to eight words that would likely cause difficulty for the students and four to six words that are likely to be familiar to the students. As a group, using the words to form sentences that relate to the major concepts in the chapter should be relatively easy. Second, the teacher writes the ten to twelve words on the board and either provides a brief definition or asks if anyone knows a definition. Third, the students are asked to think of possible sentences in the chapter or passage they will be reading that use at least two of the words in each sentence. The teacher writes their sentences on the board whether they are accurate or not. When all the words have been included in at least one sentence and the students have no further ideas, the students read the chapter or passage, which is the fourth step. Fifth, the students discuss each sentence and decide if it could or could not be true based on what they have just read. Sentences that could not be true are modified to make them true.

Assistance

A few of the models include a step designed to assist the students through questioning and discussion as they read. Only the DRA and DRTA provide opportunities for a variety of activities, such as asking questions that encourage different levels of thinking and discussion, and are flexible enough to allow the teacher to use other strategies, such as scaffolded conversations, mental imagery, and self-questioning. In the Concept-Text-Application model, the teacher is supposed to ask literal-level questions at only periodic points during reading because knowing the key details is considered important for thinking analytically and critically about the material after reading. The other models discussed previously should be chosen when deaf students do not need the teacher's support as they read. An alternative is to modify the steps and include strategies that offer assistance while the students are reading the text material.

The strategies described in Chapter 4 for asking questions and encouraging deaf children to be metacognitive are beneficial for enhancing the child's comprehension of expository text. An adjustment to the prediction strategy making it more appropriate to content material is the *Gist Strategy* developed by Schuder, Clewell, and Jackson (1989). For this strategy, the teacher uses seven prompts to model and coach students in understanding the text material they are reading. The term *gist* is used to make it clear that the goal of this strategy is for the youngsters to get an overall sense of the text.

The first two prompts are used before the reading: (a) "What do you think this material is going to be about?" "What makes you think so?" and (b) "What do you think . . . (the text) is going to tell you about . . . (the predicted topic)?" "What makes you think so?" The next three prompts occur during the reading: (c) "Did you find evidence that supports your prediction?" "What was it?" (d) "Did you find evidence that does not support your prediction?" "What was it?" and (e) "Do you want to change your prediction at this point?" "If not, why not?" "If you do, how do you want to change it?" The last two prompts are used after the reading: (f) "Do you want to make any changes in your statement of what this is about?" "If yes, what changes do you want to make?" "Why do you want to make those changes?" and (g) "What did you learn that you did not know before reading?" (p. 230).

The following strategies have been developed specifically for understanding and remembering content area material.

Writing during Reading

Content area instruction has traditionally incorporated a melange of writing activities. As he or she reads, the deaf child can take notes, write a lab, develop a time line, keep a learning log, write a journal or diary entry, conduct an interview, create a chart or graph, construct a map, or complete a chart (Armbruster, Anderson, & Meyer, 1991; Braselton & Decker, 1994; Hadaway & Young, 1994; Hennings, 1993; Rakes, Rakes, & Smith, 1995; Schroeder & Strosnider, 1997).

The *Cognitive Frame Strategy* developed by Ryder (1994) combines writing with instruction on expository text structure. In Step 1, the teacher identifies the major ideas, concepts, and principles in the text passage. In Step 2, the teacher determines which of three frames is best suited to the information—descriptive, goal, or problem–solution. The descriptive frame is designed for material that involves comparisons-contrasts, cause–effect relationships, forms-functions, or advantages-disadvantages. The goal frame is designed for material that is temporal or sequential in nature. The problem–solution frame is designed for material in which there is a problem or issue, action to address the problem, and a resolution or consequence. In Step 3, the teacher draws the frame by labeling each row with an idea, concept, or principle the teacher identified in Step 1 and each column with the characteristics or relationships of the text structure. In Step 4, the children complete the frame as they read the text.

Literature

Literature can be used as a supportive strategy during content area instruction. Novels, stories, poems, and plays that relate to the topic being studied can provide reading experiences that supplement and extend deaf children's knowledge while they are reading content area material (Guzzetti, Kowalinski, & McGowan, 1992; Sanacore, 1990). Nonfiction literature is another resource of reading material within the content areas (Young & Vardell, 1993). For teachers who theme their instruction, using literature is a natural part of units in science, social studies, health, and other areas, as described in Chapter 2. As Smith and Johnson noted, "Literature can become the lens through which content is viewed. This lens holds the young reader's attention while connecting content with the variety of human experiences" (1994, p. 198).

Study Strategies

Most content area teachers want their students not only to comprehend the material but also to remember it and be able to recall it on a test. While comprehension is an essential first step, comprehension alone is not sufficient to enable youngsters to study and learn from their texts. As Caverly and Orlando (1991) noted, being able to learn from text involves "learning how to learn when reading" (p. 86).

Study strategies are designed to help youngsters focus their attention on the important information in text material, organize this information in a way that makes sense, integrate it with other previously known information so that it can be retained, and retrieve it when needed. Each strategy tends to focus on one or a few of these goals. For youngsters to accomplish all four, they need to be able to use combinations of strategies. Furthermore, they need to be able to choose the most appropriate strategies based on the demands of the material and the nature of the expected learning outcome.

The effectiveness of any given strategy depends on four factors—the student, the material, the student's degree of knowledge about the strategy and skill in using it, and the appropriateness of the strategy. After reviewing the research on study strategies, Caverly and Orlando (1991) concluded that the question "is not whether study strategies are successful, but rather where, when, and under what conditions they are successful" (p. 88).

Students who are deaf need to know an assortment of strategies and have the skill to apply them appropriately. The strategies presented in this section are the major ones discussed in the literature. I have organized them into four categories, categories that represent the learning goals of study strategies.

Focusing Strategies.   *Focusing strategies* are study strategies designed to help youngsters focus their attention on the important information in the text. The most common focusing strategy is *underlining/highlighting*. As a matter of fact, underlining/highlighting is reported to be the most popular study strategy used by students (Blanchard, 1985; McAndrew, 1983).

Underlining/highlighting takes less time than virtually any other study strategy, which may be the reason it is used spontaneously by so many students. Although it is an efficient strategy, it is effective only under two conditions, (1) if the students take the time to review the underlined/highlighted material and (2) if they limit the amount of material they underline/highlight to higher-level general statements. The research on underlining/highlighting also indicates that it is less effective for students below the fifth grade and for students at lower reading levels (Caverly & Orlando, 1991; McAndrew, 1983; Rickards, 1980). To increase the effectiveness of this strategy, teachers should model the use of underlining/highlighting, provide guided practice, and encourage students to review what they have underlined or highlighted (Blanchard, 1985; Poostay, 1984).

Focusing and Organizing Strategies.   A few of the study strategies described in the literature are designed to help students accomplish two goals—focus on important text information and organize the information in a way that makes sense.

One of these strategies is *notetaking* while reading. According to Smith and Tompkins (1988), notetaking from text has four benefits:

■ First, students actively attend to the written message, selecting important ideas to retain in notes.

■ Second, students who paraphrase and add their own comments or examples are relating their prior knowledge to new information.

■ Third, as learners elaborate on content by paraphrasing, indicating relationships among ideas, and developing their own examples, they are processing the content more deeply.

■ Finally, in creating their own notes, students generate a transportable and permanent storage of important information that is available for review. (pp. 46–47)

From Smith, P. L., & Tompkins, G. E. (1988, October). Structured notetaking: A new strategy for content area readers. *Journal of Reading, 32*(1), 46–53. Reprinted with permission of Patricia L. Smith and the International Reading Association. All rights reserved.

The research has shown that students who profit from notetaking are those who are able to identify the central ideas in text material. Connected to this finding is the observation that notetaking is more productive for material that is relatively easy for the youngster to read and comprehend (Caverly & Orlando, 1991). It has also been found that the act of taking notes is less important than the actual studying of the notes (Smith & Tompkins, 1988), a finding that may be self-evident to teachers but not at all obvious to students.

Notetaking is one focusing and organizing study strategy. *Study guides* are another. Study guides are typically viewed as a set of questions the student must answer either during or after reading text material (Horton & Lovitt, 1989). It has been suggested that questions requiring different levels of comprehension be included in study guides. For example, Bean and Ericson (1989) recommended the use of Pearson and Johnson's taxonomy of textually explicit, textually implicit, and scriptally implicit questions.

Reading road maps were developed by Wood (1988) as elaborated versions of study guides. In a reading road map, a winding road is drawn down the left side of a page, and questions are written down the right side of the page. Road signs are drawn alongside the winding road. The signs on the left side of the road present the topics and page numbers, and the signs on the right side of the road provide the directions.

Study guides can be valuable as a study strategy with students who are deaf for three reasons. First, the questions focus the youngster's attention on key text information. Second, the questions can be designed to encourage higher-order thinking. And third, they provide a set of notes the youngsters can use for reviewing major concepts.

Focusing, Organizing, and Integrating Strategies.   Several study strategies are designed to enable students to accomplish three goals—focus their attention on important text information, organize the information into a conceptual framework, and integrate it with previously known information so that it can be retained. Strategies in this category include outlining, semantic mapping, and graphic organizers.

The major difference between these study strategies and the ones discussed previously is that these particular strategies require the student to elucidate the relationships between concepts. The strategies are different from each other in the ways that connections between relationships are drawn.

Outlining requires that the student identify superordinate concepts and relate subordinate concepts to superordinate ones. *Semantic mapping* and *graphic organizers* also require the student to relate subordinate concepts to superordinate ones but go a step further by providing a way for the student to relate subordinate concepts to one another.

Outlining and semantic mapping have been found to be effective with material that is at or only slightly above the student's reading level and with relatively lengthy material. (Caverly & Orlando, 1991; Laframboise, 1986–1987). Smith and Tompkins (1988) found that graphic organizers could be used by students, particularly low ability students, to summarize, understand, and retain information from text when the organizers reflected expository text structures.

Focusing, Organizing, Integrating, and Retrieving Strategies.   A few strategies are designed to enable youngsters to achieve all of the goals involved in studying. These study strategies incorporate activities to help the youngster select the most important information in the text material, organize this information in a way that makes sense, integrate it with previously known information, and retrieve it when needed.

It would seem that the comprehensiveness of these strategies would make them highly useful. After all, instead of learning a menu of strategies such as the ones I described previously, the youngster could learn one comprehensive strategy and use it all the time. This comprehensiveness, however, can be a drawback when specific components of the strategy do not feel comfortable to the youngster or are not appropriate for every study situation. Comprehensive study strategies are somewhat like all-symptom cold tablets; they may contain ingredients you do not need, and the side effects can leave you immobile.

SQ3R is one of these comprehensive strategies. Originally developed in 1946 by Robinson, it continues to be one of the most widely taught strategies today. SQ3R contains five steps. *S* is for survey, the step in which the student skims the material to get a general overview of the organization and content. *Q* is for question, and in this step, the student converts chapter headings and subheadings into questions. These first two steps take place before reading. The *3R* is for read, recite, and review. During reading, the student finds answers to the questions. After reading, the student recites the answers or writes them down. Lastly, the student reviews the answers until the information is fully remembered.

For the advantages of SQ3R to be realized, it has been found that teachers need to spend a substantial amount of time teaching the strategy and providing students with guided practice in applying it (Caverly & Orlando, 1991; Gustafson & Pederson, 1986).

PORPE is another study strategy that is designed to be comprehensive. It was developed by Simpson, Stahl, and Hayes (1989) and is unique from many other strategies in that it begins after the youngster has read the text material. PORPE consists of five steps: predict, organize, rehearse, practice, and evaluate.

In the predict step, the student poses several essay questions the teacher might ask about the material. The student is encouraged to develop questions requiring synthesis, discussion, comparison-and-contrast, or evaluation of major concepts presented in the text. In the organize step, the student gathers information from the text to answer the questions and organizes the information into a map, chart, or outline. In the rehearse step, the student recites the answers aloud or in sign. In the practice step, the student writes the answers. In the evaluate step, the student evaluates his or her own answers.

PLAN is a study–reading strategy that takes students through the planning, assistance, and reflection stages of reading content area text (Caverly, Mandeville, & Nicholson, 1995). In the predict step, the students create a prediction map for an upcoming chapter by using information from the chapter title and subtitles, highlighted words, and graphics. The map can be organized as a semantic map or other type of graphic organizer showing relationships between concepts. In the locate step, the students put a check next to the information on the map that is already familiar to them and a question mark by the unfamiliar concepts. In the add step, the students read the text and while reading, they add words or short phrases next to the concepts on the map. During this step, the teacher can assist with concepts that continue to remain unclear to the students. In the note step, the students review their map and reconstruct it if necessary. They then use their map to study for an exam, write a report, or complete other assignments.

Content Literacy Guides

Content literacy guides are written to provide students with summaries, questions, and other information to help them pay attention to important information in the text and to understand it more fully. Hierarchical guides, such as Earle's three-level guide (1969), consist of three types of questions—literal, interpretive, and applied. When creating a three-level guide, the teacher writes a set of questions for each level. Nonhierarchical guides (Armstrong, Patberg, & Dewitz, 1988) consist of questions following the sequential order of the text. Selective guides (Cunningham & Shablak, 1975) focus the students' attention on important sections of the text and give the students advice about which sections are less important and can be skipped, skimmed, or scanned. Many other types of literacy guides have been developed that are modifications of these patterns, such as point-of-view guides (Wood, 1988), which use questions in an interview form, and pattern guides (Vacca & Vacca, 1999), which focus students' attention on text structure, organization, and patterns.

McKenna and Robinson (1997) suggested that when creating a content literacy guide, teachers should analyze the material, be careful not to put too much print on each page, make the guide interesting, make sure it matches the purpose of the reading assignment, include page numbers and headings to assist the students in matching the guide with the text, and keep comprehension in mind so that the guide supports the student in understanding the material.

Reflection

All of the content area reading models include steps for reviewing the information in the text, synthesizing it into new knowledge structures, and extending the child's understanding. The DRA and DRTA involve discussion strategies, summarizing, and activities such as journal writing. In the Guided Reading Procedure, the students present the information they remember from the text, go back to the material to resolve inconsistencies, and organize it into a visual structure. The students also develop a visual structure for the Concept-Text-Application model, after which they discuss the information in the text. Discussion is also the culminating step of Listen-Read-Discuss and K-W-L.

In addition to the after-reading strategies discussed in Chapter 4, writing activities can help deaf children reflect on expository material. These strategies are sometimes called *writing across the curriculum.*

Writing after Reading
Innumerable writing activities have been developed for content area instruction. Research reports are typically included in the curricula from elementary through high school. Letter writing is a staple of the curriculum, and students are not only taught letter format but also use this skill to write letters of complaint, invitation, thank-you, and letters of request for information, services, or goods to peers, editors, and public officials. As a complement to reading in science and social studies, students are often asked to write actual or imaginary biographies and autobiographies. Essay writing has been a particular emphasis in the study of current events. In addition to essays, writing in the form of advertisements, web pages, newspaper articles, television reports,

book or film reviews, directions, and recipes are frequently used to extend the learning of content material.

Story Problems.   Math was traditionally viewed as an academic area of strength for deaf students, though this appears to have been largely dependent on one factor of mathematical knowledge, computational ability (Titus, 1996). One place that math and literacy development intersects is math *story problems,* and these present a particular difficulty to deaf students (Pau, 1995). Problem-writing is a writing activity that can help deaf students comprehend the nature of story problem language (Winograd & Higgins, 1995). When first introducing this strategy, textbook problems can be used as templates from which the students change a few facts to create new problems. Subsequently, the teacher encourages students to create divergent problems, using language that is consistent with story problem jargon. The class solves the problems the students have written, and they discuss the language within the problem that was helpful or confusing.

Picture Books.   Creating *picture books* can help students use writing to summarize the important concepts from content area material. In this strategy, students create picture books for younger children about a topic they are studying. To create the picture books, they must identify the major concepts and write about them in a way that will be understandable to children who are younger than themselves. Schroder (1996) used this strategy with her sixth graders and found the following steps to be helpful. First, the students read the relevant material. Second, she gathered a set of picture books that she shared with the students as exemplars, pointing out the features of the texts. Third, the students developed a flow chart for their books. In the fourth and fifth steps, they drafted and revised their books. In the last step, they published the books and shared them with younger children.

Summary Writing.   *Summary writing* traditionally has been valued as a writing activity in all subject areas because it combines reading and writing, has been found to improve comprehension and recall, and requires the student to use higher-order thinking processes (Bromley, 1985; Brown, Day, & Jones, 1983; Casazza, 1993; Rinehart, Stahl, & Erickson, 1986). It has been observed that the ability to summarize improves with age, able readers write better summaries than less able readers, and even good readers may need explicit instruction in the rules of summary writing (Englert, Raphael, Anderson, Anthony, & Stevens, 1991; Hill, 1991; Wood, Winne, & Carney, 1995).

Noyce and Christie (1989) suggested teaching the following four rules for summary writing, modeling them, and providing opportunities for students to practice applying them.

1. Select a topic sentence. If you do not see a sentence by the author that summarizes the paragraph, write your own.
2. Delete unnecessary information. Text information may be repeated in a passage, or it may be trivial. Delete both redundant and unimportant ideas.

3. Collapse list of items. Substitute a collective term for a number of things that fall into the same category, e.g., instead of bracelets, pendants, pins, and watches, you might use jewelry. Also, substitute one encompassing action for a list of subcomponents of the action.
4. Collapse paragraphs. Some paragraphs expand on others and can be combined with them. Others are unnecessary and can be deleted. (pp. 234–235)

Guido and Colwell (1987) suggested teaching the following four principles for summary writing by presenting the principles, giving examples, providing practice, sharing applications, and offering feedback.

1. Don't include unnecessary detail (even if it's interesting to you).
2. Don't repeat anything you have already said.
3. Use a general term for a list of specific items.
4. Use one word to describe a list of actions that were included in one or several sentences. (pp. 94–95)

Final Comments

It is not uncommon for teachers of the content areas to be more interested in their subject matter curriculum goals and objectives than in the children's reading, writing, and language goals. After all, at each grade level, children are expected to master specific content area material. It is extremely difficult for teachers of deaf children to pay close attention to language and literacy while they are presenting complex concepts and ideas in science, social studies, math, health, and other subject areas. The purpose of this chapter was to provide teachers of content area subjects with models and strategies designed to help them deal with the competing demands of literacy and content area instruction.

Gaskins and her colleagues from the Benchmark School (1994), which serves children who are experiencing difficulty in learning to read, used six axioms of instruction to represent the ways that reading and talking about text should be integrated into content area instruction. According to the first and most important axiom, every student must have an opportunity to respond to text every day, which they called *every-pupil-response activities*. The second axiom encourages collaboration between students and provides opportunities to discuss their responses with peers. The third axiom focuses on real-life problems by connecting information in the text to life experiences with which the children could relate. The fourth axiom emphasizes a few important concepts that represent relationships and themes within the unit being studied. The fifth axiom teaches students how to learn, and the sixth guides the construction of understanding. When the models and strategies presented in this chapter are viewed within the context of these axioms, they can be applied in ways that will enable deaf students to integrate expository material within their reading repertoires and develop increasing ability to use reading for learning.

In the next chapter, I will present approaches that teachers can use to assess the deaf child's growth in reading and writing.

Suggested Readings

Manzo, A. V., & Manzo, U. (1997). *Content area literacy: Interactive teaching for active learning* (2nd ed.). Columbus, OH: Merrill/Prentice Hall.

McKenna, M. C., & Robinson, R. D. (1997). *Teaching through text: A content literacy approach to content area reading* (2nd ed.). New York: Longman.

Ruddell, M. R. (1997). *Teaching content reading and writing* (2nd ed.). Boston: Allyn and Bacon.

Ryder, R. J., & Graves, M. F. (1998). *Reading and learning in the content areas* (2nd ed.). Columbus, OH: Merrill/Prentice Hall.

Tompkins, G. E. (2000). *Teaching writing: Balancing process and product* (3rd ed.). Upper Saddle River, NJ: Merrill/Prentice Hall.

Vacca, R. T., & Vacca, J. L. (1999). *Content area reading: Literacy and learning across the curriculum* (6th ed.). New York: Longman.

6 Monitoring the Learning Process in Reading and Writing

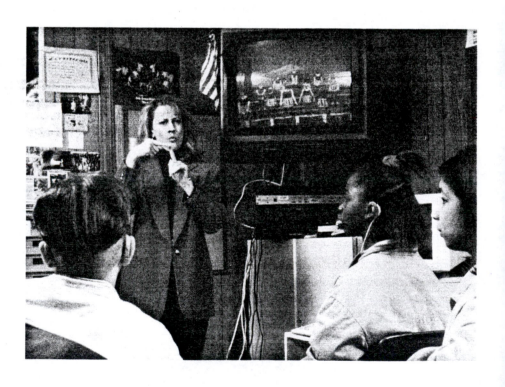

Monitoring the Learning Process in Reading and Writing

Assessment Principles

Assessment Process

Child Background

Reading and Writing Abilities

Ongoing Assessment

Assessment, diagnosis, measurement, and evaluation are terms that are used to describe the process of gathering information about each child's strengths and weaknesses in learning and then making judgments about instruction. Purposes for literacy assessment fall into distinct categories, which are related to the stakeholders who want the assessment information. Different stakeholders want different information about literacy achievement. Five assessment audiences have been identified (Farr, 1992; Salvia & Ysseldyke, 1998; Williams, 1996):

- The general public, press, and public policy makers want information related to groups of students to determine if the schools are effective, are accountable to standards of performance, and meet state and national goals.
- School administrators want information that helps them judge the effectiveness of the curriculum, the materials, and the quality of instruction.
- Teachers want information that enables them to monitor the literacy learning of individual children and provides guidance for making instructional decisions.
- Parents want information about the progress of their own child and how their child compares to other children, so they can determine whether the educational program is appropriate.
- Students want information about their own strengths and needs, so they can decide on which skills to focus their energies.

The information needed by administrators, the public, public policy makers, and the press is important, but this chapter will focus on the information that is most beneficial to teachers, students, and parents. With this perspective in mind, I will concentrate on the informal approaches to literacy assessment rather than the formal, standardized approaches.

Assessment Principles

The following set of principles should guide teachers in monitoring the literacy development of children who are deaf.

1. *Assessment and Teaching Are Bound Together.* Assessment should be grounded in what children are learning, assessment should be linked with authentic reading and writing activities, assessment should enhance the teacher's ability to observe and understand learning. Teaching goals should be focused enough to be assessed.

2. *Assessment Is a Continuous, Systematic, and Evolving Process.* This principle means that some types of assessment take place moment-by-moment and some on a regularly scheduled basis. It also means that assessment changes over time as children demonstrate the ability to engage in new kinds of literacy tasks.

3. *Assessment Is Multidimensional.* Assessment techniques and instruments must be varied, and diverse contexts should be used to gather information on the full spectrum of knowledge and skills possessed by the youngsters.

   4. *Assessment Should Include a Balance of Formative and Summative Measures.* Formative evaluation is ongoing during instruction whereas summative evaluation is completed at the end of instruction.
   5. *Assessment Is a Shared Endeavor between Teacher and Student.* According to this principle, the goal of assessment is to inform the teacher and the student mutually so that they can make joint decisions about what to do next.

Assessment Process

The assessment process in literacy is not unlike the process used to assess language ability described in Chapter 2. First, the teacher obtains information about the child's background. Next, reading and writing abilities are assessed. In keeping with the principles above, both informal and formal approaches are used. The information is summarized and interpreted, literacy goals are determined, instructional models and strategies are identified, and instruction is implemented with ongoing assessment.

Child Background

When we look into the child's background for the purposes of a language assessment, we are interested in information such as developmental milestones, degree of hearing loss, presence of disabilities that might affect learning, relevant medical history, language(s) used at home, profile of the family structure, age at which the hearing loss was diagnosed, age at which the child began receiving educational services, and school progress reports.

   We are equally interested in this information when we are conducting an assessment of the child's literacy development. However, we also want to know the nature of the child's previous reading and writing instruction. For example, it is extremely important to know the kinds of reading materials the child used in the past, the types of writing the child did, the teaching models and strategies the teacher used, and the previous teacher's evaluation of the child's progress.

Reading and Writing Abilities

Regardless of the richness of background data available to the teacher, when the child is new to the classroom, there is a need to obtain information about the child's current reading and writing abilities, the genres the child typically reads, and the child's attitude toward reading.

Informal Approaches
The advantages and disadvantages of informal approaches in literacy assessment are similar to the advantages and disadvantages of informal approaches in language assessment discussed in Chapter 1. Informal approaches offer the best potential for providing a link between literacy assessment and instruction because the assessment tasks

closely resemble actual instruction, and they engage the child in authentic reading and writing. The disadvantage of informal approaches is that the accuracy and completeness of the information depends heavily on the skill of the teacher.

Informal Reading Inventory.   An *informal reading inventory* is one type of informal approach to reading assessment. In an informal reading inventory, the teacher begins by choosing reading passages at easy to progressively more difficult levels. Two equivalent passages are chosen at each level. Passage length is typically twenty-five to fifty words for the preprimer and primer levels, fifty words for first- and second-grade levels, and one hundred to two hundred words for third-grade level and above. The teacher then develops six to ten factual and inferential questions for each passage.

It is usually recommended that teachers begin the procedure with passages the child would find easy to read. Child background information can be very helpful at this time for indicating a starting point. The teacher should mark the location of the passage in the actual book for the child to use and make a photocopy of the passage for his or her own use.

The child is asked to read the first passage aloud or in sign. During this reading, the teacher records any inaccuracies the child makes such as substituting, adding, or omitting words. It is important for teachers of children who are deaf to record the places in which the child uses a sign that is not conceptual or fingerspells a word because these responses sometimes indicate that the child does not recognize the word concept. During this reading, the teacher also makes note of the child's reading behaviors. Observations focus on the child's effort, concentration, expression, and strategies for identifying unknown words. After the passage is read, the teacher asks the comprehension questions and records the child's answers.

The child is asked to read the second passage silently. During this reading, the teacher can make note of reading behaviors such as signing to oneself or subvocalizing, rereading words and phrases, and tracking with a finger or pencil. When the child finishes reading the passage, the teacher asks the comprehension questions and records the child's answers.

This procedure is repeated with increasingly more difficult passages until the passage the child is reading is clearly at his or her frustration level. At that point, the teacher reads the passage aloud or in sign to the child and then asks the comprehension questions.

After completing the procedure, the teacher examines the child's reading inaccuracies, behaviors, and answers to the comprehension questions to determine the child's independent, instructional, frustration, and capacity reading levels. The *independent reading level* is considered to be the level at which the child recognizes 98 percent of the words, answers 90 percent of the comprehension questions correctly, and reads in a relaxed and fluent manner. The *instructional level* is considered to be the level at which the child recognizes 95 percent of the words, answers 75 percent of the comprehension questions correctly, and demonstrates a few behaviors that indicate the child is having some difficulty reading the material. At the *frustration level,* the child is only able to recognize 90 percent of the words and if forced to complete reading the passage, answers no more than 50 percent of the comprehension questions correctly. Furthermore, the child demonstrates the desire to avoid reading the material by exhibiting behaviors such as fidgeting and looking up constantly. The *capacity level* is the level at which the child can answer 75 percent of the comprehension questions correctly when the material is read to him or her.

Creating informal reading inventories is obviously time-consuming for the teacher. It is tempting for teachers to use one of the commercially available informal reading inventories, a couple of which are described in the appendix. However, a published informal reading inventory no longer embodies all of the advantages of an informal approach because it will not include the material that the teacher will use for instruction. When teachers create their own informal reading inventories, they can learn a great deal about how well children can perform on material used in the classroom.

Diagnostic Reading Lesson. In a *diagnostic reading lesson,* the teacher develops a lesson implementing a reading model and strategies thought to be appropriate for the child, with reading material likely to be at the child's independent or instructional reading level. If a parent or administrator happened to be watching the teacher and child, it would probably be assumed that this was an ordinary teaching lesson and not an assessment procedure. The teacher conducts the lesson as a typical reading lesson, but the purpose is to gather information about the child's reading abilities.

Any of the strategies discussed in Chapter 4 could be used to develop a diagnostic teaching lesson. One example is a Directed Reading Thinking Activity. A teacher who wants to use a DRTA as a diagnostic teaching lesson would choose a story or chapter at a level believed to be at the child's independent to instructional reading level. The teacher would develop and teach a lesson incorporating the steps in a DRTA—concept development, sight vocabulary, guided reading (prediction, silent reading, questions, purposeful oral or sign rereading), and discussion.

If the child demonstrated prior knowledge of most or all of the sight vocabulary, showed few difficulties with recognizing words in the selection, answered comprehension questions fully with little help from the teacher, and seemed relaxed during the reading, the teacher could assume that the text material could be read independently by the child. If the child did not previously know most of the sight vocabulary but was able to learn the words relatively quickly, could recognize most words in the selection but needed assistance with a few words or figurative expressions, and demonstrated good comprehension with help from the teacher, the teacher could assume that the text material would be appropriate for instruction with a model such as the DRTA that offers the child considerable teacher support. The teacher would have also learned the kinds of word identification strategies and comprehension strategies that the child used and whether these strategies were being used effectively.

Analytical Writing Scoring. Assessing the writing abilities of a child who is deaf can be extremely frustrating because it can be difficult to sort out the child's abilities to manipulate English sentence structures from other aspects of the child's writing. One of the techniques used to gather information about the child's writing that can avoid the problem of focusing too intensely on one aspect of writing is *analytical writing scoring*. In this technique, separate writing traits are assessed individually, and each trait is given equal weight.

In Figure 6.1, criteria for analytical writing scoring are presented. Six writing traits are included—ideas and content, organization, voice, word choice, sentence structures, and mechanics. For each trait, the teacher evaluates the child's writing on a scale from one to five.

The usefulness of this technique as a measure of the deaf child's writing abilities depends on how representative the child's composition is of the child's writing in general. For example, a child who writes prolifically and creatively about sports may write with no enthusiasm when asked to write a mystery. If the teacher chooses to evaluate the mystery using analytical writing scoring, the results might indicate false problems with the child's writing.

Analytical writing scoring provides more reliable assessment information if the teacher applies it to several different pieces of writing and with at least some pieces that are based on self-selected topics. This guideline should be followed not only at the beginning of the school year but also at intervals during the year when the teacher wants to assess the child's writing.

In a study conducted with middle school deaf children, a writing assessment rubric similar to the one in Figure 6.1 was used as an instructional strategy (Schirmer, Bailey, & Fitzgerald, 1999). For one year, the language arts teacher at a state school for the deaf taught the students the qualities of writing and evaluated their compositions using the rubric, which defined levels of performance for each quality. Results indicated that by the end of the school year, the students showed improvement in four of the qualities—topic, content, story development, and organization—but no improvement in the other qualities—text structure, voice/audience, word choice, sentence structures, and mechanics. The compositions also reflected changes in the ways the students used language functionally both interpersonally and intrapersonally during the school year. As an instructional strategy, rubrics would appear to be most effective when individualized by students, class, age level, genre, or assignment to target the development needs of students who are deaf.

Standardized Assessment Instruments

In Chapter 1, the advantages and disadvantages of standardized tests of language were discussed. Standardized tests of reading offer similar advantages and disadvantages. On the plus side, they are relatively easy to administer, and results are not influenced by the skill or bias of the examiner. Also on the plus side, these tests offer data regarding reliability, validity, representativeness, and standard error of measurement. On the minus side, standardized reading tests tend to focus heavily on isolated reading skills such as phonic analysis and structural analysis, comprehension is measured with relatively short passages unrelated to one another, and knowledge of vocabulary is often assessed with words that are out of context.

It is an understatement to say that there is a fair amount of discussion regarding the usefulness of standardized tests to measure reading ability and reading growth.

FIGURE 6.1   Analytical Writing Scoring

I. Ideas and Content

5 *Paper:* The topic is clear, there is a good balance between central ideas and details, and the paper is interesting.

3 *Paper:* Some ideas are clear and others are unclear or not appropriate; and there is too much emphasis on the central idea and not enough supporting details, or vice versa.

1 *Paper:* The topic is unclear and ideas seem unrelated to one another, or very few ideas are presented.

II. Organization

5 *Paper:* Presentation of ideas is logical, relationships between ideas are clearly drawn, and details and examples fit in well with central ideas.

3 *Paper:* The presentation of ideas is unclear or not logical, connections between ideas are not made, and details and examples are sometimes not appropriate.

1 *Paper:* There is no obvious order to the presentation of ideas, and it is difficult to figure our how ideas relate to one another.

III. Voice

5 *Paper:* The writer demonstrates genuine interest in the topic, a desire to express ideas in an original way, and a concern that the reader respond to the writing.

3 *Paper:* The writer demonstrates knowledge but no deep interest in the topic, expresses him- or herself in routinized ways, and seems aware of his or her audience but does not engage them in the writing.

1 *Paper:* The writer demonstrates no sincere interest in the topic and seems unaware of an audience.

IV. Word Choice

5 *Paper:* The writer chooses words carefully and with creativity.

3 *Paper:* The writer chooses words that are clear but ordinary, and may use inappropriate or overused words or phrases.

1 *Paper:* The writer uses a limited variety of words, the words used are not always clear, and some words are inappropriately used.

V. Sentence Structures

5 *Paper:* Sentences are easy to read and understand, structures are grammatically correct, and a variety of structures are used.

3 *Paper:* Most sentences are understandable, but some structures are incorrect and similar structures are often used.

1 *Paper:* Sentence structure errors are frequent, and it is a difficult paper to read and understand.

VI. Mechanics (Grammar, Capitalization, Punctuation, Spelling, and Paragraphing)

5 *Paper:* Errors in mechanics are few, and they do not interfere with the reading flow.

3 *Paper:* Errors in mechanics sometimes draw the reader's attention away from the ideas being presented.

1 *Paper:* Errors in mechanics are so glaring that it is extremely tedious to read the paper.

Diagnostic reading tests can give the teacher valuable information about the deaf child's current reading abilities when used in conjunction with informal approaches, although standardized reading tests should not be used as a sole measure of the child's current abilities. Furthermore, many school administrators require standardized tests to be given at periodic intervals and if the teacher must administer these tests, the information should be interpreted and used.

One way to elicit information from standardized tests beyond the grade equivalent score is to use a procedure referred to as *probing*. Probing takes place after the teacher has administered and scored the test. In probing, the teacher chooses a few items from the test that were answered correctly and a few that were answered incorrectly by the child. The teacher gives the child a clean copy of the test and asks the child to read and answer the marked items aloud or in sign. For each item, the teacher asks why the child chose that particular answer.

I have described several diagnostic reading tests and academic achievement tests in the appendix. With the exception of the Stanford Achievement Test, none have been normed on students who are deaf. It is common knowledge that youngsters who are deaf tend to obtain depressed scores on standardized tests of reading, probably because these tests focus largely on the surface structure features of the reading process.

Attitude and Interest

Attitude toward reading and writing is an important factor in performance. Deaf students with negative attitudes toward literacy can become reluctant readers and writers. The reasons often include frustration with the difficulty involved in reading and the frequent failure that many deaf students experience. Finding out about the child's attitudes and interests is an important part of a literacy assessment. One approach involves observing them during classroom activities, free time, as well as reading and writing instruction. During these observations, the teacher can ask questions such as the following. Does the child:

- Approach reading and writing with enthusiasm?
- Demonstrate confidence about reading and writing abilities?
- Participate willingly in reading and writing activities?
- Read text material thoroughly?
- Use books as resources?
- Read a variety of genres?
- Read independently?
- Write independently?

Is the child:

- Relaxed when reading and writing?
- Able to concentrate?
- Able to read and write for more than a few minutes?

Another approach for assessing attitudes and interests is a questionnaire or survey. The following open-ended questions are one type of reading questionnaire.

1. I think reading is . . .
2. My favorite place to read is . . .
3. When my mom or dad reads to me . . .
4. When my teacher reads to me . . .
5. My parents read because . . .
6. My favorite kind of reading is . . .
7. I would rather read than . . .
8. The reasons that people read are . . .
9. The reason that I read is . . .
10. The hardest thing about reading is . . .
11. The easiest thing about reading is . . .
12. If I got a book for a present, I would . . .
13. My friends think that reading is . . .
14. When I am grown-up . . .
15. If I were the teacher, I would teach reading by . . .

Understanding the child's attitudes can help the teacher figure out models, strategies, materials, and activities that can capitalize on the child's interests and motivations.

Ongoing Assessment

By conducting ongoing assessment, teachers of deaf children can obtain continuous information about individual children's progress. Many educators recommend curriculum-based assessment or portfolio assessment for this purpose. Curriculum-based assessment for literacy involves assessing specific curriculum skills by examining the component areas of the literacy curriculum, such as word recognition, reading comprehension, written expression, and spelling. Portfolio assessment involves assessing literacy by collecting items that reflect the student's strengths, growth, and goals in literacy.

In a balanced literacy program, multiple sources of assessment information should be obtained on an ongoing basis. The following procedures and items can provide teachers with a comprehensive picture of deaf children's progress as they become readers and writers.

Literacy Development Checklists
Reading and writing development checklists can be constructed from two possible sources of information. One source is the yearly goals and objectives developed by the teacher in the areas of reading and writing. These goals and objectives are typically based on the teacher's evaluation of the child's current abilities along with the teacher's own perspective regarding the important milestones and attributes of literacy development. *Literacy development checklists* can also be curriculum-based. The

teacher who is expected to conduct curriculum-based assessment can transfer the learning objectives from the school district, statewide, or basal curriculum into a literacy development checklist.

Teachers usually record their observations on literacy development checklists at regularly scheduled intervals such as monthly or quarterly. Examples of three literacy development checklists are provided in Figures 6.2, 6.3, and 6.4. One is a reading development checklist, one is a writing development checklist, and the third is an emergent literacy checklist.

Portfolio Items

The following items are frequently suggested for literacy portfolios because they illustrate the child's growth in areas that are crucial to literacy development. These items do not exhaust all of the possibilities but rather represent the core items within a deaf child's literacy portfolio.

Reading Records.   One item usually suggested for a portfolio is a *reading record.* In a reading record, the student records the title and author of each book he or she has read and the date it was completed. Au, Scheu, Kawakami, and Herman (1990) commented that teachers can use the reading record for periodic conferences with the child regarding the amount he or she is reading, the appropriateness of the material, the child's preferences, the child's reading habits, and books the child might be interested in reading next. The teacher's notes on these conferences can also become a part of the child's portfolio.

Writing Samples.   *Writing samples* constitute another element typically recommended for a portfolio. It is suggested that the choice of writing samples from the body of work the youngster is producing should be a collaborative decision between the student and teacher. Simmons (1990) proposed a Theirs/Mine/Ours system in which students choose a piece, teachers choose a piece, and they collaborate on a piece for every three pieces that are selected. Writing samples should be collected periodically, with the frequency dependent on the amount and diversity of writing produced by the child.

Progress Notes, Observation Notes, and Anecdotes.   *Progress notes, observation notes, and anecdotes* can be additional items in a portfolio. Even though they can provide an important dimension to assessment, they can also be the most difficult to manage. Cambourne and Turbill (1990) observed that conference time, both formal teacher–student conferences and informal conferences carried out as the teacher moved around the classroom, provided pivotal time for taking notes on individual student learning.

Rhodes and Nathenson-Mejia (1992) reminded teachers that analyzing notes must be the companion activity to taking notes. They suggested that effective analysis involves making inferences, identifying trends and patterns in the child's literacy behaviors, and recognizing both strengths and weaknesses in teaching and learning.

FIGURE 6.2   Reading Development Checklist

	Most of the time	Some-times	Not yet noticed	Not applicable
Comprehension Strategies				
Uses content schema				
Uses textual schema				
Story schema				
Schema for expository text				
Predicts				
Uses metacognition				
Self-questions				
Uses mental imagery				
Summarizes/Retells				
Determines central idea or theme				
Engages in higher-level thinking				
Engages in critical reading				
Uses vocabulary knowledge				
Uses study strategies				
Uses knowledge of writing				
Strategies for Understanding Words and Sentences				
Uses word recognition strategies				
Uses lexical cues				
Uses graphophonic cues				
Uses structural cues				
Uses context cues				
Uses text cohesion devices				
Understands sentence transformations				
Understands figurative language				
Demonstrates flexibility in using strategies				
Types of Reading				
Short stories				
Comic books				
Poetry				
Magazine articles				
Newspaper articles				
Scripts/Plays				
Books				
Fiction (e.g., fables and folktales, mystery, adventure)				
_____				
Nonfiction (e.g., biography, science, history)				
_____				
Attitudes toward Reading				
Approaches reading with enthusiasm				
Demonstrates confidence in reading ability				
Reads text material thoroughly				
Reads a variety of genres				
Is relaxed when reading				
Reads independently				

FIGURE 6.3   Writing Development Checklist

	Most of the time	Some-times	Not yet noticed	Not applicable
Writing Process				
Engages in planning				
Chooses own topic				
Identifies a purpose				
Considers the audience				
Engages in rehearsal activities				
Engages in writing/drafting				
Places emphasis on content over form				
Uses spelling strategies				
Considers first draft as a rough draft				
Engages in revising				
Revises at the word level				
Revises at the sentence level				
Revises at the paragraph level				
Makes substantive changes in the text				
Proofreads for final editing				
Shares writing with others				
Revises based on peer review				
Publishes				
Publishes some writing pieces				
Shares publications with others				
Writing Traits				
Ideas and content are clear				
Organization is logical				
Voice demonstrates sincerity				
Words are chosen carefully				
Sentence structures are correct and clear				
Mechanics do not interfere with content				
Grammar				
Capitalization				
Punctuation				
Spelling				
Paragraphing				
Writing Topics				
Dialogue journals				
Stories				
Reports				
Summaries				
Learning logs				
Letters				
Biographies/Autobiographies				
Poems				
Essays				
Advertisements				
Attitudes toward Writing				
Approaches writing with enthusiasm				
Demonstrates confidence in writing abilities				
Writes extensively				
Takes risks in types of writing				
Writes independently				
Shares writing with others				

FIGURE 6.4   Emergent Literacy Checklist

	Most of the time	Some-times	Not yet noticed	Not applicable
Literacy Concepts				
Recognizes the purposes, functions, and uses of literacy				
Is aware that print conveys a message				
Realizes that ideas and feelings are communicated through reading and writing				
Demonstrates story schema				
Retells a story				
Creates a story about pictures				
Understands the connection between written and spoken words				
Understands print concepts such as first-last-end				
Conventions and Decoding				
Understands directionality in reading				
Front to back				
Left to right				
Return sweep for each line				
Top to bottom				
Page to page				
Recognizes the differences between letters, words, spaces, numbers, and pictures				
Recognizes punctuation				
Identifies letters				
Capital				
Lower case				
Demonstrates phonemic awareness				
Recognizes word repetitions and patterns				
Identifies environmental print				
Identifies words in stories				
Writing				
Engages in drawing as writing				
Engages in scribble writing				
Writes letter-like units				
Uses nonphonetic letter strings				
Copies from environmental print				
Uses conventional writing				

A CASE STUDY

Juan is an eleven-year-old boy who is currently in the sixth grade. He has a profound hearing loss. He is mainstreamed for many content area subjects and is in Ms. Lim's resource room for one hour and fifteen minutes daily along with three other youngsters who are deaf. Ms. Lim also has other groups of youngsters who are deaf or hard of hearing who come to her resource room for scheduled periods of time daily.

At the beginning of the school year, Ms. Lim had looked through Juan's cumulative file and learned that the etiology of his hearing loss was unknown, his parents and siblings were hearing, his hearing loss had been identified at nineteen months of age, and he and his parents had begun participating in an early intervention program when he was almost two years old. She also learned that Juan's previous school progress reports indicated that his former teacher felt he was progressing satisfactorily in reading, and his SAT-HI score from the spring indicated that he was reading at the second-grade level. Ms. Lim wrote a note to herself that at the fall parent-teacher conferences, she would ask Juan's parents about the kinds of reading he does at home, the parents' own reading habits, and whether they read to him on a regular basis, and the language they speak at home.

The first week of school, Ms. Lim administered the Gates-MacGinitie Reading Test, Level 2, Form K, and Juan received a grade equivalent score of 2.5 on vocabulary, 1.8 on comprehension, and 2.2 overall. She probed the test with Juan and learned that in the vocabulary section, Juan made a couple of errors because he had spelled the key words incorrectly, and one of his mistakes was a misinterpretation of the target concept. The picture was a boy looking at his reflection in the mirror. The correct answer was "reflection," but Juan chose "affection," which an eleven-year-old boy with high self-esteem might feel when he looks at himself in the mirror.

Ms. Lim learned several things about Juan's thinking when she probed the comprehension section also. For most of the questions he answered incorrectly, there were one or two words that were pivotal for determining the correct answer, and these words were in the last part of the sentence or last sentence of the paragraph. For example, in one item, Juan chose a picture of twins dressed identically for the statement, "The girls looked exactly alike, but they wore different kinds of clothes." In another item, he chose a picture of two-holed, lined paper for the paragraph, "Inez bought a three-ring notebook and some paper for it. But the paper had only two holes. Which paper should she have bought?"

After probing the test, Ms. Lim realized that his score probably underestimated Juan's reading ability, particularly in the area of comprehension. She considered it likely that when given meaningful reading material that was longer than a few sentences, and when asked questions that relied less heavily on the surface structure of individual sentences, that Juan would demonstrate much better comprehension than the test results indicated. Ms. Lim put the test and her observation notes about the probing into Juan's portfolio.

Ms. Lim decided to teach a diagnostic reading lesson. She had already planned that fables and folktales would be the reading topic for the first month of school. For the first diagnostic reading lesson, she chose "The Elves and the Shoemaker" because with a 2.0 readability, she felt it would be relatively easy for Juan to read. She conducted a Directed Reading Thinking Activity and found that Juan read the story with good literal and inferential comprehension, and when he retold it, he included all the major story structure components.

For a second diagnostic reading lesson, she chose "The Cat and the Fiddler," which had a readability of 2.8. She conducted a Directed Reading Thinking Activity and found that Juan learned the sight vocabulary presented prior to reading fairly quickly, although he was initially unfamiliar with several of the words. She also noticed that he struggled with a few of the words and phrases in the story that she had not presented prior to the reading. She made note of the strategies that he used to figure out unknown words so that she could decide which strategies to teach in her reading strategy lessons. For example, she observed that Juan did not use context clues effectively. She also paid close attention to the answers Juan gave to the comprehension questions she asked. She found that even brief discussions helped him to more fully understand major concepts in the story.

Ms. Lim briefly recorded her observations regarding the diagnostic reading lessons and put this paper into Juan's portfolio, along with her conclusion that she would choose folktales and fables written at the late second- and early third-grade levels to use with Juan as instructional reading materials for the first month of school. She also chose several fables and folktales written at the fourth- and fifth-grade levels to read to Juan for daily read-aloud during the month. She decided to use a Directed Reading Thinking Activity for her method of instruction but also planned to shift to a more student-directed approach, such as reciprocal teaching, by the second half of the school year.

Ms. Lim gathered books containing fables and folktales to include in her small classroom library so that Juan and the other youngsters in her resource room could choose to read some additional stories independently. She put a sheet in each child's portfolio with "Reading Record" written at the top. She explained to the students that each time they completed reading a story or book, they should arrange to have a conference with her, and at that conference, the child could record the title, author, and date on the Reading Record. She told them that they could read books, stories, magazine articles, and newspaper articles on any topic of their choosing unless there were particular topics, books, or authors their parents did not want them to read.

Ms. Lim then developed a literacy development checklist for Juan. She decided to record her observations on the checklist once each month by writing the date in the appropriate column next to each characteristic.

Ms. Lim planned to teach reading five days each week for approximately thirty minutes of the one and one-half hour period Juan spends in the resource room. She also planned to include sustained silent reading for approximately fifteen minutes three days each week and read-aloud for fifteen minutes daily. For writing instruction, she decided to incorporate Writing Workshop for thirty minutes at least three days each week, dialogue journal writing for ten to fifteen minutes two days each week, and writing across the curriculum for thirty minutes two days each week. During the writing across the curriculum period, Ms. Lim planned to include writing projects from Juan's sixth grade teacher; if there were no current projects, she would use the time to teach summary writing during the first month of school.

Ms. Lim recognized that the writing Juan accomplished the first week or two of school might not be representative of his writing abilities. So, she decided to postpone evaluating his writing but planned to keep several early pieces to place in his portfolio. She felt that by the beginning of the second month of school, she could use the analytical writing scoring procedure on one or two pieces of his writing, share her observations with Juan, and include her evaluation in Juan's portfolio. In the meantime, she included her goals for Juan's writing development on the literacy development checklist, recognizing that these goals might need to be modified once she was able to gather more information about Juan's current writing abilities.

Ms. Lim decided to keep informal notes on Juan's progress and the progress of her other students in a notebook. She purchased a three-ring binder, put dividers in it, wrote each student's name on one of the dividers, and put notebook paper into each section. She planned to leave the notebook on her desk during the day so that she could jot down her observations easily. She also decided that once each week, she would regularly schedule time to write about any student on whom she had not entered notes in the past week.

Ms. Lim then discussed the portfolio with Juan. She explained that the responsibility for maintaining the portfolio was with both of them. She suggested to him that he could include work he completed in the resource room, at home, and in his classroom as long as he felt that the item he put into the portfolio showed how much he was learning.

Final Comments

This chapter began with a discussion of the purposes for literacy assessment. The general public, press, public policy makers, and school administrators are clearly more interested in norm- and criterion-referenced test results than any other type of assessment information whereas teachers, parents, and students are more interested in information gathered through informal approaches because it directly relates to the child's progress in meeting literacy goals. No single assessment can serve all of the purposes. MacGinitie (1993) offered the following caution about the uses of literacy assessment information.

> Reflecting on the limits of assessment, we discover that no matter how careful we are, we will be biased in many of our judgments; that we cannot hope to assess many things

that are important; that our assessment procedures, however realistic we try to make them, will have limited validity; and that we can never be sure what our assessments will mean to the students who are assessed. Since our assessments are fallible and limited, the decisions based on them should be tentative. There are not many decisions about students that need to be final. Nearly every decision should be reconsidered periodically. A program that seemed right at one time should eventually be reevaluated. A diagnosis that once seemed correct should be reexamined. Above all, a student who didn't make it on one try should have another. (p. 559)

Teachers of deaf children must strive to stay continuously aware of the progress their students are making. No one assessment procedure, technique, or test is sufficient; these only provide a snapshot of a few literacy abilities and skills. Assessment conducted at one point in time simply provides information about the child's current learning at that point in time. It tells the teacher, parent, and child very little about tomorrow, next week, next month, or next year. Assessment information gathered informally and formally, at regularly scheduled times and minute-by-minute during learning activities, form a corpus of information that the teacher can use to make choices about what and how to teach by building on the child's current strengths and providing a scaffold for new learning.

Suggested Readings

Cohen, L. G., & Spenciner, L. J. (1998). *Assessment of children and youth.* New York: Longman.

Gunning, T. G. (1998). *Assessing and correcting reading and writing difficulties.* Boston: Allyn and Bacon.

Lipson, M. Y., & Wixson, K. K. (1997). *Assessment and instruction of reading and writing disability: An interactive approach* (2nd ed.). New York: Longman.

Salvia, J., & Ysseldyke, J. E. (1998). *Assessment* (7th ed.). Boston: Houghton Mifflin.

Walker, B. J. (1996). *Diagnostic teaching of reading* (3rd ed.). Englewood Cliffs, NJ: Prentice Hall.

7 Language and Literacy Development through Parent–Child–Teacher Partnerships

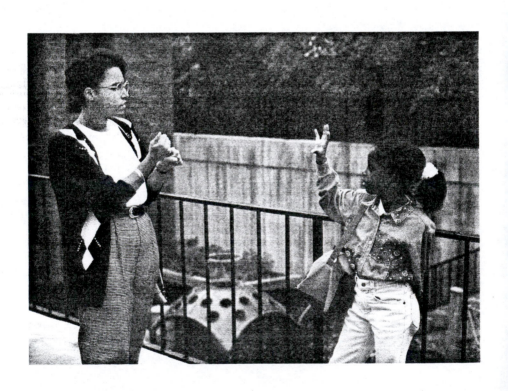

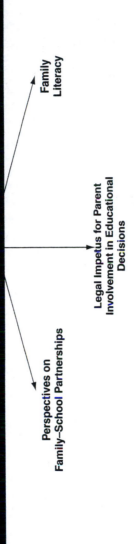

Language and Literacy Development through Parent–Child–Teacher Partnerships

Perspectives on
Family–School Partnerships

Legal Impetus for Parent
Involvement in Educational
Decisions

Family
Literacy

Throughout this book, I have discussed current theories and suggested practices regarding the language and literacy development in children who are deaf. The discussion has been directed to classroom teachers because this text is designed to be used by teachers of deaf students from preschool through high school. Yet, although the classroom is certainly an important place for language learning to happen, this final chapter will acknowledge the place and the individuals that are much more important to the child's language and literacy development than the classroom. I am, of course, referring to the home and to the child's parents.

I begin with a set of statements that reflect assumptions about the roles and responsibilities of teachers and parents in the language and literacy development of children who are deaf:

1. To develop language, children need to be immersed within an environment in which language is used consistently by individuals who are fluent users of the language. Whether children are learning English or ASL, it is the responsibility of teachers to help their students develop that language in face-to-face communication. Whether children are learning English or ASL, it is the responsibility of teachers to help their students develop their ability to read and write English.

2. Parents are the first and most salient models of language acquisition for their children. Their influence and importance to their children's language development should not be overlooked or diminished.

3. Regardless of which language system any particular educational program decides to use in the classroom, the program must include parents in all educational decisions about their children.

As Meadow-Orlans and Sass-Lehrer (1995) wrote:

> Professionals need to assess their views and practices in designing and implementing support to families. Family-centered professionals encourage active involvement of families in all aspects of a program, recognizing that families with different interests and resources will participate in different ways at different times. . . . Families whose children are deaf and hard of hearing face a complex educational system with multiple options and professional opinions. Navigating the educational maze demands skillful decision making and advocacy. These families need full knowledge about their options and how to procure appropriate services. Families with a sense of control are better equipped to seek information and services for themselves and their children. (pp. 328–329)

Families who are full partners will be much more likely to work collaboratively with teachers in supporting the child's language and literacy goals.

Perspectives on Family–School Partnerships

Partnerships do not always work smoothly. The mutual respect, good will, and shared interests that bring partners together are difficult to sustain when there is disagreement about goals, priorities, and specific actions. It is an understatement to say that parents and professionals do not necessarily work in harmony with one another. Trout and Foley (1989) captured a major source of the conflict in the following questions:

> Why, indeed, do families keep "distracting" us from our roles as language specialists or special educators with their endless questions, complaints, and stories about recently born healthy children of neighbors or siblings; with unsettling descriptions of marital strife; and with expressions of hopelessness or helplessness? Why are these parents unable to "accept" the illness or handicapping condition? Why do they claim to want help and then fail to "cooperate" with us, or even appear to sabotage our plans by failing to show up for appointments or to carry out homework assignments? And why must there be so much guilt (in spite of our protestations that there is nothing to feel guilty about), not to mention the rage, defensiveness, and sorrow? (p. 58)

I would like to add a set of questions that parents might ask:

> Why, indeed, do teachers keep "distracting" us from our roles as parents with their endless questions, complaints, and stories about the other children in class; with unsettling descriptions of school problems; and with expressions of frustration and disappointment? Why are these teachers unable to "accept" the school system's condition? Why do they overestimate or underestimate our children's abilities? Why do they claim to want to help and then fail to "cooperate" with us, or even appear to sabotage our plans by saying things at meetings that make no sense to the average person and sending homework that requires our undivided attention when we have a million things to do and no energy left by the end of the day? And why must there be so much blame, not to mention the anger, defensiveness, and sorrow?

For partnership to be more than a catchword, parents and professionals must be able to find a common set of principles guiding their interactions. The following principles represent a point for beginning a partnership and avoiding the kind of blaming that all too often has characterized the relationship between home and school.

1. **The child is part of a family system.** When we intervene with the child, we impact on every other member of the child's family. In family systems theory, the family is viewed as a whole, and each member understood by looking at the interactions and relationships among all the family members (Bailey & Simeonsson, 1988; Dunst, Trivette, & Deal, 1988; Turnbull, Summers, & Brotherson, 1983).

Viewing the child as an interdependent member of a family system is important for two reasons. First, it helps us realize that anything we do educationally for the child will influence the interactions and relationships between the child and his or her family members and among the mother, father, siblings, as well as perhaps the grandparents and others in the extended family.

Second, viewing the child within the family context forces us to recognize and be sensitive to the many demands on families. It has been observed that when the family unit is supported, each member is strengthened. When the family unit is ignored, the result is often a weakening of every member and a lack of cooperation with the educational system that is purporting to help the child (Winton, 1986).

As we seek to understand each child's unique family structure, it is crucial to remember that traditional definitions of family structures and notions regarding the roles of family members no longer apply as families have changed in response to social, political, and economic pressures. Teachers must recognize that they will work with children from families with one parent, foster families, families with two adults of the same gender, homeless families, families that migrate frequently for work, blended families, extended families, families with multiple ethnicities, and families with two biological parents. Teachers need to demonstrate awareness and sensitivity to the values, attitudes, beliefs, and customs of each child's family.

2. Parents need to be encouraged to develop the skills and knowledge that will enable them to become competent and capable. The traditional relationship between parents of deaf children and professionals has been paternalistic. Professionals have taken responsibility for the educational needs of the child, and often social and emotional needs as well, without expecting much more than cooperation from the parents. This principle suggests that the child benefits when parents are confident of their knowledge and skills and respected for their contributions to educational decision making.

The implication is that educators need to help parents to identify and build on their strengths and capabilities. It also means that educators need to spend less time helping parents to identify and correct family weaknesses and deficiencies.

3. Families experience a life cycle in much the same way that individuals do, and the changes inherent in major family events need to be understood by individuals working with any family member. The shifts experienced by families during transition times disrupt the interactions and relationships among family members. When individuals pass from one stage to another, they experience anxiety and stress. When families pass from one stage to another, the whole family experiences anxiety and stress (Winton, 1986).

Complicating this picture is that while the family undergoes passages through developmental phases, family members undergo their own individual life passages. Furthermore, mothers and fathers undergo change as they develop their parental abilities.

4. Educational decisions should be made collaboratively between parents and professionals. There is a great difference between soliciting parent input for the purposes of making educational decisions and jointly making educational decisions. Collaboration is crucial to any partnership. It recognizes that both partners have essential insights to contribute. When decisions are made collaboratively, both partners are vested in the implementation and results.

Ultimately, there are two arguments in favor of family–school partnerships. One is that it is the rightful role of parents to decide what is best for their child. The second is that decisions made as a result of an equal sharing of ideas will be fully supported by the parents and therefore are more likely to result in positive outcomes for the child.

Legal Impetus for Parent Involvement in Educational Decisions

The legal impetus for parent involvement in educational decisions was a result of parent activism. The beginning of this impetus can be found in the civil rights movement of the 1950s and 60s. As Heward (2000) noted, the 1954 *Brown v. Board of Education of Topeka* decision in which the U.S. Supreme Court established the right of all children to equal opportunity to an education "began a period of intense concern and questioning among parents of children with disabilities, who asked why the same principles of equal access to education did not apply to their children" (p. 15).

Parents initiated a number of court cases, which resulted in decisions and publicity that directly led to legislation aimed at guaranteeing the rights of exceptional children. Public Law 94-142, the Education for All Handicapped Children Act, passed by the U.S. Congress in 1975, not only mandated a free, appropriate public education for all children with disabilities between the ages of three and twenty-one regardless of the type or degree of severity of their disability, but it also protected the rights of parents. One of the provisions of this law was a mandatory inclusion of parents in educational decisions regarding evaluation, placement, and delivery of instruction.

Since 1975, Congress has amended this federal special education law several times. The most recent was the reauthorization of the Individuals with Disabilities Education Act (IDEA) in 1997. In reauthorizing the act, Congress found, in part, that parents were not participating as real partners with educators in making decisions about the education of their children and that strengthening their roles and opportunities would improve educational programs.

Family Literacy

Family literacy is an approach to developing partnerships between families and schools for the purpose of improving the literacy of children through their families. In 1988, the Barbara Bush Foundation for Family Literacy was organized to promote family literacy initiatives. In 1995, Barbara Bush wrote:

> Common sense tells us and the experts agree: the home is the child's first school and the parent (or adult who fills the role of primary caregiver) is the child's first and most important teacher. This is one of the main reasons that improving the literacy skills of adults is so critical to our future. Children who are read to and who grow up in print-rich environments learn to read more easily than those who do not. This link between the literacy level and practices of the parent and a child's success in school seems clear; however, we all know the success stories of children whose parents lack formal literacy skills. Often literacy is valued in those homes, and the parent finds ways to support the child's educational development. Where literacy is valued, it is nurtured. That's why an important

part of our mission at the Foundation is to help make literacy a value in every home. (Morrow, 1995, p. x)

Family literacy initiatives have tended to focus on three areas. One area has involved examining the uses of literacy within families. In one study, researchers observed the literacy experiences of children from low-socioeconomic status urban communities and found that the families engaged in a number of print-embedded family activities involving daily living routines, entertainment, school-related activities, interpersonal communication, literacy for the sake of teaching or learning literacy, storybook reading, religion, participation in information networks, and work (Purcell-Gates, L'Allier, & Smith, 1995). Studies such as this suggest that teachers should find out how the families of their students use literacy in their homes so that these home literacies can be used as a foundation for classroom literacy.

A second area of family literacy has involved intergenerational literacy programs that are designed to help family members improve their own literacy skills and to teach parents how to help their children develop literacy. Teachers are urged to learn about adult literacy and adult basic education programs that are available in their communities so that they can refer parents to these resources. Intergenerational literacy programs also involve having teachers set up parent volunteer opportunities in the classroom and working with parents in identifying topics for evening workshops, lectures, demonstrations, or support group meetings.

Home-school programs comprise the third area of family literacy initiatives. In these programs, parents learn about school literacy activities, and teachers learn about home literacy activities. Examples include parent read-aloud or storytelling at school, dialogue journal writing between parents and teachers, setting up a classroom lending library for parents, and establishing a school resource center in which information and items are donated by the school, teachers, and parents.

Final Comments

Years ago, I was a teacher at a school for the deaf in the northeast region of the United States. One of my students was a twelve-year-old boy who exhibited what I thought were emotional problems that were interfering with his ability to benefit from instruction in my language class. I talked to my supervisor about him, and after observing him in my class and talking with the other teachers in our department, she brought her concerns about this boy to the school psychologist. After observing him in several of his classes, the school psychologist concluded that this boy would benefit from professional counseling. She arranged for a conference with his parents, and the suggestion for professional counseling was presented and discussed. Nothing happened. Several months later, this boy's father came to school for an evening open house. I chatted with him for quite a while, and during our conversation, I broached the topic of counseling for his son. To my surprise, the father was quite receptive, and I went home feeling pleased with myself. The boy did not come back to our school.

After several days, my supervisor received a request that his school records be forwarded to a school in a different part of the city.

For a long time afterwards, I believed that the boy's parents, and particularly his mother, were in denial about their son's problems. It took me many years to realize the extent of my own denial. I had been unable to recognize that my student was their son; that while I knew things about him they did not know, they knew many things about him that I did not know. They knew about their family, and I knew only about their son.

Actually, I did not learn this lesson until I was a parent myself, and I became the recipient of unsolicited advice from my children's teachers. Then, I learned that parent-child-teacher partnerships can work only when we express sensitivity and respect toward one another.

I want to stress that I have only touched on some of the important issues involved in family-school partnerships. These and other issues are dealt with extensively in other sources, and it is my hope that the reader will use some of these sources for developing skills in working with families.

It is important to emphasize that teachers of children who are deaf need to be knowledgeable about many areas. This text has focused on language and literacy development specifically. The information in this text should help enable teachers to create classroom environments that foster the development of face-to-face language, reading, and writing in children who are deaf.

Suggested Readings

Marschark, M. (1997). *Raising and educating a deaf child.* New York: Oxford University Press.

Moles, O. C. (1996). *Reaching all families: Creating family-friendly schools.* Washington, DC: U.S. Department of Education *www.ed.gov/pubs/ReachFam/*

Morrow, L. M. (Ed.). (1995). *Family literacy: Connections in schools and communities.* Newark, DE: International Reading Association.

APPENDIX

Standardized and Criterion-Referenced Tests

Norm- and criterion-referenced tests can serve as one part of a language and literacy assessment program. While naturalistic assessment strategies such as language sampling and diagnostic reading lessons can provide teachers with a wealth of information for making educational decisions, standardized tests can also provide valuable supplementary information. Much has been written regarding the limitations of standardized tests and the misuse of standardized test scores. Some educators even advocate the elimination of standardized testing. This stance ignores two realities. First, standardized tests can be used in ways that are productive to educational decision making. Second, standardized tests will not disappear in the near future. I agree with Pikulski's (1990) point that "it seems imperative as responsible professionals we reduce the amount of time that we spend railing against standardized tests in an unproductive way and that we concentrate our efforts on three things: curtailing specific misuses and misinterpretations of standardized tests, improving existing tests, and proposing alternative assessment procedures that place standardized test scores in a broader context or begin to substitute for them" (p. 686).

Listed in this appendix are the basic characteristics of a selected group of published tests in the areas of language, literacy, and academic achievement. All of these tests meet three criteria: (a) they were published for the first time or substantially revised within the last fifteen years, (b) they received relatively positive reviews in the literature, and (c) they are reportedly used with regularity by teachers throughout the United States. This list of tests is not exhaustive nor does it provide enough information for teachers to decide specifically which tests are appropriate for their students who are deaf. These descriptions are intended to narrow the choices from among the hundreds of standardized and criterion-referenced tests on the market today.

Language Screening

Test of Early Language Development (2nd Ed.)

Authors: Wayne P. Hresko, D. Kim Reid, and Donald D. Hammill
Copyright Date: 1991
Publisher: Pro-Ed (8700 Shoal Creek Blvd., Austin, TX 78757 / www.proedinc.com)

Age Range: 2–0 to 7–11 years
Administration Time: approximately 20 minutes
Purpose: To measure the early development of expressive and receptive oral language, syntax, and semantics
Description: The test consists of 38 items designed to measure form, content, and interpretation of meaning. Form includes syntax, semantics, and morphology. Content includes word and concept knowledge.

The normative sample is reported as 1,329 youngsters representative, where possible, of the U.S. population on a number of variables. No norms for deaf students are provided. Reliability is reported as excellent, and validity as adequate.

Vocabulary

Carolina Picture Vocabulary Test

Authors: Thomas L. Layton and David W. Holmes
Copyright Date: 1985
Publisher: Butte Publications (P. O. Box 1328, Hillsboro, OR 97123)
Age Range: 2.5 to 16 years
Administration Time: 10–30 minutes
Purpose: To assess the receptive sign vocabulary of deaf and hearing impaired children
Description: The test consists of 130 plates, each of which contains four line drawings. The child's task is to identify the correct picture from the examiner's sign.

The normative sample is reported as 767 hearing impaired youngsters from a nationwide population of children using manual communication as their primary means of communicating. Reliability is reported as adequate, and evidence for validity is provided. The examiner needs to be familiar with the sign system used by the child to use the appropriate signs (e.g., an ASL sign may be quite different from a SEE sign for the same word). When signs are iconic, vocabulary knowledge may not be assessed accurately.

Peabody Picture Vocabulary Test—3

Authors: Lloyd M. Dunn, Leota M. Dunn, Gary J. Robertson, and Jay L. Eisenberg
Copyright Date: 1997
Publisher: American Guidance Service (4201 Woodland Road, Circle Pines, MN 55014-1796 / www.agsnet.com)
Age Range: 2.5 to 90+ years
Administration Time: 10–20 minutes approximately

Purpose: To assess the youngster's receptive vocabulary in face-to-face communication. It is intended to provide a quick estimate of verbal ability and scholastic aptitude.

Description: The test consists of a list of vocabulary words and a series of plates with four pictures per plate. The examiner reads each word aloud, and the child points to the most appropriate picture.

The normative sample is reported as 4,200 youngsters between 2 ½ and 24 years of age from 268 states in 4 regions who were representative of the U.S. population on a number of variables. Norms for students who are deaf are provided. Reliability and validity are reported as adequate.

The Word Test—Elementary (Revised) and the Word Test—Adolescent

Authors: Rosemary Huisingh, Mark Barrett, Linda Zachman, Carolyn Blagden, and Jane Orman

Copyright Date: 1990

Publisher: LinguiSystems, Inc. (3100 4th Ave., East Moline, IL 61244-9700 / www.linguisystems.com)

Age Range: 7 to 11 years for the elementary level and 12 to 17 years for the adolescent level

Administration Time: approximately 30 minutes

Purpose: To assess student knowledge about the critical features of words and about the relationships between words for the elementary level. To assess semantic and vocabulary tasks reflective of school assignments as well as language usage in everyday life for the adolescent level.

Description: The elementary level tests six essential vocabulary and semantic areas: associations, multiple definitions, semantic absurdities, antonyms, definitions, and synonyms. The adolescent level includes four tasks: brand names (explaining why a semantically descriptive name of a product or company is appropriate), synonyms, signs of the times (telling what a sign or message means and why it is important), and definitions.

The normative sample is reported as more than 2,000 youngsters for the elementary level, and more than 1,500 youngsters for the adolescent level gathered nationwide. No norms for deaf students are provided. Reliability is reported as adequate, and evidence for validity is provided for both levels.

Syntax and Semantics

Clinical Evaluation of Language Fundamentals—3

Authors: Eleanor Semel, Elisabeth Wiig, and Wayne Secord

Copyright Date: 1995

Publisher: The Psychological Corp. (555 Academic Ct., San Antonio, TX 78293 / www.psychorp.com)
Age Range: 6–21 years
Administration Time: 30–45 minutes
Purpose: To assess the language processing and production of children
Description: The diagnostic battery includes subtests designed to measure the child's morphology, syntax, semantics, and memory.

The normative sample is reported as 2,450 youngsters. No norms for students who are deaf are provided. Reliability is reported as adequate, and evidence for validity is provided.

Test of Language Development—3, Primary and Test of Language Development—3, Intermediate

Authors: Phyllis L. Newcomer and Donald D. Hammill
Copyright Date: 1996
Publisher: Pro-Ed (8700 Shoal Creek Blvd., Austin, TX 78757 / www.proedinc.com)
Age Range: 4–0 to 8–11 for the primary level and 8–0 to 12–11 for the intermediate level
Administration Time: 30–60 minutes
Purpose: To identify specific receptive and expressive language skills of primary age and intermediate level youngsters
Description: Subtests for the primary level are picture vocabulary, oral vocabulary, grammatic understanding, grammatic completion, sentence imitation, word articulation, and word discrimination. Subtests for the intermediate level are sentence combining, vocabulary, word ordering, generals, grammatic comprehension, and malapropisms.

The normative sample for the primary level is reported as more than 1,000 youngsters and for the intermediate level as more than 700 youngsters who were representative of the U.S. population on a number of variables. No norms for students who are deaf are provided. Reliability is reported as adequate, and evidence for validity is reported.

Test of Adolescent Language—3

Authors: Donald D. Hammill, Virginia L. Brown, Stephen C. Larsen, and J. Lee Wiederholt
Copyright Date: 1994
Publisher: Pro-Ed (8700 Shoal Creek Blvd., Austin, TX 78757 / www.proedinc.com)
Age Range: 12 to 25 years
Administration Time: 60–180 minutes

Purpose: To assess the spoken and written vocabulary and grammar of adolescents and identify students for language intervention

Description: The test includes eight subtests: listening/vocabulary, listening/grammar, speaking/vocabulary, writing/vocabulary, speaking/grammar, reading/vocabulary, reading/grammar, and writing/grammar.

The normative sample is reported as 3,050 adolescents who were representative of the U.S. population on a number of variables. No norms for deaf students are provided. Reliability is reported as adequate, and evidence for validity is provided though criterion validity is suspect.

Reading

Gates-MacGinitie Reading Tests (3rd Ed.)

Authors: Walter H. MacGinitie and Ruth K. MacGinitie
Copyright Date: 1989
Publisher: The Riverside Publishing Co. (425 Spring Lake Dr., Itasca, IL 60143-2079 / www.riverpub.com)
Age Range: emergent literacy to grade 12
Administration Time: approximately 55 minutes for all levels except the prereading and readiness levels
Purpose: To measure reading readiness skills and language concepts, beginning reading skills at grade 1, and vocabulary and comprehension at grades 1.5 to 12
Description: The prereading test assesses language skills, letter knowledge, and auditory discrimination of letter sounds. The grade 1 test assesses phonic skills and use of context clues. The grade 1.5 through 12 tests assess vocabulary and comprehension.

The normative sample is reported as 77,413 youngsters who were representative of the U.S. population on a number of variables. No norms for deaf students are provided. Reliability is reported as adequate, and limited evidence for validity is provided.

Gray Oral Reading Test—3

Authors: J. Lee Wiederholt and Brian R. Bryant
Copyright Date: 1992
Publisher: Pro-Ed (8700 Shoal Creek Blvd., Austin, TX 78757 / www.proedinc.com)
Age Range: 7–0 to 18–11 years
Administration Time: 15–30 minutes
Purpose: To assess reading skill development through oral reading

Description: Each form of the test contains 13 progressively more difficult oral reading passages. Oral miscues are noted by the examiner. The youngster is also asked a set of 5 comprehension questions after reading each paragraph.

The normative sample is reported as 1,485 youngsters from 18 states who were representative of the U.S. population on a number of variables. No norms for students who are deaf are provided. Reliability is reported as adequate, and evidence for satisfactory validity is provided.

Metropolitan Achievement Tests—7

Authors: Roger C. Farr, George A. Prescott, Irving H. Balow, and Thomas P. Hogan
Copyright Date: 1992
Publisher: The Psychological Corp. (555 Academic Ct., San Antonio, TX 78293 / www.psychcorp.com)
Age Range: grades K–5 to 9–9
Administration Time: 1½–2½ hours
Purpose: To assess the child's reading strengths and weaknesses
Description: The test includes subtests in word recognition, reading vocabulary, reading comprehension, and prereading.

For the MAT-7, the normative sample is reported as 100,000 youngsters who were representative of the U.S. population on a number of variables. No norms are provided for deaf students. Reliability is reported as adequate, and limited evidence for validity is provided.

Woodcock Diagnostic Reading Battery

Author: Richard W. Woodcock
Copyright Date: 1997
Publisher: The Riverside Publishing Co. (425 Spring Lake Dr., Itasca, IL 60143-2079 / www.riverpub.com)
Age Range: 4 to 90+ years
Administration Time: 50–60 minutes
Purpose: To measure readiness skills, word recognition skills, and reading comprehension skills
Description: The test consists of 10 subtests: letter–word identification, passage comprehension, word attack, reading vocabulary, incomplete words, sound blending, oral vocabulary, listening comprehension, memory for sentences, and visual matching.

The normative sample is reported as over 6,000 youngsters from 100 different communities who were representative of the U.S. population on a number of variables. No norms are provided for students who are deaf. Reliability is reported as good, and evidence for good validity is provided.

Informal Reading Inventories

Analytical Reading Inventory (5th Ed.)

Authors: Mary Lynn Woods and Alden J. Moe
Copyright Date: 1995
Publisher: Merrill/PrenticeHall (Upper Saddle River, NJ 07458 / www.prenhall.com)
Age Range: primer to grade 9 reading level
Administration Time: approximately 30 minutes
Purpose: To identify the youngster's independent, instructional, frustration, and capacity (listening level) reading levels and to assess strengths and weaknesses in word recognition and comprehension
Description: The test contains three narrative and two expository forms for each grade level that are equivalent in terms of content, format, and readability. Each form consists of graded word lists and graded passages.

The test is not normed. No reliability or validity data are provided.

Standardized Reading Inventory

Author: Phyllis L. Newcomer
Copyright Date: 1986
Publisher: Pro-Ed (8700 Shoal Creek Blvd., Austin, TX 78757 / www.proedinc.com)
Age Range: grades 1 to 8 reading level
Administration Time: 15–60 minutes
Purpose: To assess word recognition and comprehension, diagnose reading strengths and weaknesses, and determine the youngster's independent, instructional, and frustration reading levels
Description: The test consists of a set of graded word lists and graded passages for each of two forms.

The test is not normed. It is a criterion-referenced test that the author argues is standardized because the content was selected and checked empirically, administration procedures are defined, scoring is objective and consistent, and guidelines are provided for interpreting results. Reliability is reported as adequate; however, it is based on a limited sample of students. Limited evidence for validity is provided.

Writing

Test of Written Language—3

Author: Donald D. Hammill and Stephen C. Larsen
Copyright Date: 1996

Publisher: Pro-Ed (8700 Shoal Creek Blvd., Austin, TX 78757 / www.proedinc.com)
Age Range: 7.0 to 17–11
Administration Time: approximately 1½ hours
Purpose: To assess competency in written language
Description: The test includes five subtests in vocabulary, spelling, style, logical sentences, and sentence combining.

The normative sample is reported as 2,217 youngsters who were representative of the U.S. population on a number of variables, though the sample is distributed somewhat unevenly across age groups. No norms are provided for students who are deaf. Reliability is reported as good, and very limited evidence for validity is provided.

Academic Achievement

California Achievement Tests

Author: California Test Bureau
Copyright Date: 1993
Publisher: CTB/McGraw-Hill (Del Monte Research Park, Monterey, CA 93940)
Age Range: kindergarten to grade 12
Administration Time: From 1 hour-27 minutes for kindergarten to 5 hours-16 minutes at highest levels
Purpose: To assess skill development in content areas
Description: The test is a battery of seven tests: reading, spelling, language, mathematics, study skills, science, and social studies. The reading test includes subtests in visual recognition, sound recognition, word analysis, vocabulary, and comprehension. The language test includes subtests in language mechanics and language expression.

The normative sample is reported as 300,000 youngsters in 1984 and 230,000 in 1985 who were representative of the U.S. population on a number of variables. No norms are provided for students who are deaf. Very limited evidence is provided for reliability and validity.

Iowa Tests of Basic Skills

Authors: H. D. Hoover, A. N. Hieronymus, D. A. Frisbie, and S. B. Dunbar
Copyright Date: 1990
Publisher: The Riverside Publishing Co. (425 Spring Lake Dr., Itasca, IL 60143-2079 / www.riverpub.com)
Age Range: kindergarten to grade 9
Administration Time: 3–6 hours

Purpose: To assess general functioning and growth in the skills essential to academic success

Description: The test includes subtests in listening, writing, word analysis, vocabulary, reading comprehension, language skills (spelling, capitalization, punctuation), reference materials, mathematics skills (math concepts, math problem solving, math computation), science, social studies, maps, and diagrams.

The normative sample is reported as several hundred thousand youngsters who were representative of the U.S. population on a number of variables. No norms are provided for students who are deaf. Reliability is reported as adequate, and evidence for validity is provided.

Stanford Achievement Test (9th Ed.)

Authors: Harcourt Brace Educational Measurement
Copyright Date: 1997
Publisher: The Psychological Corp. (555 Academic Court, San Antonio, TX 78293 / www.psychcorp.com)
Age Range: grades 1 through 9
Administration Time: 4½–6½ hours
Purpose: To assess skill development in major content areas
Description: The test is divided by grade levels and includes 5 to 11 subtests at each level. Subtests include sounds and letters, word study skills, word reading, sentence reading, reading comprehension, reading vocabulary, listening to words and stories, listening comprehension, spelling, language, mathematics, study skills, science, social studies, and environment.

The normative sample is reported as more than 250,000 youngsters who were representative of the U.S. population on a number of variables. Norms are provided for deaf students enrolled in special education programs throughout the United States. Reliability is reported as adequate, and evidence for validity is provided.

Woodcock-Johnson Psychoeducational Battery (Revised)

Authors: Richard W. Woodcock and Associates
Copyright Date: 1991
Publisher: The Riverside Publishing Co. (425 Spring Lake Dr., Itasca, IL 60143-2079 / www.riverpub.com)
Age Range: 2 to 90 years
Administration Time: 2 hours +
Purpose: To assess cognitive ability, scholastic aptitude, academic achievement, and interests
Description: The test consists of two parts. Part One, the Tests of Cognitive Ability, includes 21 subtests measuring 7 cognitive factors: long-term re-

trieval, short-term memory, visual processing, comprehension-knowledge, processing speed, auditory processing, and fluid reasoning. Part Two, the Tests of Achievement, includes 18 subtests in 5 achievement clusters: reading, mathematics, written language, knowledge, and early development/skills.

The normative sample is reported as 6,359 individuals. No norms are provided for students who are deaf. Reliability is reported as adequate, and evidence for validity is provided.

REFERENCES

Abraham, S., & Stoker, R. (1988). Language assessment of hearing-impaired children and youth: Patterns of test use. *Language, Speech, and Hearing Services in Schools, 19,* 160–174.

Acredolo, L., & Goodwyn, S. (1988). Symbolic gesturing in normal infants. *Child Development, 59,* 450–466.

Adams, M. J. (1990). *Beginning to read: Thinking and learning about print.* Cambridge, MA: MIT.

Aguirre, A. (1982). *In search of a paradigm for bilingual education.* Los Angeles: Evaluation, Dissemination, and Assessment Center, California State University, Los Angeles.

Ainsworth, D. (1987). What century is this anyway? A critical look at technology in education and training. *Educational Technology, 27*(9), 26–28.

Akamatsu, C. T. (1988). Summarizing stories: The role of instruction in text structure in learning to write. *American Annals of the Deaf, 133,* 294–302.

Alessi, S., & Trollop, S. (1991). *Computer-based instruction: Methods and development.* Englewood Cliffs, NJ: Prentice Hall.

Almasi, J. F. (1995). The nature of fourth graders' sociocognitive conflicts in peer-led and teacher-led discussions of literature. *Reading Research Quarterly, 30,* 314–351.

Altwerger, B., Diehl-Faxon, J., & Dockstader-Anderson, K. (1985). Read-aloud events as meaning construction. *Language Arts, 62,* 476–484.

Alvarez, M. C. (1983). Using a thematic pre-organizer and guided instruction as aids to concept learning. *Reading Horizons, 24,* 51–58.

Alvermann, D. E., & Boothby, P. R. (1986). Children's transfer of graphic organizer instruction. *Reading Psychology, 7,* 87–100.

Alvermann, D. E., & Swafford, J. (1989). Do content area strategies have a research base? *Journal of Reading, 32,* 388–394.

Anders, P. L., & Bos, C. S. (1986). Semantic feature analysis: An interactive strategy for vocabulary development and text comprehension. *Journal of Reading, 29,* 610–616.

Anderson, R. C., Spiro, R. J., & Anderson, M. C. (1978). Schemata as scaffolding for the representation of information in connected discourse. *American Educational Research Journal, 15,* 433–440.

Andrews, J. F. (1988). Deaf children's acquisition of prereading skills using the reciprocal teaching procedure. *Exceptional Children, 54,* 349–355.

Andrews, J. F., Ferguson, C., Roberts, S., & Hodges, P. (1997). What's up, Billy Jo? Deaf children and bilingual-bicultural instruction in east-central Texas. *American Annals of the Deaf, 142,* 16–25.

Andrews, J. F., & Mason, J. M. (1986). How do deaf children learn about prereading? *American Annals of the Deaf, 131,* 210–217.

Andrews, J. F., Winograd, P., & DeVille, G. (1994). Deaf children reading fables: Using ASL summaries to improve reading comprehension. *American Annals of the Deaf, 139,* 378–386.

Andrews, J. F., Winograd, P., & DeVille, G. (1996). Using sign language summaries during prereading lessons. *Teaching Exceptional Children, 28,* 30–34.

Ankney, P., & McClurg, P. (1981). Testing Manzo's guided reading procedure. *The Reading Teacher, 34,* 681–685.

Applebee, A. N. (1978). *The child's concept of story: Ages two to seventeen.* Chicago: University of Chicago.

Applebee, A. N. (1980). Children's narratives: New directions. *The Reading Teacher, 34,* 137–142.

Armbruster, B. B., Anderson, T. H., & Meyer, J. L. (1991). Improving content-area reading using instructional graphics. *Reading Research Quarterly, 26,* 393–416.

Armbruster, B. B., Anderson, T. H., & Ostertag, J. (1987). Does text structure/summarization instruction facilitate learning from expository text? *Reading Research Quarterly, 22,* 331–346.

Armstrong, D. P., Patberg, J. P., & Dewitz, P. (1988). Reading guides: Helping students understand. *Journal of Reading, 31,* 154–156.

Atwell, N. (1998). *In the middle: New understandings about writing, reading, and learning* (2nd ed.). Portsmouth, NH: Heinemann.

Au, K. H., & Scheu, J. A. (1989). Guiding students to interpret a novel. *The Reading Teacher, 43,* 104–110.

Au, K. H., Scheu, J. A., Kawakami, A. J., & Herman, P. A. (1990). Assessment and accountability in a whole literacy curriculum. *The Reading Teacher, 43,* 574–578.

Ausubel, D. P. (1960). The use of advance organizers in the learning and retention of meaningful material. *Journal of Educational Psychology, 51,* 267–272.

Babbs, P. J., & Moe, A. J. (1983). Metacognition: A key for independent learning from text. *The Reading Teacher, 36,* 422–426.

Bailey, D. B., & Simeonsson, R. J. (1988). *Family assessment in early intervention.* New York: Merrill/Macmillan.

Baker, C. (1996). *Foundations of bilingual education and bilingualism.* Clevedon, England: Multilingual Matters.

Baker, K. A., & deKanter, A. A. (1983). Federal policy and the effectiveness of bilingual education. In K. A. Baker & A. A. deKanter (Eds.), *Bilingual education* (pp. 33–86). Lexington, MA: Lexington Books.

Baker-Shenk, C., & Cokely, D. (1994). *American Sign Language.* Washington, DC: Gallaudet University.

Barnes, B. L. (1997). But teacher you went right on: A perspective on Reading Recovery. *The Reading Teacher, 50,* 284–292.

Barrett, T. C. (1976). Taxonomy of reading comprehension. In R. Smith & T. C. Barrett (Eds.), *Teaching reading in the middle grades* (pp. 51–58). Reading, MA: Addison-Wesley.

Barron, R. F. (1969). The use of vocabulary as an advance organizer. In H. L. Herber & P. L. Sanders (Eds.), *Research in reading in the content areas: First year report* (pp. 29–39). Syracuse, NY: Syracuse University, Reading and Language Arts Center.

Bates, E., Bretherton, I., Snyder, L., Shore, C., & Volterra, V. (1980). Vocal and gestural symbols at 13 months. *Merrill-Palmer Quarterly, 26,* 407–423.

Bates, E., Thal, D., Whitesell, K., Fenson, L., & Oakes, L. (1989). Integrating language and gesture in infancy. *Developmental Psychology, 25,* 1004–1019.

Baumann, J. F. (1988). Direct instruction reconsidered. *Journal of Reading, 31,* 716–718.

Bean, T. W., & Ericson, B. O. (1989). Test previews and three level study guides for content area critical reading. *Journal of Reading, 32,* 337–341.

Bear, D. R., & Templeton, S. (1998). Explorations in developmental spelling: Foundations for learning and teaching phonics, spelling, and vocabulary. *The Reading Teacher, 52,* 222–242.

Bebko, J. M. (1998). Learning, language, memory, and reading: The role of language automization and its impact on complex cognitive activities. *Journal of Deaf Studies and Deaf Education, 3,* 4–14.

Beck, I. L. (1989). Improving practice through understanding reading. In L. B. Resnick & L. E. Klopfer (Eds.), *Toward the thinking curriculum: Current cognitive research* (pp. 40–58). Alexandria, VA: Association for Supervision and Curriculum Development.

Beed, P. L., Hawkins, E. M., & Roller, C. M. (1991). Moving learners toward independence: The power of scaffolded instruction. *The Reading Teacher, 44,* 648–655.

Beers, T. (1987). Schema-theoretic models of reading: Humanizing the machine. *Reading Research Quarterly, 22,* 369–377.

Bensinger, J., Santomen, L., & Volpe, M. (1987). From fear to fluency: The writing process. In D. S. Copeland & D. C. Fletcher (Eds.), *Proceedings of the 1987 National Conference on Innovative Writing Programs and Research for Deaf and Hearing Impaired Students, Removing the writing barrier: A dream?* (pp. 18–29). New York: Lehman College, The City University of New York.

Berger, L. R. (1996). Reader response journals: You make the meaning . . . and how. *Journal of Adolescent and Adult Literacy, 39,* 380–385.

Bergman, J. L. (1992). SAIL—A way to success and independence for low-achieving readers. *The Reading Teacher, 45,* 598–602.

Berk, L. E., & Garvin, R. A. (1984). Development of private speech among low-income Appalachian children. *Developmental Psychology, 20,* 271–286.

Betts, E. A. (1946). *Foundations of reading instruction.* New York: American Book.

Bidwell, S. M. (1990). Using drama to increase motivation, comprehension, and fluency. *Journal of Reading, 34,* 38–41.

Billingsley, B. S., & Wildman, T. M. (1988). The effects of prereading activities on the comprehension monitoring of learning disabled adolescents. *Learning Disabilities Research, 4,* 36–44.

Birnbaum, J. C. (1982). The reading and composing behaviors of selected fourth- and seventh-grade students. *Research in the Teaching of English, 16,* 241–260.

Blachowicz, C. L. Z. (1984). Reading and remembering: A constructivist perspective on reading comprehension and its disorders. *Visible Language, 18,* 391–403.

Blachowicz, C., & Fisher, P. (1996). *Teaching vocabulary in all classrooms.* Englewood Cliffs, NJ: Merrill/Prentice Hall.

Blanchard, J. S. (1985). What to tell students about underlining . . . and why. *Journal of Reading, 29,* 199–203.

Blanchard, J. S., & Rottenberg, C. J. (1990). Hypertext and hypermedia: Discovering and creating meaningful learning environments. *The Reading Teacher, 43,* 656–661.

Bloom, B. (1986). Automaticity. *Educational Leadership, 43*(5), 70–77.

Bloom, B. S., Engelhart, M. D., Furst, E. J., Hill, W. H., & Krathwohl, D. R. (1956). *Taxonomy of educational objectives. The classification of educational goals. Handbook I: Cognitive domain.* New York: David McKay.

Bloom, K., Russell, A., & Wassenberg, K. (1987). Turn taking affects the quality of infant vocalizations. *Journal of Child Language, 14,* 211–227.

Bloom, L., & Lahey, M. (1978). *Language development and language disorders.* New York: Wiley.

Bock, J. K., & Brewer, W. F. (1985). Discourse structure and mental models. In T. H. Carr (Ed.), *The development of reading skills* (pp. 55–75). San Francisco: Jossey-Bass.

Bode, B. A. (1989). Dialogue journal writing. *The Reading Teacher, 42,* 568–571.

Bohannon, J. N., & Stanowicz, L. (1988). The issue of negative evidence: Adult responses to children's language errors. *Developmental Psychology, 24,* 684–689.

Bonvillian, J. D., & Siedlecki, T. (1996). Young children's acquisition of the location aspect of American Sign Language signs: Parental report findings. *Journal of Communication Disorders, 29,* 13–35.

Bouffler, C. (1984). Predictability: A redefinition of readability. *Australian Journal of Reading, 7,* 125–134.

Braselton, S., & Decker, B. C. (1994). Using graphic organizers to improve the reading of mathematics. *The Reading Teacher, 48,* 276–281.

Brennan, A. D., Bridge, C. A., & Winograd, P. N. (1986). The effects of structural variation on children's recall of basal reader stories. *Reading Research Quarterly, 21,* 91–103.

Bretherton, I., Bates, E., McNew, S., Shore, C., Williamson, C., & Beeghly-Smith, M. (1981). Comprehension and production of symbols in infancy: An experimental study. *Developmental Psychology, 17,* 728–736.

Brinton, B., & Fujiki, M. (1984). Development of topic manipulation skills in discourse. *Journal of Speech and Hearing Research, 27,* 350–358.

Britton, J., Burgess, T., Martin, N., McLeod, A., & Rosen, H. (1975). *The development of writing abilities (11–18).* London: Macmillan Education.

Bromley, K. D. (1985). Precis writing and outlining enhance content learning. *The Reading Teacher, 38,* 406–411.

Brown, A. L. (1980). Metacognitive development and reading. In R. J. Spiro, B. C. Bruce, & W. F. Brewer (Eds.), *Theoretical issues in reading comprehension* (pp. 453–481). Hillsdale, NJ: Lawrence Erlbaum.

Brown, A. L., Day, J. D., & Jones, R. S. (1983). The development of plans for summarizing texts. *Child Development, 54,* 968–979.

Brown, M. H., Cromer, P. S., & Weinberg, S. H. (1986). Shared book experiences in kindergarten: Helping children come to literacy. *Early Childhood Research Quarterly, 1,* 397–405.

Brown, M. J. M. (1981). What does the author say, what does the author mean? Reading in the social studies. *Theory into Practice, 20,* 199–205.

Brown, P. M., & Brewer, L. C. (1996). Cognitive processes of deaf and hearing skilled and less skilled readers. *Journal of Deaf Studies and Deaf Education, 1,* 263–270.

Brown, R. (1973). *A first language: The early stages.* Cambridge, MA: Harvard University.

Brown, R., & Hanlon, C. (1970). Derivational complexity and order of acquisition in child speech. In J. R. Hayes (Ed.), *Cognition and the development of language* (pp. 11–53). New York: Wiley.

Bruner, J. (1983). *Child's talk: Learning to use language.* New York: Wiley.

Bullard, C. S., & Schirmer, B. R. (1991). Understanding questions: Hearing impaired children with learning problems. *The Volta Review, 93,* 235–245.

Buss, R. R., Yussen, S. R., Mathews, S. R., Miller, G. E., & Rembold, K. L. (1983). Development of children's use of a story schema to retrieve information. *Developmental Psychology, 19,* 22–28.

Butler, C. (1980). When the pleasurable is measurable: Teachers reading aloud. *Language Arts, 57,* 882–885.

Buttery, T. J., & Parks, D. (1988). Instructive innovation: Interactive videodisc system. *Reading Improvement, 25,* 56–59.

Cairney, T. H. (1987). Story frames—story cloze. *The Reading Teacher, 41,* 239–241.

Calkins, L. M. (1994). *The art of teaching writing* (2nd ed.). Portsmouth, NH: Heinemann.

Callahan, D., & Drum, P. A. (1984). Reading ability and prior knowledge as predictors of eleven and twelve year olds' text comprehension. *Reading Psychology, 5,* 145–154.

Cambourne, B., & Turbill, J. (1990). Assessment in whole-language classrooms: Theory into practice. *The Elementary School Journal, 90,* 337–349.

Cambra, C. (1994). An instructional program approach to improve hearing-impaired adolescents' narratives: A pilot study. *The Volta Review, 96,* 237–246.

Caniglia, J., Cole, N. J., Howard, W., Krohn, E., & Rice, M. (1975). *Apple tree.* Beaverton, OR: Dormac.

Canney, G., & Neuenfield, C. (1993). Teachers' preferences for reading materials. *Reading Improvement, 30,* 238–245.

Carnine, D., & Kinder, D. (1985). Teaching low-performing students to apply generative and schema strategies to narrative and expository material. *Remedial and Special Education, 6,* 20–30.

Carroll, J. J., & Gibson, E. J. (1986). Infant perception of gestural contrasts: Prerequisites for the acquisition of a visually specified language. *Journal of Child Language, 13,* 31–49.

Casazza, M. E. (1993). Using a model of direct instruction to teach summary writing in a college reading class. *Journal of Reading, 37,* 202–208.

Caselli, M. C. (1983). Communication to language: Deaf children's and hearing children's development compared. *Sign Language Studies, 39,* 113–144.

Caverly, D. C., Mandeville, T. F., & Nicholson, S. A. (1995). PLAN: A study–reading strategy for informational text. *Journal of Adolescent and Adult Literacy, 39,* 190–199.

Caverly, D. C., & Orlando, V. P. (1991). Textbook study strategies. In R. F. Flippo & D. C. Caverly (Eds.), *Teaching reading & study strategies at the college level* (pp. 86–165). Newark, DE: International Reading Association.

Cazden, C. B. (1988). *Classroom discourse: The language of teaching and learning.* Portsmouth, NH: Heinemann.

Center, Y., Wheldall, K., Freeman, L., Outhred, L., & McNaught, M. (1995). An evaluation of Reading Recovery. *Reading Research Quarterly, 30,* 240–263.

Chall, J. S., Bissex, G. L., Conard, S. S., & Harris-Sharples, S. H. (1996). *Qualitative assessment of text difficulty.* Cambridge, MA: Brookline.

Chall, J. S., & Dale, E. (1995). *Readability revisited: The new Dale-Chall readability formula.* Cambridge, MA: Brookline.

Chaplin, M. T. (1982). Rosenblatt revisited: The transaction between reader and text. *Journal of Reading, 26,* 150–154.

Chapman, J. (1979). Confirming children's use of cohesive ties in text: Pronouns. *The Reading Teacher, 33,* 317–322.

Christie, J. F. (1990). Dramatic play: A context for meaningful engagements. *The Reading Teacher, 43,* 542–545.

Christie, J., Enz, B., & Vukelich, C. (1997). *Teaching language and literacy: Preschool through the elementary grades.* New York: Addison Wesley Longman.

Ciocci, S. R., & Morrell-Schumann, M. (1987). The writing process: Applications in a program for deaf and hearing-impaired students. In D. S. Copeland & D. C. Fletcher (Eds.), *Proceedings of the 1987 National Conference on Innovative Writing Programs and Research for Deaf and Hearing Impaired Students, Removing the writing barrier: A dream?* (pp. 120–150). New York: Lehman College, The City University of New York.

Clarke, B. R. (1983). Competence in communication for hearing impaired children: A conversation, activity, experience approach. *B. C. Journal of Special Education, 7,* 15–27.

Clarke, B. R., & Stewart, D. A. (1986). Reflections on language programs for the hearing impaired. *The Journal of Special Education, 20,* 153–165.

Clarke, L. K. (1988). Invented versus traditional spelling in first graders' writings: Effects on learning to spell and read. *Research in the Teaching of English, 22,* 281–309.

Clay, M. M. (1985). *The early detection of reading difficulties* (3rd ed.). Portsmouth, NH: Heinemann.

Cohen, L. G., & Spenciner, L. J. (1998). *Assessment of children and youth.* New York: Longman.

Collins, C. (1980). Sustained silent reading period: Effect on teachers' behaviors and students' achievement. *The Elementary School Journal, 81,* 109–114.

Colman, P. (1989). Utilizing interactive instructional systems. *Media & Methods, 25*(4), 18, 48–50.

The Commission on Reading, National Council of Teachers of English. (1989). Basal readers and the state of American reading instruction: A call for action. *Language Arts, 66,* 896–898.

Conway, D. (1985). Children (re)creating writing: A preliminary look at the purposes of free-choice writing of hearing-impaired kindergartners. *The Volta Review, 87,* 91–126.

Conway, D. F. (1990). Semantic relationships in the word meanings of hearing-impaired children. *The Volta Review, 92,* 339–349.

Conway, D. F., Mettler, R., Downs, K., Loverin, J., Bush, R., Hurrell, M., Robertson, D., & Truax, R. (1988, July). *Literature, language, and learning. Part I: Dialogue journals.* Paper presented at the International Convention of the Alexander Graham Bell Association for the Deaf, Orlando, FL.

Cooke, N. L., Heron, T. E., & Heward, W. L. (1983). *Peer tutoring: Implementing classwide programs in the primary grades.* Columbus, OH: Special Press.

Cooper, D. C., & Anderson-Inman, L. (1988). Language and socialization. In M. A. Nippold (Ed.), *Later language development: Ages nine through nineteen* (pp. 225–245). San Diego: Singular.

Copra, E. R. (1990). Using interactive video discs for bilingual education. *Perspectives in Education and Deafness, 8*(5), 9–11.

Cox, B., & Sulzby, E. (1982). Evidence of planning in dialogue and monologue by five-year-old emergent readers. In J. A. Niles & L. A. Harris (Eds.), *New inquiries in reading research and instruction* (pp. 124–130). Rochester, NY: The National Reading Conference.

Crowell, D. C., Kawakami, A. J., & Wong, J. L. (1986). Emerging literacy: Reading-writing experiences in a kindergarten classroom. *The Reading Teacher, 40,* 144–149.

Crowson, K. (1994). Errors made by deaf children acquiring sign language. *Early Child Development and Care, 99,* 63–78.

Cudd, E. T., & Roberts, L. L. (1987). Using story frames to develop reading comprehension in a 1st grade classroom. *The Reading Teacher, 41,* 74–79.

Cummins, J. (1979). *Linguistic interdependence and the educational development of bilingual children.* Los Angeles: National Dissemination and Assessment Center, California State University, Los Angeles.

Cummins, J. (1984). *Bilingualism and special education: Issues in assessment and pedagogy.* Clevedon, England: Multilingual Matters.

Cummins, J. (1987). Bilingualism, language proficiency, and metalinguistic development. In P. Homel, M. Palij, & D. Aaronson (Eds.), *Childhood bilingualism: Aspects of linguistic, cognitive, and social development* (pp. 57–73). Hillsdale, NJ: Lawrence Erlbaum.

Cummins, J., Harley, B., Swain, M., & Allen, P. (1990). Social and individual factors in the development of bilingual proficiency. In B. Harley, P. Allen, J. Cummins, & M. Swain (Eds.), *The development of second language proficiency* (pp. 119–133). Cambridge, England: Cambridge University.

Cunningham, D., & Shablak, S. L. (1975). Selective reading guide-o-rama: The content teachers' best friend. *Journal of Reading, 18,* 380–382.

Curtiss, S., Prutting, C. A., & Lowell, E. L. (1979). Pragmatic and semantic development in young children with impaired hearing. *Journal of Speech and Hearing Research, 22,* 534–552.

Daines, D. (1986). Are teachers asking higher level questions? *Education, 106,* 368–374.

Darch, C. B., Carnine, D. W., & Kameenui, E. J. (1986). The role of graphic organizers and social structure in content area instruction. *Journal of Reading Behavior, 18,* 275–295.

Davey, B., & King, S. (1990). Acquisition of word meanings from context by deaf readers. *American Annals of the Deaf, 135,* 227–234.

Davis, Z. T., & McPherson, M. D. (1989). Story map instruction: A road map for reading comprehension. *The Reading Teacher, 43,* 232–240.

Davison, A., & Kantor, R. N. (1982). On the failure of readability formulas to define readable texts: A case study for adaptations. *Reading Research Quarterly, 17,* 187–209.

Delquadri, J., Greenwood, C. R., Whorton, D., Carta, J. J., & Hall, R. V. (1986). Classwide peer tutoring. *Exceptional Children, 52,* 535–542.

Demetrus, M. J., Post, K. N., & Snow, C. E. (1986). Feedback to first language learners: The role of repetitions and clarification questions. *Journal of Child Language, 13,* 275–292.

DePaulo, B. M., & Bonvillian, J. D. (1978). The effect on language development of the special characteristics of speech addressed to children. *Journal of Psycholinguistic Research, 7,* 189–211.

deVilliers, P. A., & deVilliers, J. G. (1979). *Early language.* Cambridge, MA: Harvard University.

deVilliers, P. A., & Pomerantz, S. B. (1992). Hearing-impaired students learning new words from written context. *Applied Psycholinguistics, 13,* 409–431.

Diaz, R. M. (1986). Issues in the empirical study of private speech: A response to Frawley and Lantolf's commentary. *Developmental Psychology, 22,* 709–711.

Dillon, D. (1990). Dear readers. *Language Arts, 67,* 7–9.

Dobson, L. (1989). Connections in learning to write and read: A study of children's development through kindergarten and first grade. In J. M. Mason (Ed.), *Reading and writing connections* (pp. 83–103). Boston: Allyn and Bacon.

Donaldson, J. (1984). Bookwebbing across the curriculum. *The Reading Teacher, 37,* 435–437.

Donin, J., Doehring, D. G., & Browns, F. (1991). Text comprehension and reading achievement in orally educated hearing-impaired children. *Discourse Processes, 14,* 307–337.

Dreher, M. J., & Singer, H. (1980). Story grammar instruction unnecessary for intermediate grade students. *The Reading Teacher, 34,* 261–268.

Dreher, M. J., & Singer, H. (1989). The teacher's role in students' success. *The Reading Teacher, 42,* 612–617.

Dreyer, L. G. (1984). Readability and responsibility. *Journal of Reading, 27,* 334–338.

Dry, E., & Earle, P. T. (1988). Can Johnny have time to read? *American Annals of the Deaf, 133,* 219–222.

Duffelmeyer, F. A. (1994). Effective anticipation guide statements for learning from expository prose. *Journal of Reading, 37,* 452–457.

Duffelmeyer, F. A., & Banwart, B. H. (1993). Word maps for adjectives and verbs. *The Reading Teacher, 46*, 351–352.

Dunst, C. J., Trivette, C. M., & Deal, A. G. (1988). *Enabling and empowering families: Principles and guidelines for practice.* Cambridge, MA: Brookline.

Dyson, A. H. (1983). The role of oral language in early writing processes. *Research in the Teaching of English, 17*, 1–30.

Dyson, A. H. (1984). "N spell my Grandmama": Fostering early thinking about print. *The Reading Teacher, 38*, 262–271.

Dyson, A. H. (1986). Transitions and tensions: Interrelationships between the drawing, talking, and dictating of young children. *Research in the Teaching of English, 20*, 379–409.

Earle, R. A. (1969). Developing and using study guides. In H. L. Herber & P. L. Sanders (Eds.), *Research in reading in the content areas: First year report* (pp. 71–92). Syracuse, NY: Syracuse University.

Earle, R. A. (1969). Use of the structured overview in mathematics classes. In H. L. Herber & P. L. Sanders (Eds.), *Research in reading in the content areas: First year report* (pp. 49–58). Syracuse, NY: Syracuse University, Reading and Language Arts Center.

Earle, R. A., & Barron, R. F. (1973). An approach for teaching vocabulary in content subjects. In H. L. Herber & P. L. Sanders (Eds.), *Research in reading in the content areas: Second year report* (pp. 84–100). Syracuse, NY: Syracuse University, Reading and Language Arts Center.

Echevarria, J. (1995). Interactive reading instruction: A comparison of proximal and distal effects of instructional conversations. *Exceptional Children, 61*, 536–552.

Eeds, M., & Cockrum, W. A. (1985). Teaching word meanings by expanding schemata vs. dictionary work vs. reading in context. *Journal of Reading, 28*, 492–497.

Eldredge, J. L., Reutzel, D. R., & Hollingsworth, P. M. (1996). Comparing the effectiveness of two oral reading practices: Round-robin reading and the shared book experience. *Journal of Literacy Research, 28*, 201–225.

Ely, R. (1997). Language and literacy in the school years. In J. B. Gleason (Ed.), *The development of language* (4th ed.) (pp. 122–158). Boston: Allyn and Bacon.

Emery, D. W. (1996). Helping readers comprehend stories from the characters' perspectives. *The Reading Teacher, 49*, 534–541.

Emig, J. (1971). *The composing process of twelfth graders.* Urbana, IL: National Council of Teachers of English.

Englert, C. S., Raphael, T. E., Anderson, L. M., Anthony, H. M., & Stevens, D. D. (1991). Making strategies and self-talk visible: Writing instruction in regular and special education classrooms. *American Educational Research Journal, 28*, 337–372.

Erickson, M. E. (1987). Deaf readers reading beyond the literal. *American Annals of the Deaf, 132*, 291–294.

Ewoldt, C. (1978). Reading for the hearing or hearing impaired: A single process. *American Annals of the Deaf, 123*, 945–948.

Ewoldt, C. (1984). Problems with rewritten materials, as exemplified by "To Build a Fire." *American Annals of the Deaf, 129*, 23–28.

Ewoldt, C. (1987). Emerging literacy in three- to seven-year-old deaf children. In D. S. Copeland & D. C. Fletcher (Eds.), *Proceedings of the 1987 National Conference on Innovative Writing Programs and Research for Deaf and Hearing Impaired Students, Removing the writing barrier: A dream?* (pp. 5–17). New York: Lehman College, The City University of New York.

Ewoldt, C., & Hammermeister, F. (1986). The language-experience approach to facilitating reading and writing for hearing-impaired students. *American Annals of the Deaf, 131,* 271–274.

Farr, R. (1992). Putting it all together: Solving the reading assessment puzzle. *The Reading Teacher, 46,* 26–37.

Farrar, J. (1992). Negative evidence and grammatical morpheme acquisition. *Developmental Psychology, 28,* 90–98.

Feldman, M. J. (1985). Evaluating pre-primer basal readers using story grammar. *American Educational Research Journal, 22,* 527–547.

Fischler, I. (1985). Word recognition, use of context, and reading skill among deaf college students. *Reading Research Quarterly, 20,* 203–218.

Fitzgerald, E. (1949). *Straight language for the deaf.* Washington, DC: The Volta Bureau.

Fitzgerald, J. (1984). The relationship between reading ability and expectations for story structures. *Discourse Processes, 7,* 21–41.

Fitzgerald, J. (1987). Research on revision in writing. *Review of Educational Research, 57,* 481–506.

Fitzgerald, J. (1988). Helping young writers to revise: A brief review for teachers. *The Reading Teacher, 42,* 124–129.

Fitzgerald, J. (1989). Enhancing two related thought processes: Revision in writing. *The Reading Teacher, 43,* 42–48.

Fitzgerald, J., Spiegel, D. L., & Webb, T. B. (1985). Development of children's knowledge of story structure and content. *Journal of Educational Research, 79,* 101–108.

Fivush, R., & Fromhoff, F. A. (1988). Style and structure in mother-child conversations about the past. *Discourse Processes, 11,* 337–355.

Flower, L., & Hayes, J. R. (1980). The dynamics of composing: Making plans and juggling constraints. In L. W. Gregg & E. R. Steinberg (Eds.), *Cognitive processes in writing* (pp. 31–50). Hillsdale, NJ: Lawrence Erlbaum.

Forcier, R. C. (1999). *The computer as an educational tool: Productivity and problem solving* (2nd ed.). Columbus, OH: Merrill/Prentice Hall.

Foster, S. (1983). Topic and the development of discourse structure. *The Volta Review, 85,* 44–54.

Frauenglass, M. H., & Diaz, R. M. (1985). Self-regulatory functions of children's private speech: A critical analysis of recent challenges to Vygotsky's theory. *Developmental Psychology, 21,* 357–364.

Frawley, W., & Lantolf, J. P. (1986). Private speech and self-regulation: A commentary on Frauenglass and Diaz. *Developmental Psychology, 22,* 706–708.

Freedman, G., & Reynolds, E. G. (1980). Enriching basal reader lessons with semantic webbing. *The Reading Teacher, 33,* 677–684.

French, L., & Pak, M. K. (1995). Young children's play dialogues with mothers and peers. In K. E. Nelson & Z. Reger (Eds.), *Children's language* (Vol. 8, pp. 65–101). Hillsdale, NJ: Lawrence Erlbaum.

French, M. M. (1988). Story retelling for assessment and instruction. *Perspectives for Teachers of the Hearing Impaired, 7*(2), 20–22.

Fry, E. B. (1989). Reading formulas—maligned but valid. *Journal of Reading, 32,* 292–297.

Furman, L. N., & Walden, T. A. (1990). Effect of script knowledge on preschool children's communicative interactions. *Developmental Psychology, 26,* 227–233.

Furrow, D., & Nelson, K. (1986). A further look at the motherese hypothesis: A reply to Gleitman, Newport, & Gleitman. *Journal of Child Language, 13,* 163–176.

Fusaro, J. A., & Slike, S. B. (1979). The effect of imagery on the ability of hearing-impaired children to identify words. *American Annals of the Deaf, 124,* 829–832.

Galda, L. (1982). Playing about a story: Its impact on comprehension. *The Reading Teacher, 36,* 52–55.

Galda, L. (1984). Narrative competence: Play, storytelling, and story comprehension. In A. D. Pellegrini & T. D. Yawkey (Eds.), *The development of oral and written language in social contexts* (pp. 105–117). Norwood, NJ: Ablex.

Gambrell, L. B. (1980). Think-time: Implications for reading instruction. *The Reading Teacher, 34,* 143–146.

Gambrell, L. B. (1983). The occurrence of think-time during reading comprehension instruction. *The Journal of Educational Research, 77,* 77–80.

Gambrell, L. B. (1985). Dialogue journals: Reading-writing interaction. *The Reading Teacher, 38,* 512–515.

Gambrell, L. B., & Bales, R. J. (1986). Mental imagery and the comprehension-monitoring performance of fourth- and fifth-grade poor readers. *Reading Research Quarterly, 21,* 454–464.

Gambrell, L. B., & Jawitz, P. B. (1993). Mental imagery, text illustrations, and children's story comprehension and recall. *Reading Research Quarterly, 28,* 264–276.

Gambrell, L. B., Pfeiffer, W. R., & Wilson, R. M. (1985). The effects of retelling upon reading comprehension and recall of text information. *The Journal of Educational Research, 78,* 216–220.

Gardner, R. C. (1979). Attitudes and motivation: Their role in second-language acquisition. In H. T. Trueba & C. Barnett-Mizrahi (Eds.), *Bilingual multicultural education and the professional: From theory to practice* (pp. 319–327). Rowley, MA: Newbury House.

Garrison, W., Long, G., & Dowaliby, F. (1997). Working memory capacity and comprehension processes in deaf readers. *Journal of Deaf Studies and Deaf Education, 2,* 78–94.

Gartner, G. M., Trehub, S. E., & Mackay-Soroka, S. (1993). Word awareness in hearing-impaired children. *Applied Psycholinguistics, 14,* 61–73.

Garton, A., & Pratt, C. (1998). *Learning to be literate: The development of spoken and written language.* Oxford, England: Basil Blackwell.

Gaskins, I. W., Satlow, E., Hyson, D., Ostertag, J., & Six, L. (1994). Classroom talk about text: Learning in the science class. *Journal of Reading, 37,* 558–565.

Geers, A., & Moog, J. (1989). Factors predictive of the development of literacy in profoundly hearing-impaired adolescents. *The Volta Review, 91,* 69–86.

Genesee, F. (1989). Early bilingual development: One language or two? *Journal of Child Language, 16,* 161–179.

Geoffrion, L. D. (1982). An analysis of teletype conversation. *American Annals of the Deaf, 127,* 747–752.

Gersten, R., Woodward, J., & Darch, C. (1986). Direct instruction: A research-based approach to curriculum design and teaching. *Exceptional Children, 53,* 17–31.

Gilbertson, M., & Kamhi, A. G. (1995). Novel word learning in children with hearing impairment. *Journal of Speech and Hearing Research, 38,* 630–642.

Gillespie, C. W., & Twardosz, S. (1997). A group storybook–reading intervention with children at a residential school for the deaf. *American Annals of the Deaf, 142,* 320–332.

Gillet, J. W., & Gentry, J. R. (1983). Bridges between Nonstandard and Standard English with extensions of dictated stories. *The Reading Teacher, 36,* 360–364.

Gipe, J. P. (1980). Use of a relevant context helps kids learn new word meanings. *The Reading Teacher, 33,* 398–402.

Gipe, J. P., & Arnold, R. D. (1979). Teaching vocabulary through familiar associations and contexts. *Journal of Reading Behavior, 11,* 281–284.

Gleason, J. B. (Ed.). (1997). *The development of language* (4th ed.). Boston: Allyn and Bacon.

Gleitman, L. R., Newport, E. L., & Gleitman, H. (1984). The current status of the motherese hypothesis. *Journal of Child Language, 11,* 43–79.

Glenn, C. G. (1978). The role of episodic structure and of story length in children's recall of simple stories. *Journal of Verbal Learning and Verbal Behavior, 17,* 229–247.

Goatley, V. J., Brock, C. H., & Raphael, T. E. (1995). Diverse learners participating in regular education "Book Clubs." *Reading Research Quarterly, 30,* 352–380.

Golden, J. M. (1984). Children's concept of story in reading and writing. *The Reading Teacher, 37,* 578–584.

Goldenberg, C. (1993). Instructional conversations: Promoting comprehension through discussion. *The Reading Teacher, 46,* 316–326.

Goldin-Meadow, S., Butcher, C., Mylander, C., & Dodge, M. (1994). Nouns and verbs in a self-styled gesture system: What's in a name? *Cognitive Psychology, 27,* 259–319.

Goldin-Meadow, S., & Morford, M. (1985). Gesture in early child language: Studies of deaf and hearing children. *Merrill-Palmer Quarterly, 31,* 145–176.

Goldin-Meadow, S., Mylander, C., & Butcher, C. (1995). The resilience of combinatorial structure at the word level: Morphology in self-styled gesture systems. *Cognition, 56,* 195–262.

Gonzalez, E., & Hamra, M. K. (1995). Connecting the nation: Classrooms, libraries and health care organizations in the information age. Washington, DC: U.S. Department of Commerce. Available *www.ntia.doc.gov/connect.html*

Gonzalez, V., & Schallert, D. L. (1999). An integrative analysis of the cognitive development of bilingual and bicultural children and adults. In V. Gonzalez (Ed.), *Language and cognitive development in second language learning* (pp. 19–55). Boston: Allyn and Bacon.

Goodman, K. S. (1989). Whole-language research: Foundations and development. *The Elementary School Journal, 90,* 207–221.

Goodman, Y. M. (1982). Retellings of literature and the comprehension process. *Theory into Practice, 21,* 301–307.

Goodman, Y. M. (1989). Roots of the whole-language movement. *The Elementary School Journal, 90,* 113–127.

Goodman, Y. M., & Burke, C. L. (1972). *Reading miscue inventory.* New York: Richard C. Owen.

Gormley, K. A. (1981). On the influence of familiarity on deaf students' text recall. *American Annals of the Deaf, 126,* 1024–1030.

Gourley, J. W. (1978). The basal is easy to read—or is it? *The Reading Teacher, 32,* 174–182.

Graves, D. H. (1975). An examination of the writing process of seven-year-old children. *Research in the Teaching of English, 9,* 227–241.

Graves, D. H. (1983). *Writing: Teachers and children at work.* Portsmouth, NH: Heinemann.

Graves, M. F. (1986). Vocabulary learning and instruction. In E. Z. Rothkopf (Ed.), *Review of research in education* (pp. 49–89). Washington, DC: American Educational Research Association.

Graves, M. F., Cooke, C. L., & Laberge, M. J. (1983). Effects of previewing difficult short stories on low ability junior high school students' comprehension, recall, and attitudes. *Reading Research Quarterly, 17,* 262–276.

Gray, M. A. (1986). Let them play! *Reading Instruction Journal, 30,* 19–22.

Greenlaw, M. J. (1990). The basal's new clothes. *Learning, 18*(8), 33–36.

Grieser, D. L., & Kuhl, P. K. (1988). Maternal speech to infants in a tonal language: Support for universal prosodic features in motherese. *Developmental Psychology, 24,* 14–20.

Griffith, P. L., Johnson, H. A., & Dastoli, S. L. (1985). If teaching is conversation, can conversation be taught? Discourse abilities in hearing impaired children. In D. N. Ripich & F. M. Spinelli (Eds.), *School discourse problems* (pp. 149–177). San Diego, CA: College-Hill.

Griffith, P. L., & Ripich, D. N. (1988). Story structure recall in hearing-impaired learning-disabled and nondisabled children. *American Annals of the Deaf, 133,* 43–50.

Guido, B., & Colwell, C. G. (1987). A rationale for direct instruction to teach summary writing following expository text reading. *Reading Research and Instruction, 26,* 89–98.

Gustafson, D. J., & Pederson, J. (1986). SQ3R and the strategic reader. *Wisconsin State Research Association Journal, 31*(1), 25–28.

Guthrie, J. T. (1982). Metacognition: Up from flexibility. *The Reading Teacher, 35,* 510–512.

Guzzetti, B. J., Kowalinski, B. J., & McGowan, T. (1992). Using a literature-based approach to teaching social studies. *Journal of Reading, 36,* 114–122.

Hacker, C. J. (1980). From schema theory to classroom practice. *Language Arts, 57,* 866–871.

Hadaway, N. L., & Young, T. A. (1994). Content literacy and language learning: Instructional decisions. *The Reading Teacher, 47,* 522–527.

Haggard, M. R. (1988). Developing critical thinking with the Directed Reading-Thinking Activity. *The Reading Teacher, 41,* 526–533.

Hakuta, K. (1986). *Mirror of language: The debate on bilingualism.* New York: Basic Books.

Hakuta, K. (1987). The second-language learner in the context of the study of language acquisition. In P. Homel, M. Palij, & D. Aaronson (Eds.), *Childhood bilingualism: Aspects of linguistic, cognitive, and social development* (pp. 31–55). Hillsdale, NJ: Lawrence Erlbaum.

Hall, N. (1987). *The emergence of literacy.* Portsmouth, NH: Heinemann.

Halliday, M. A. K. (1975). *Learning how to mean: Explorations in the development of language.* New York: Elsevier North-Holland.

Halliday, M. A. K. (1984). Three aspects of children's language development: Learning language, learning through language, and learning about language. In Y. M. Goodman, M. Haussler, & D. Strickland (Eds.), *Oral and written language development research: Impact on the schools* (pp. 165–192). Urbana, IL: National Council of Teachers of English.

Hammermeister, F. K., & Israelite, N. K. (1983). Reading instruction for the hearing impaired: An integrated language arts approach. *The Volta Review, 85,* 136–148.

Hancock, M. R. (1993a). Character journals: Initiating involvement and identification through literature. *Journal of Reading, 37,* 42–50.

Hancock, M. R. (1993b). Exploring and extending personal response through literature journals. *The Reading Teacher, 46,* 466–474.

Hansen, E. J. (1989). Interactive video for reflection: Learning theory and a new use of the medium. *Educational Technology, 29*(7), 7–15.

Hansen, J. (1981). The effects of inference training and practice on young children's reading comprehension. *Reading Research Quarterly, 16,* 391–417.

Hansen, J. (1987). *When writers read.* Portsmouth, NH: Heinemann.

Hansen, J., & Pearson, P. D. (1983). An instructional study: Improving the inferential comprehension of good and poor fourth-grade readers. *Journal of Educational Psychology, 75,* 821–829.

Hanson, V. (1989). Phonology and reading: Evidence from profoundly deaf readers. In D. Shankweiler & I. Liberman (Eds.), *Phonology and reading disability: Solving the reading puzzle* (pp. 69–89). Ann Arbor: University of Michigan.

Hanson, V. L., & Padden, C. (1989, May). *Computers and videodisc for bilingual ASL/English instruction.* Paper presented at the annual meeting of the International Reading Association, New Orleans, LA.

Hanson, V. L., & Wilkenfeld, D. (1985). Morphophonology and lexical organization in deaf readers. *Language and Speech, 28,* 269–280.

Harding, E., & Riley, P. (1986). *The bilingual family: A handbook for parents.* Cambridge, England: Cambridge University.

Hare, V. C., Rabinowitz, M., & Schieble, K. M. (1989). Text effects on main idea comprehension. *Reading Research Quarterly, 24,* 72–88.

Harris, T. L., & Hodges, R. E. (Eds.). (1995). *The literacy dictionary.* Newark, DE: International Reading Association.

Harrison, M. F., Layton, T. L., & Taylor, T. D. (1987). Antecedent and consequent stimuli in teacher-child dyads. *American Annals of the Deaf, 132,* 227–231.

Harste, J. C. (1989). The future of whole language. *The Elementary School Journal, 90,* 243–249.

Harste, J. C., Short, K. G., & Burke, C. (1988). *Creating classrooms for authors: The reading-writing connection.* Portsmouth, NH: Heinemann.

Harste, J. C., Woodward, V. A., & Burke, C. L. (1984). *Language stories and literacy lessons.* Portsmouth, NH: Heinemann.

Hartson, E. K. (1984). The effects of story structure in texts on the reading comprehension of 1st and 2nd grade students. *The California Reader, 17*(3), 6–10.

Hayes, P., & Arnold, P. (1992). Is hearing-impaired children's reading delayed or different? *Journal of Research in Reading, 15,* 104–116.

Heald-Taylor, B. G. (1984). Scribble in first grade writing. *The Reading Teacher, 38,* 4–8.

Heimlich, J. E., & Pittelman, S. D. (1986). *Semantic mapping: Classroom applications.* Newark, DE: International Reading Association.

Heller, M. F. (1988). Comprehending and composing through language experience. *The Reading Teacher, 42,* 130–135.

Hennings, D. G. (1993). On knowing and reading history. *Journal of Reading, 36,* 362–370.

Hertzog, M., Stinson, M. S., & Keiffer, R. (1989). Effects of caption modification and instructor intervention on comprehension of a technical film. *Educational Technology Research & Development, 37*(2), 59–68.

Heward, W. L. (2000). *Exceptional children* (6th ed.). New York: Merrill/Prentice Hall.

Hiebert, E. H. (1994). Reading Recovery in the United States: What difference does it make to an age cohort? *Educational Researcher, 23*(9), 15–25.

Hiebert, E. H., & Colt, J. (1989). Patterns of literature-based reading instruction. *The Reading Teacher, 43,* 14–20.

Hiebert, E. H., & Raphael, T. E. (1998). *Early literacy instruction.* Fort Worth, TX: Harcourt Brace.

Hill, M. (1991). Writing summaries promotes thinking and learning across the curriculum—but why are they so difficult to write? *Journal of Reading, 34,* 536–539.

Hirsh-Pasek, K. (1987). The metalinguistics of fingerspelling: An alternate way to increase reading vocabulary in congenitally deaf readers. *Reading Research Quarterly, 22,* 455–474.

Hirsh-Pasek, K., & Golinkoff, R. (1993). Skeletal supports for grammatical learning: What the infant brings to the language learning task. In C. Rovee-Collier & L. Lipsitt (Eds.), *Advances in infancy research* (Vol. 8). Norwood, NJ: Ablex.

Hirsh-Pasek, K., Treiman, R., & Schneiderman, M. (1984). Brown & Hanlon revisited: Mothers' sensitivity to ungrammatical forms. *Journal of Child Language, 11*, 81–88.

Hoff-Ginsberg, E. (1986). Function and structure in maternal speech: Their relation to the child's development of syntax. *Developmental Psychology, 22*, 155–163.

Hoff-Ginsberg, E. (1990). Maternal speech and the child's development of syntax: A further look. *Journal of Child Language, 17*, 85–99.

Hoffman, S., & McCully, B. (1984). Oral language functions in transaction with children's writing. *Language Arts, 61*, 41–50.

Holdaway, D. (1979). *The foundations of literacy.* Sydney, Australia: Ashton Scholastic.

Holdaway, D. (1982). Shared book experience: Teaching reading using favorite books. *Theory into Practice, 21*, 293–300.

Holdgrafer, G. (1987). Getting children to talk: A model of natural adult teaching/child learning strategies for language. *Canadian Journal for Exceptional Children, 3*(3), 71–76.

Holmes, B. C. (1985). The effect of four different modes of reading on comprehension. *Reading Research Quarterly, 20*, 575–585.

Holmes, K. M., & Holmes, D. W. (1981). Normal language acquisition: A model for language programming for the deaf. *American Annals of the Deaf, 126*, 23–31.

Holt, J. (1993). Stanford Achievement Test—8th edition: Reading comprehension subgroup results. *American Annals of the Deaf, 138*, 172–175.

Holt, S. B., & O'Tuel, F. S. (1989). The effect of sustained silent reading and writing on achievement and attitudes of seventh and eighth grade students reading two years below grade level. *Reading Improvement, 26*, 290–297.

Horowitz, R. (1985a). Text patterns: Part I. *Journal of Reading, 28*, 448–454.

Horowitz, R. (1985b). Text patterns: Part II. *Journal of Reading, 28*, 534–541.

Horton, S. V., & Lovitt, T. C. (1989). Using study guides with three classifications of secondary students. *The Journal of Special Education, 22*, 447–462.

Hosie, P. (1987). Adopting interactive videodisc technology for education. *Educational Technology, 27*(7), 5–10.

Howe, S. F. (1985). Interactive video: Salt & pepper technology. *Media & Methods, 21*(5), 8–14.

Hubbard, R. (1985). Second graders answer the question "Why publish?" *The Reading Teacher, 38*, 658–662.

Huck, C. S. (1987). Literature as the content of reading. *Theory into Practice, 26*, 374–382.

Hull, G. A. (1989). Research on writing: Building a cognitive and social understanding of composing. In L. B. Resnick & L. E. Klopfer (Eds.), *Toward the thinking curriculum: Current cognitive research* (pp. 104–128). Alexandria, VA: Association for Supervision and Curriculum Development.

Humes, A. (1983). Research on the composing process. *Review of Educational Research, 53*, 201–216.

Humphries, T., & Padden, C. (1992). *Learning American Sign Language.* Englewood Cliffs, NJ: Prentice Hall.

Idol, L. (1987). Group story mapping: A comprehension strategy for both skilled and unskilled readers. *Journal of Learning Disabilities, 20*, 196–205.

Ingram, D. (1989). *First language acquisition: Method, description, and explanation.* Cambridge, England: Cambridge University.

Irwin, J. W., & Davis, C. A. (1980). Assessing readability: The checklist approach. *Journal of Reading, 24*, 124–130.

Isenberg, J., & Jacob, E. (1983). Literacy and symbolic play: A review of the literature. *Childhood Education, 59,* 272–274, 276.

Isenhath, J. O. (1990). *The linguistics of American Sign Language.* Jefferson, NC: McFarland & Co.

Isom, B. A., & Casteel, C. P. (1986). Prereaders' understanding of function of print: Characteristic trends in the process. *Reading Psychology, 7,* 261–266.

Israelite, N. K. (1988). On readability formulas: A critical analysis for teachers of the deaf. *American Annals of the Deaf, 133,* 14–18.

Israelite, N. K., & Helfrich, M. A. (1988). Improving text coherence in basal readers: Effects of revisions on the comprehension of hearing-impaired and normal-hearing readers. *The Volta Review, 90,* 261–273.

Jackson, D. W., Paul, P. V., & Smith, J. C. (1997). Prior knowledge and reading comprehension ability of deaf adolescents. *Journal of Deaf Studies and Deaf Education, 2,* 172–184.

Jacobs, H. H. (1989a). The growing need for interdisciplinary curriculum content. In H. H. Jacobs (Ed.), *Interdisciplinary curriculum: Design and implementation* (pp. 1–11). Alexandria, VA: Association for Supervision and Curriculum Development.

Jacobs, H. H. (1989b). Design options for an integrated curriculum. In H. H. Jacobs (Ed.), *Interdisciplinary curriculum: Design and implementation* (pp. 13–24). Alexandria, VA: Association for Supervision and Curriculum Development.

Jacobs, H. H. (1989c). The interdisciplinary concept model: A step-by-step approach for developing units of study. In H. H. Jacobs (Ed.), *Interdisciplinary curriculum: Design and implementation* (pp. 53–65). Alexandria, VA: Association for Supervision and Curriculum Development.

James, S. L., & Seebach, M. A. (1982). The pragmatic function of children's questions. *Journal of Speech and Hearing Research, 25,* 2–11.

Jamieson, J. R. (1995a). Interactions between mothers and children who are deaf. *Journal of Early Intervention, 19,* 108–117.

Jamieson, J. R. (1995b). Visible thought: Deaf children's use of signed and spoken private speech. *Sign Language Studies, 86,* 63–80.

Jenkins, J. R., & Heliotis, J. G. (1981). Reading comprehension instruction: Findings from behavioral and cognitive psychology. *Topics in Language Disorders, 1*(2), 25–41.

Jenkins, J. R., Stein, M. L., & Wysocki, K. (1984). Learning vocabulary through reading. *American Educational Research Journal, 21,* 767–787.

Johnson, D. D., Pittelman, S. D., & Heimlich, J. E. (1986). Semantic mapping. *The Reading Teacher, 39,* 778–783.

Johnson, D. W., & Johnson, R. T. (1986). Mainstreaming and cooperative learning strategies. *Exceptional Children, 52,* 553–561.

Johnson, D. W., Johnson, R. T., & Holubec, E. J. (1993). *Circles of learning: Cooperation in the classroom* (4th ed.). Edina, MN: Interaction.

Johnson, G. S., & Bliesmer, E. P. (1983). Effects of narrative schema training and practice in generating questions on reading comprehension of seventh grade students. In G. H. McNinch (Ed.), *Reading research to reading practice* (pp. 91–94). Athens, GA: The American Reading Forum.

Johnson, H. A. (1997, June). *Internet use within deaf education: Current status, trends and applications.* Paper presented at the CAID/CEASD Conference, Hartford, CT.

Johnson, H. A., & Barton, L. E. (1988). TDD conversations: A context for language sampling. *American Annals of the Deaf, 133,* 19–25.

Johnson, H. A., Padak, N. D., & Barton, L. E. (1994). Developmental spelling strategies of hearing-impaired children. *Reading and Writing Quarterly, 10,* 359–367.

Johnson, J. M., & Rash, S. J. (1990). A method for transcribing signed and spoken language. *American Annals of the Deaf, 135,* 343–351.

Johnson, K. L. (1987). Improving reading comprehension through prereading and post-reading exercises. *Reading Improvement, 24,* 81–83.

Johnson, M. A., & Roberson, G. F. (1988). The language experience approach: Its use with young hearing-impaired students. *American Annals of the Deaf, 133,* 223–225.

Johnson, M. J. (1992). What's basic in a student-centered reading, writing, and thinking approach: One teacher's perspective. *The Volta Review, 94,* 389–394.

Johnson, N. S., & Mandler, J. M. (1980). A tale of two structures: Underlying and surface forms in stories. *Poetics, 9,* 51–86.

Jones, L. L. (1982). An interactive view of reading: Implications for the classroom. *The Reading Teacher, 35,* 772–777.

Joyce, B. R. (1987). Learning how to learn. *Theory into Practice, 26,* 416–428.

Joyce, B., & Weil, M. (1996). *Models of teaching* (5th ed.). Boston: Allyn and Bacon.

Kaisen, J. (1987). SSR/Booktime: Kindergarten and 1st grade sustained silent reading. *The Reading Teacher, 40,* 532–536.

Kapinus, B. A., Gambrell, L. B., & Koskinen, P. S. (1987). Effects of practice in retelling upon the reading comprehension of proficient and less proficient readers. In J. E. Readence & R. S. Baldwin (Eds.), *Research in literacy: Merging perspectives* (pp. 135–141). Rochester, NY: The National Reading Conference.

Karnowski, L. (1989). Using LEA with process writing. *The Reading Teacher, 42,* 462–465.

Kauchak, D. P., & Eggen, P. D. (1997). *Learning and teaching: Research-based methods.* (3rd ed.). Boston: Allyn and Bacon.

Keeler, M. A. (1993). Story map game board. *The Reading Teacher, 46,* 626–628.

Kelly, L. (1996). The interaction of syntactic competence and vocabulary during reading by deaf students. *Journal of Deaf Studies and Deaf Education, 1,* 75–90.

Kelly, L. P. (1995). Processing of bottom-up and top-down information by skilled and average deaf readers and implications for whole language instruction. *Exceptional Children, 61,* 318–334.

Kessler, C. (1984). *Language acquisition processes in bilingual children.* Los Angeles: Evaluation, Dissemination and Assessment Center, California State University, Los Angeles.

Kibby, M. W. (1995). The organization and teaching of things and the words that signify them. *Journal of Adolescent and Adult Literacy, 39,* 208–223.

Kletzien, S. B., & Baloche, L. (1994). The shifting muffled sound of the pick: Facilitating student-to-student discussion. *The Reading Teacher, 37,* 540–545.

Klima, E., & Bellugi, U. (1979). *The signs of language.* Cambridge, MA: Harvard University.

Kluwin, T. N. (1996). Getting hearing and deaf students to write to each other through dialogue journals. *Teaching Exceptional Children, 28,* 50–53.

Kluwin, T. N., & Kelly, A. B. (1991). The effectiveness of dialogue journal writing in improving the writing skills of young deaf writers. *American Annals of the Deaf, 136,* 284–291.

Kluwin, T. N., & Kelly, A. B. (1992). Implementing a successful writing program in public schools for students who are deaf. *Exceptional Children, 59,* 41–53.

Koenke, K. (1987). Readability formulas: Use and misuse. *The Reading Teacher, 40,* 672–674.

Koskinen, P. S., Gambrell, L. B., Kapinus, B. A., & Heathington, B. S. (1988). Retelling: A strategy for enhancing students' reading comprehension. *The Reading Teacher, 41,* 892–896.

Koskinen, P. S., & O'Flahavan, J. F. (1995). Teacher role options in peer discussions about literature. *The Reading Teacher, 48,* 354–356.

Koskinen, P. S., Wilson, R. M., Gambrell, L. B., & Neuman, S. B. (1993). Captioned video and vocabulary learning: An innovative practice in literacy instruction. *The Reading Teacher, 47,* 36–43.

Koskinen, P. S., Wilson, R. M., & Jensema, C. J. (1986). Using closed-captioned television in the teaching of reading to deaf students. *American Annals of the Deaf, 131,* 43–46.

Krein, E. L., & Zaharias, J. A. (1986). Analysis of able and disabled sixth-grade readers' knowledge of story structure: A comparison. *Reading Horizons, 27,* 45–53.

Kretschmer, R. R., & Kretschmer, L. W. (1979). The acquisition of linguistic and communicative competence: Parent-child interactions. *The Volta Review, 81,* 306–322.

Kretschmer, R. R., & Kretschmer, L. W. (1995). Communication-based classrooms. *The Volta Review, 97*(5), 1–18.

Laframboise, K. L. (1986–1987). The use of study techniques with young and less-able students. *Journal of Reading Education, 12*(2), 23–31.

Laine, C., & Schultz, L. (1985). Composition theory and practice: The paradigm shift. *The Volta Review, 87*(5), 9–20.

Lane, H., Hoffmeister, R., & Bahan, B. (1996). *A journey into the Deaf-World.* San Diego, CA: Dawn Sign Press.

Lange, B. (1981). Making sense with schemata. *Journal of Reading, 24,* 442–445.

Lange, B. (1982). Readability formulas: Second looks, second thoughts. *The Reading Teacher, 35,* 858–861.

Langer, J. A. (1985). Children's sense of genre. *Written Communication, 2,* 157–187.

Langer, J. A. (1994). A response-based approach to reading literature. *Language Arts, 71,* 203–211.

Langer, J. A., & Applebee, A. N. (1986). Reading and writing instruction: Toward a theory of teaching and learning. In E. Z. Rothkopf (Ed.), *Review of research in education* (pp. 171–194). Washington, DC: American Educational Research Association.

Larking, L. (1984). ReQuest helps children comprehend: A study. *Australian Journal of Reading, 7,* 135–139.

LaSasso, C., Davey, B. (1987). The relationship between lexical knowledge and reading comprehension for prelingually, profoundly hearing impaired students. *The Volta Review, 89,* 211–220.

LaSasso, C. J., & Mobley, R. T. (1997). National survey of reading instruction for deaf or hard-of-hearing students in the U.S. *The Volta Review, 99,* 31–58.

Leal, D. J. (1993). The power of literacy peer-group discussions: How children collaboratively negotiate meaning. *The Reading Teacher, 47,* 114–120.

Lee, L. (1974). *Developmental sentence analysis.* Evanston, IL: Northwestern University.

Lentz, E. M., Mikos, K., & Smith, C. (1988). *Signing naturally, level 1.* San Diego, CA: Dawn Sign Press.

Lenz, B. K., Alley, G. R., & Schumaker, J. B. (1987). Activating the inactive learner: Advance organizers in the secondary content classroom. *Learning Disability Quarterly, 10,* 53–67.

Leu, D. J., & Kinzer, C. K. (1999). *Effective reading instruction, K–8* (4th ed.). Columbus, OH: Prentice Hall.

Levy, A. K., Schaefer, L., & Phelps, P. C. (1986). Increasing preschool effectiveness: Enhancing the language abilities of 3- and 4-year-old children through planned sociodramatic play. *Early Childhood Research Quarterly, 1,* 133–140.

Lewis, E. G. (1981). *Bilingualism and bilingual education.* Oxford, England: Pergamon.

Leybaert, J. (1993). Reading in the deaf: The roles of phonological codes. In M. Marschark & M. D. Clark (Eds.), *Psychological perspectives on deafness* (pp. 269–309). Hillsdale, NJ: Erlbaum.

Lillo-Martin, D. C., Hanson, V. L., & Smith, S. T. (1992). Deaf readers' comprehension of relative clause structures. *Applied Psycholinguistics, 13,* 13–30.

Limbrick, E. A. (1991). The reading development of deaf children: Critical factors associated with success. *Teaching English to Deaf and Second-Language Students, 9*(1), 4–9.

Limbrick, E. A., McNaughton, S., & Clay, M. M. (1992). Time engaged in reading: A critical factor in reading achievement. *American Annals of the Deaf, 137,* 309–314.

Lindberg, B. (1988). Teaching literature: The process approach. *Journal of Reading, 31,* 732–735.

Lindholm, K. J., & Padilla, A. M. (1978). Language mixing in bilingual children. *Journal of Child Language, 5,* 327–335.

Livingston, S. (1997). *Rethinking the education of deaf students.* Portsmouth, NH: Heinemann.

Long, S. A., Winograd, P. N., & Bridge, C. A. (1989). The effects of reader and text characteristics on imagery reported during and after reading. *Reading Research Quarlerly, 24,* 353–372.

Lucariello, J., & Nelson, K. (1987). Remembering and planning talk between mothers and children. *Discourse Processes, 10,* 219–235.

Luetke-Stahlman, B. (1988). Assessing the semantic language development of hearing impaired students. *A.C.E.H.I. Journal, 14*(1), 5–12.

Luetke-Stahlman, B. (1993). Research-based language intervention strategies adapted for deaf and hard of hearing children. *American Annals of the Deaf, 138,* 404–410.

Luetke-Stahlman, B., Griffith, C., & Montgomery, N. (1998). Development of text structure knowledge as assessed by spoken and signed retellings of a deaf second-grade student. *American Annals of the Deaf, 143,* 337–346.

MacGinitie, W. H. (1993). Some limits of assessment. *Journal of Reading, 36,* 556–560.

MacGregor, S. K., & Thomas, L. B. (1988). A computer-mediated text system to develop communication skills for hearing-impaired students. *American Annals of the Deaf, 133,* 280–284.

Mandler, J. M. (1978). A code in the node: The use of story schema in retrieval. *Discourse Processes, 1,* 14–35.

Mandler, J. M. (1987). On the psychological reality of story structure. *Discourse Processes, 10,* 1–29.

Mandler, J. M., & Johnson, N. S. (1977). Remembrance of things parsed: Story structure and recall. *Cognitive Psychology, 9,* 111–151.

Manson, M. (1982). Explorations in language arts for preschoolers (who happen to be deaf). *Language Arts, 59,* 33–39, 45.

Manzo, A. V. (1969). The ReQuest procedure. *Journal of Reading, 13,* 123–126, 163.

Manzo, A. V. (1975). Guided reading procedure. *Journal of Reading, 18,* 287–291.

Manzo, A. V., & Casale, U. P. (1985). Listen-read-discuss: A content reading heuristic. *Journal of Reading, 28,* 732–734.

Marr, M. B., & Gormley, K. (1982). Children's recall of familiar and unfamiliar text. *Reading Research Quarterly, 18,* 89–104.

Marshall, N. (1979). Readability and comprehensibility. *Journal of Reading, 22,* 542–544.

Marshall, N. (1984). The effects of differential instruction on story comprehension. *Florida Reading Quarterly, 20*(3), 3–7.

Martinez, M., & Roser, N. (1985). Read it again: The value of repeated readings during story-time. *The Reading Teacher, 38,* 782–786.

Marvin, C., & Kasal, K. R. (1996). A semantic analysis of signed communication in an activity-based classroom for preschool children who are deaf. *Language, Speech, and Hearing Services in Schools, 27,* 57–67.

Masataka, N. (1992). Motherese in a signed language. *Infant Behavior and Development, 15,* 453–460.

Masataka, N. (1996). Perception of motherese in a signed language by 6-month-old deaf infants. *Developmental Psychology, 32,* 874–879.

Mason, J. M., & Allen, J. (1986). A review of emergent literacy with implications for research and practice in reading. In E. T. Rothkopf (Ed.), *Review of research in education* (pp. 3–47). Washington, DC: American Educational Research Association.

Mason, J. M., Peterman, C. L., Powell, B. M., & Kerr, B. M. (1989). Reading and writing attempts by kindergartners after book reading by teachers. In J. M. Mason (Ed.), *Reading and writing connections* (pp. 105–120). Boston: Allyn and Bacon.

Mavrogenes, N. A. (1983). Teaching implications of the schemata theory of comprehension. *Reading World, 22,* 295–305.

Mavrogenes, N. A. (1986). What every reading teacher should know about emergent literacy. *The Reading Teacher, 40,* 174–178.

Mayer, C., & Moskos, E. (1998). Deaf children learning to spell. *Research in the Teaching of English, 33,* 158–180.

McAnally, P. L., Rose, S., & Quigley, S. P. (1998). *Language learning practices with deaf children* (2nd ed.). Austin, TX: Pro-Ed.

McAndrew, D. A. (1983). Underlining and notetaking: Some suggestions from research. *Journal of Reading, 27,* 103–108.

McCaslin, M. M. (1989). Whole language: Theory, instruction, and future implementation. *The Elementary School Journal, 90,* 223–229.

McCauley, R. J., & Swisher, L. (1984). Psychometric review of language and articulation tests for preschool children. *Journal of Speech and Hearing Disorders, 49,* 34–42.

McClure, E., Mason, J., & Barnitz, J. (1979). An exploratory study of story structure and age effects on children's ability to sequence stories. *Discourse Processes, 2,* 213–249.

McCollum, P. A. (1981). Concepts in bilingualism and their relationship to language assessment. In J. G. Erickson & D. R. Omark (Eds.), *Communication assessment of the bilingual bicultural child: Issues and guidelines* (pp. 25–41). Baltimore: University Park.

McConaughy, S. H. (1980). Using story structure in the classroom. *Language Arts, 57,* 157–165.

McConaughy, S. H. (1982). Developmental changes in story comprehension and levels of questioning. *Language Arts, 59,* 580–589.

McGee, L. M. (1982). Awareness of text structure: Effects on children's recall of expository text. *Reading Research Quarterly, 17,* 581–590.

McGee, L. M., & Richgels, D. J. (1985). Teaching expository text structure to elementary students. *The Reading Teacher, 38,* 739–748.

McKenna, M. C., & Robinson, R. D. (1997). *Teaching through text* (2nd ed.). New York: Longman.

McKeown, M. G. (1993). Creating effective definitions for young word learners. *Reading Research Quarterly, 28,* 16–31.

McKeown, M. G., Beck, I. L., Omanson, R. C., & Pople, M. T. (1985). Some effects of the nature and frequency of vocabulary instruction on the knowledge and use of words. *Reading Research Quarterly, 20,* 522–535.

McKnight, T. K. (1989). The use of cumulative cloze to investigate contextual build-up in deaf and hearing readers. *American Annals of the Deaf, 134,* 268–272.

McLaughlin, B. (1990). The relationship between first and second languages: Language proficiency and language aptitude. In B. Harley, P. Allen, J. Cummins, & M. Swain (Eds.), *The development of second language proficiency* (pp. 158–174). Cambridge, England: Cambridge University.

McLaughlin, B., White, D., McDevitt, T., & Raskin, R. (1983). Mothers'and fathers' speech to their young children: Similar or different? *Journal of Child Language, 10,* 245–252.

McMahon, S. I., & Raphael, T. E. (1997). *The book club connection.* New York: Teachers College.

McNeil, J. D. (1992). *Reading comprehension: New directions for classroom practice* (3rd ed.). New York: HarperCollins.

McNergney, R., Lloyd, J., Mintz, S., & Moore, J. (1988). Training for pedagogical decision making. *Journal of Teacher Education, 39*(5), 37–43.

Meadow-Orlans, K. P., & Sass-Lehrer, M. (1995). Support services for families with children who are deaf: Challenges for professionals. *Topics in Early Childhood Special Education, 15,* 314–334.

Menyuk, P. (1971). *The acquisition and development of language.* Englewood Cliffs, NJ: Prentice Hall.

Menyuk, P. (1988). *Language development: Knowledge and use.* Glenview, IL: Scott, Foresman.

Meyer, B. J. F. (1975). *The organization of prose and its effects on memory.* Amsterdam, Holland: North-Holland.

Meyer, B. J. F., & Freedle, R. O. (1984). Effects of discourse type on recall. *American Educational Research Journal, 21,* 121–143.

Mezynski, K. (1983). Issues concerning the acquisition of knowledge: Effects of vocabulary training on reading comprehension. *Review of Educational Research, 53,* 253–279.

Miller, L. C., Lechner, R. E., & Rugs, D. (1985). Development of conversational responsiveness: Preschoolers' use of responsive listener cues and relevant comments. *Developmental Psychology, 21,* 473–480.

Minton, M. J. (1980). The effect of sustained silent reading upon comprehension and attitudes among ninth graders. *Journal of Reading, 23,* 498–502.

Mohay, H. (1982). A preliminary description of the communication systems evolved by two deaf children in the absence of a sign language model. *Sign Language Studies, 34,* 73–90.

Moldofsky, P. B. (1983). Teaching students to determine the central story problem: A practical application of schema theory. *The Reading Teacher, 36,* 740–745.

Monteith, M. K. (1979). Schemata: An approach to understanding reading comprehension. *Journal of Reading, 22,* 368–371.

Moore, D. W., & Moore, S. A. (1986). Possible sentences. In E. K. Dishner, T. W. Bean, J. E. Readence, & D. W. Moore (Eds.), *Reading in the content areas* (pp. 174–178). Dubuque, IA: Kendall-Hunt.

Moore, P. (1987). On the incidental learning of vocabulary. *Australian Journal of Reading, 10,* 12–19.

Moore, P. J. (1988). Reciprocal teaching and reading comprehension: A review. *Journal of Research in Reading, 11,* 3–14.

Moores, D. F. (1996). *Education the deaf: Psychology, principals, and practices* (4th ed.). Boston: Houghton Mifflin.

Moorman, G. B., & Blanton, W. E. (1990). The Information Text Reading Activity (ITRA): Engaging students in meaningful learning. *Journal of Reading, 34,* 183.

Moorman, G. B., Blanton, W. E., & McLaughlin, T. (1994). The rhetoric of whole language. *Reading Research Quarterly, 29,* 308–329.

Morford, J. P. (1996). Insights to language from the study of gesture: A review of research on the gestural communication of non-signing deaf people. *Language and Communication, 16,* 165–178.

Morford, J. P., & Goldin-Meadow, S. (1997). From here and now to there and then: The development of displaced reference in homesign and English. *Child Development, 68,* 420–435.

Morrow, L. M. (1985). Retelling stories: A strategy for improving young children's comprehension, concept of story structure, and oral language complexity. *The Elementary School Journal, 85,* 647–661.

Morrow, L. M. (1986). Effects of structural guidelines in story retelling on children's dictation of original stories. *Journal of Reading Behavior, 18,* 135–152.

Morrow, L. M. (1987). The effects of one-to-one story readings on children's questions and responses. In J. E. Readence & R. S. Baldwin (Eds.), *Research in literacy: Merging perspectives* (pp. 75–83). Rochester, NY: The National Reading Conference.

Morrow, L. M. (1988). Young children's responses to one-to-one story readings in school settings. *Reading Research Quarterly, 23,* 89–107.

Morrow, L. M. (1989). *Literacy development in the early years: Helping children read and write.* Englewood Cliffs, NJ: Prentice Hall.

Morrow, L. M. (Ed.). (1995). *Family literacy: Connections in schools and communities.* Newark, DE: International Reading Association.

Morrow, L. M., & Weinstein, C. S. (1982). Increasing children's use of literature through program and physical design changes. *The Elementary School Journal, 83,* 131–137.

Muffoletto, R. (1994). Technology and restructuring education: Constructing a context. *Educational Technology, 34*(2), 24–28.

Mulcahy, P. I., & Samuels, S. J. (1987). Problem-solving schemata for text types: A comparison of narrative and expository text structures. *Reading Psychology, 8,* 247–256.

Muth, K. D. (1987). Teachers' connection questions: Prompting students to organize text ideas. *Journal of Reading, 31,* 254–259.

Nagy, W. E., Herman, P. A., & Anderson, R. C. (1985). Learning words from context. *Reading Research Quarterly, 20,* 233–253.

Nelson, C. E., Prosser, T., & Tucker, D. (1987). The decline of traditional media and materials in the classroom. *Educational Technology, 27*(1), 48–49.

Nelson, K. E., Welsh, J., Camarata, S., & Butkovsky, N. (1995). Available input for language-impaired children and younger children of matched language levels. *First Language, 15,* 1–17.

Nelson, O. (1989). Storytelling: Language experience for meaning making. *The Reading Teacher, 42,* 386–390.

Newkirk, T. (1987). The non-narrative writing of young children. *Research in the Teaching of English, 21,* 121–144.

Newton, L. (1985). Linguistic environment of the deaf child: A focus on teachers' use of non-literal language. *Journal of Speech and Hearing Research, 28,* 336–344.

Nippold, M. A. (1998). *Later language development: The school-age and adolescent years.* Austin, TX: Pro-Ed.

Nolen, S. B., & Wilbur, R. B. (1985). The effects of context on deaf students' comprehension of difficult sentences. *American Annals of the Deaf, 130,* 231–235.

Norton, D. E. (1982). Using a webbing process to develop children's literature units. *Language Arts, 59,* 348–356.

Nower, B. (1985). Scratching the itch: High school students and their topic choices for writing. *The Volta Review, 87*, 171–185.

Noyce, R. M., & Christie, J. F. (1989). *Integrating reading and writing instruction in grades K–8.* Boston: Allyn and Bacon.

Obler, L. K. (1997). Development and loss: Changes in the adult years. In J. B. Gleason (Ed.), *The development of language* (4th ed.) (pp. 440–472). Boston: Allyn and Bacon.

Ogle, D. M. (1986). K-W-L: A teaching model that develops active reading of expository text. *The Reading Teacher, 39*, 564–570.

Ohlhausen, M. M., & Roller, C. M. (1988). The operation of text structure and content schemata in isolation and in interaction. *Reading Research Quarterly, 23*, 70–88.

Olson, M. W. (1984). A dash of story grammar and . . . Presto! A book report. *The Reading Teacher, 37*, 458–461.

Olson, R. C. (1987). Writing across the curriculum program at Gallaudet. In D. S. Copeland & D. C. Fletcher (Eds.), *Proceedings of the 1987 National Conference on Innovative Writing Programs and Research for Deaf and Hearing Impaired Students, Removing the writing barrier: A dream?* (pp. 151–179). New York: Lehman College, The City University of New York.

Orlich, D. C., Harder, R. J., Callahan, R. C., & Gibson, H. W. (1998). *Teaching strategies: A guide to better instruction* (5th ed.). Boston: Houghton Mifflin.

Owens, R. E. (1996). *Language development: An introduction* (4th ed.). Boston: Allyn and Bacon.

Palincsar, A. S. (1986). Metacognitive strategy instruction. *Exceptional Children, 53*, 118–124.

Palincsar, A. S., & Brown, A. L. (1986). Interactive teaching to promote independent learning from text. *The Reading Teacher, 39*, 771–777.

Palincsar, A. S., & Brown, A. L. (1988). Teaching and practicing thinking skills to promote comprehension in the context of group problem solving. *Remedial and Special Education, 9*, 53–59.

Pan, B. A., & Gleason, J. B. (1997). Semantic development: Learning the meaning of words. In J. B. Gleason (Ed.), *The development of language* (4th ed.) (pp. 122–158). Boston: Allyn and Bacon.

Pappas, C. C., & Brown, E. (1987). Young children learning story discourse: Three case studies. *The Elementary School Journal, 87*, 455–466.

Pasch, M., Moody, C. D., & Langer, G. (1995). *Teaching as decision making* (2nd ed.). New York: Longman.

Pau, C. S. (1995). The deaf child and solving problems of arithmetic: The importance of comprehensive reading. *American Annals of the Deaf, 140*, 287–290.

Paul, P. V. (1996). Reading vocabulary knowledge and deafness. *Journal of Deaf Studies and Deaf Education, 1*, 3–15.

Paul, P. V. (1998). *Literacy and deafness: The development of reading, writing, and literate thought.* Boston: Allyn and Bacon.

Pearson, P. D. (1989). Reading the whole-language movement. *The Elementary School Journal, 90*, 231–241.

Pearson, P. D., & Johnson, D. D. (1978). *Teaching reading comprehension.* New York: Holt, Rinehart and Winston.

Pearson, P. D., & Spiro, R. J. (1982). Toward a theory of reading comprehension instruction. In K. G. Butler & G. P. Wallach (Eds.), *Language disorders and learning disabilities* (pp. 71–88). Rockville, MD: Aspen.

Peck, J. (1989). Using storytelling to promote language and literacy development. *The Reading Teacher, 43,* 138–141.

Pehrsson, R. S., & Denner, P. R. (1988). Semantic organizers: Implications for reading and writing. *Topics in Language Disorders, 8*(3), 24–37.

Pellegrini, A. D. (1984). The development of the functions of private speech: A review of the Piaget-Vygotsky debate. In A. D. Pellegrini & T. D. Yawkey (Eds.), *The development of oral and written language in social contexts* (pp. 57–69). Norwood, NJ: Ablex.

Pellegrini, A. D., & Galda, L. (1982). The effects of thematic-fantasy play training on the development of children's story comprehension. *American Educational Research Journal, 19,* 443–452.

Perez, B. (1996). Instructional conversations as opportunities for English language acquisition for culturally and linguistically diverse students. *Language Arts, 73,* 173–181.

Petitto, L. A. (1987). On the autonomy of language and gesture: Evidence from the acquisition of personal pronouns in American Sign Language. *Cognition, 27,* 1–52.

Piaget, J. (1926). *The language and thought of the child.* London, England: Kegan, Paul, Trench, & Trubner.

Pikulski, J. J. (1990). The role of tests in a literacy assessment program. *The Reading Teacher, 43,* 686–688.

Pikulski, J. J. (1994). Preventing reading failure: A review of five effective programs. *The Reading Teacher, 48,* 30–39.

Pinnell, G. S., Lyons, C. A., DeFord, D. E., Bryk, A. S., & Seltzer, M. (1994). Comparing instructional models for the literacy education of high-risk first graders. *Reading Research Quarterly, 29,* 8–39.

Pogoda-Ciccone, N. (1994). The writing process in 55 minutes. *Perspectives in Education and Deafness, 13*(1), 6–9.

Poostay, E. J. (1984). Show me your underlines: A strategy to teach comprehension. *The Reading Teacher, 37,* 828–830.

Pressley, M. (1998). *Reading instruction that works: The case for balanced teaching.* New York: Guilford.

Pressley, M., & Afflerbach, P. (1995). *Verbal protocols of reading: The nature of constructively responsive reading.* New York: Springer-Verlag.

Prince, A. T., & Mancus, D. S. (1987). Enriching comprehension: A schema altered basal reading lesson. *Reading Research and Instruction, 27,* 45–54.

Prinz, P. M. (1991). Literacy and language development within microcomputer-videodisc-assisted interactive contexts. *Journal of Childhood Communication Disorders, 14,* 67–80.

Prinz, P. M., & Masin, L. (1985). Lending a helping hand: Linguistic input and sign language acquisition in deaf children. *Applied Psycholinguistics, 6,* 357–370.

Prinz, P. M., & Prinz, E. A. (1985). If only you could hear what I see: Discourse development in sign language. *Discourse Processes, 8,* 1–19.

Probst, R. E. (1988). Transactional theory in the teaching of literature. *Journal of Reading, 31,* 378–381.

Propp, G., Nugent, G., Stone, C., & Nugent, R. (1981). Videodisc for the hearing impaired. *The Volta Review, 83,* 321–327.

Prutting, C. A. (1982). Pragmatics as social competence. *Journal of Speech and Hearing Disorders, 47,* 123–134.

Pugh, B. L. (1955). *Steps in language development for the deaf.* Washington, DC: The Volta Bureau.

Purcell-Gates, V. (1989). What oral/written language differences can tell us about beginning instruction. *The Reading Teacher, 42,* 290–294.

Purcell-Gates, V., L'Allier, S., & Smith, D. (1995). Literacy at the Harts' and the Larsons': Diversity among poor, innercity families. *The Reading Teacher, 48,* 572–578.

Rahman, T., & Bisanz, G. L. (1986). Reading ability and use of a story schema in recalling and reconstructing information. *Journal of Educational Psychology, 78,* 323–333.

Rakes, G. C., Rakes, T. A., & Smith, L. J. (1995). Using visuals to enhance secondary students' reading comprehension of expository texts. *Journal of Adolescent and Adult Literacy, 39,* 46–54.

Ramsey, J., & Conway, D. F. (1995). Time and time again: Using mini-lessons within thematic units. *The Volta Review, 97*(5), 95–116.

Raphael, T. E. (1982). Question-answering strategies for children. *The Reading Teacher, 36,* 186–190.

Raphael, T. E. (1984). Teaching learners about sources of information for answering comprehension questions. *Journal of Reading, 27,* 303–311.

Raphael, T. E. (1986). Teaching question-answer relationships, revisited. *The Reading Teacher, 39,* 516–522.

Raphael, T. E., & McKinney, J. (1983). An examination of fifth- and eighth-grade children's question-answering behavior: An instructional study in metacognition. *Journal of Reading Behavior, 15*(3), 67–86.

Raphael, T. E., & McMahon, S. I. (1994). Book club: An alternative framework for reading instruction. *The Reading Teacher, 48,* 102–116.

Raphael, T. E., Myers, A. C., Tirre, W. C., Fritz, M., & Freebody, P. (1981). The effects of some known sources of reading difficulty on metacomprehension and comprehension. *Journal of Reading Behavior, 13,* 325–334.

Raphael, T. E., & Pearson, P. D. (1985). Increasing students' awareness of sources of information for answering questions. *American Educational Research Journal, 22,* 217–235.

Raphael, T. E., & Wonnacott, C. A. (1985). Heightening fourth-grade students' sensitivity to sources of information for answering comprehension questions. *Reading Research Quarterly, 20,* 282–296.

Rasinski, T. V. (1995). On the effects of Reading Recovery: A response to Pinnell, Lyons, DeFord, Bryk, and Seltzer. *Reading Research Quarterly, 30,* 264–270.

Rasinski, T. V., & Fredericks, A. D. (1990). The best reading advice for parents. *The Reading Teacher, 43,* 344–345.

Ray, S. (1989). Context and the psychoeducational assessment of hearing impaired children. *Topics in Language Disorders, 9*(4), 33–44.

Reading/Language in Secondary Schools Subcommittee of the International Reading Association. (1989). Developing strategic learners. *Journal of Reading, 33,* 61–63.

Reagan, T. (1985). The deaf as a linguistic minority: Educational considerations. *Harvard Educational Review, 55,* 265–277.

Reagan, T. (1988). Multiculturalism and the deaf: An educational manifesto. *Journal of Research and Development in Education, 22,* 1–6.

Recht, D. R., & Leslie, L. (1988). Effect of prior knowledge on good and poor readers' memory of text. *Journal of Educational Psychology, 80,* 16–20.

Redlinger, W. E., & Park, T. (1980). Language mixing in young bilinguals. *Journal of Child Language, 7,* 337–352.

Reed, S. K., (1996). *Cognition: Theory and applications* (4th ed.). Pacific Grove, CA: Brooks/Cole.

Reid, J. (1994). Responding to ESL students' texts: The myths of appropriation. *TESOL Quarterly, 28,* 273–292.

Reilly, J. S., & Bellugi, U. (1996). Competition on the face: Affect and language in ASL motherese. *Journal of Child Language, 23,* 219–239.

Reutzel, D. R. (1985a). Reconciling schema theory and the basal reading lesson. *The Reading Teacher, 39,* 194–197.

Reutzel, D. R. (1985b). Story maps improve comprehension. *The Reading Teacher, 38,* 400–404.

Reutzel, D. R., Hollingsworth, P. M., & Eldredge, J. L. (1994). Oral reading instruction: The impact on student reading development. *Reading Research Quarterly, 29,* 40–62.

Reutzel, D. R., & Larsen, N. S. (1995). Look what they've done to real children's books in the new basal readers! *Language Arts, 72,* 495–507.

Rhodes, L. K., & Nathenson-Mejia, S. (1992). Anecdotal records: A powerful tool for ongoing literacy assessment. *The Reading Teacher, 45,* 502–509.

Rice, M. L., & Kemper, S. (1984). *Child language and cognition.* Baltimore: University Park.

Richards, J. C., & Gipe, J. P. (1993). Getting to know story characters: A strategy for young and at-risk readers. *The Reading Teacher, 47,* 78–79.

Richardson, J. S., & Morgan, R. F. (1997). *Reading to learn in the content areas* (3rd ed.). Belmont, CA: Wadsworth.

Richgels, D. J. (1982). Schema theory, linguistic theory, and representations of reading comprehension. *Journal of Educational Research, 76,* 54–62.

Richgels, D. J., McGee, L. M., Lomax, R. G., & Sheard, C. (1987). Awareness of four text structures: Effects on recall of expository text. *Reading Research Quarterly, 22,* 177–196.

Richgels, D. J., McGee, L. M., & Slaton, E. A. (1989). Teaching expository text structure in reading and writing. In K. D. Muth (Ed.), *Children's comprehension of text* (pp. 167–184). Newark, DE: International Reading Association.

Rickards, J. P. (1980). Notetaking, underlining, inserted questions, and organizers in text: Research conclusions and educational implications. *Educational Technology, 20*(6), 5–11.

Rinehart, S. D., Stahl, S. A., & Erickson, L. G. (1986). Some effects of summarization training on reading and studying. *Reading Research Quarterly, 21,* 422–438.

Risko, V. J., & Alvarez, M. C. (1983). Thematic organizers: Application to remedial reading. In G. H. McNinch (Ed.), *Reading research to reading practice* (pp. 85–87). Athens, GA: The American Reading Forum.

Risko, V. J., & Alvarez, M. C. (1986). An investigation of poor readers' use of a thematic strategy to comprehend text. *Reading Research Quarterly, 21,* 298–316.

Rittenhouse, R. K., & Kenyon, P. L. (1987). Educational and social language in deaf adolescents: TDD and school-produced comparisons. *American Annals of the Deaf, 132,* 210–212.

Robinshaw, H. M. (1996). The pattern of development from non-communicative behavior to language by hearing-impaired and hearing infants. *Early Child Development and Care, 120,* 67–93.

Robinson, F. P. (1946). *Effective study* (2nd ed.). New York: Harper & Row.

Roblyer, M. D., Edwards, J., & Havriluk, M. A. (1997). *Integrating educational technology into teaching.* Columbus, OH: Prentice Hall.

Rockler, M. J. (1988). *Innovative teaching strategies.* Scottsdale, AZ: Gorsuch, Scarisbrick.

Rogers, D. (1989). "Show-me bedtime reading": An unusual study of the benefits of reading to deaf children. *Perspectives for Teachers of the Hearing Impaired, 8*(1), 2–5.

Rogers, D. L., Perrin, M. S., & Waller, C. B. (1987). Enhancing the development of language and thought through conversations with young children. *Journal of Research in Childhood Education, 2,* 17–29.

Roller, C. M., & Schreiner, R. (1985). The effects of narrative and expository organizational instruction on sixth-grade children's comprehension of expository and narrative prose. *Reading Psychology, 6,* 27–42.

Romaine, S. (1989). *Bilingualism.* Oxford, England: Basil Blackwell.

Roney, R. C. (1989). Back to the basics with storytelling. *The Reading Teacher, 42,* 520–523.

Rosenblatt, L. M. (1978). *The reader, the text, the poem.* Carbondale: Southern Illinois University.

Rosenblatt, L. M. (1989). Writing and reading: The transactional theory. In J. M. Mason (Ed.), *Reading and writing connections* (pp. 153–176). Boston: Allyn and Bacon.

Rosenshine, B., & Meister, C. (1994). Reciprocal Teaching: A review of the research. *Review of Educational Research, 64,* 479–530.

Rosenthal, M. K. (1982). Vocal dialogues in the neonatal period. *Developmental Psychology, 18,* 17–21.

Roser, N., & Juel, C. (1982). Effects of vocabulary instruction on reading comprehension. In J. A. Niles & L. A. Harris (Eds.), *New inquiries in reading research and instruction* (pp. 110–118). Rochester, NY: The National Reading Conference.

Roth, F. P., & Spekman, N. J. (1984). Assessing the pragmatic abilities of children: Part 1. Organizational framework and assessment parameters. *Journal of Speech and Hearing Disorders, 49,* 2–11.

Rottenberg, C. J., & Searfoss, L. W. (1992). Becoming literate in a preschool class: Literacy development of hearing-impaired children. *Journal of Reading Behavior, 24,* 463–479.

Rowe, M. B. (1974). Wait-time and rewards as instructional variables, their influence on language, logic and fate control: Part one—wait-time. *Journal of Research in Science Teaching, 11,* 81–94.

Rowe, M. B. (1986). Wait time: Slowing down may be a way of speeding up. *Journal of Teacher Education, 37*(1), 43–50.

Rumelhart, D. E. (1975). Notes on a schema for stories. In D. G. Bobrow & A. Collins (Eds.), *Representation and understanding: Studies in cognitive science* (pp. 211–236). New York: Academic.

Rumelhart, D. E. (1977). Understanding and summarizing brief stories. In D. LaBerge & S. J. Samuels (Eds.), *Basic processes in reading: Perception and comprehension* (pp. 265–303). Hillsdale, NJ: Lawrence Erlbaum.

Rumelhart, D. E. (1980). Schemata: The building blocks of cognition. In R. J. Spiro, B. C. Bruce, & W. F. Brewer (Eds.), *Theoretical issues in reading comprehension* (pp. 33–58). Hillsdale, NJ: Lawrence Erlbaum.

Rupley, W. H., Logan, J. W., & Nichols, W. D. (1999). Vocabulary instruction in a balanced reading program. *The Reading Teacher, 52,* 336–346.

Rush, R. T. (1985). Assessing readability: Formulas and alternatives. *The Reading Teacher, 39,* 274–283.

Rutter, D. R., & Durkin, K. (1987). Turn-taking in mother-infant interaction: An examination of vocalizations and gaze. *Developmental Psychology, 23,* 54–61.

Ryder, R. J. (1991). The directed questioning activity for subject matter text. *Journal of Reading, 34,* 606–612.

Ryder, R. J. (1994). Using frames to promote critical writing. *Journal of Reading, 38,* 210–218.

Sachs, J., Goldman, J., & Chaille, C. (1984). Planning in pretend play: Using language to coordinate narrative development. In A. D. Pellegrini & T. D. Yawkey (Eds.), *The development of oral and written language in social contexts* (pp. 119–128). Norwood, NJ: Ablex.

Sadoski, M. (1983). An exploratory study of the relationship between reported imagery and the comprehension and recall of a story. *Reading Research Quarterly, 19,* 110–123.

Sadoski, M. (1985). The natural use of imagery in story comprehension and recall: Replication and extension. *Reading Research Quarterly, 20,* 658–667.

Sadoski, M. C. (1980). Ten years of uninterrupted sustained silent reading. *Reading Improvement, 17,* 153–156.

Salvia, J., & Ysseldyke, J. E. (1998). *Assessment* (7th ed.). Boston: Houghton Mifflin.

Sanacore, J. (1990). Creating the lifetime reading habit in social studies. *Journal of Reading, 33,* 414–418.

Satterfield, J., & Powers, A. (1996). Write on! Journals open to success. *Perspectives in Education and Deafness, 15*(2), 2–5.

Saunders, J. (1997). Educating deaf and hearing children in a bilingual/bicultural environment. *The CAEDHH Journal, 23*(1), 61–68.

Savage, J. F. (1998). *Teaching reading and writing: Combining skills, strategies, and literature.* Boston: McGraw-Hill.

Saville-Troike, M. (1979a). First- and second-language acquisition. In H. T. Trueba & C. Barnett-Mizrahi (Eds.), *Bilingual multicultural education and the professional: From theory to practice* (pp. 104–119). Rowley, MA: Newbury House.

Saville-Troike, M. (1979b). Culture, language, and education. In H. T. Trueba & C. Barnett-Mizrahi (Eds.), *Bilingual multicultural education and the professional: From theory to practice* (pp. 139–156). Rowley, MA: Newbury House.

Sawyer, W. (1987). Literature and literacy: A review of research. *Language Arts, 64,* 33–39.

Schaper, M. W., & Reitsma, P. (1993). The use of speech-based recoding in reading by prelingually deaf children. *American Annals of the Deaf, 138,* 46–54.

Schatz, E. K., & Baldwin, R. S. (1986). Context clues are unreliable predictors of word meanings. *Reading Research Quarterly, 21,* 439–453.

Schewe, A., & Froese, V. (1987). Relating reading and writing via comprehension, quality, and structure. In J. E. Readence & R. S. Baldwin (Eds.), *Research in literacy: Merging perspectives* (pp. 273–279). Rochester, NY: The National Reading Conference.

Schirmer, B. R. (1984). Dynamic model of oral and/or signed language diagnosis. *Language, Speech, and Hearing Services in Schools, 15,* 76–82.

Schirmer, B. R. (1985). An analysis of the language of young hearing-impaired children in terms of syntax, semantics, and use. *American Annals of the Deaf, 130,* 15–19.

Schirmer, B. R. (1989). Framework for using a language acquisition model in assessing semantic and syntactic development and planning instructional goals for hearing-impaired children. *The Volta Review, 91,* 87–94.

Schirmer, B. R. (1993). Constructing meaning from narrative text: Cognitive processes of deaf children. *American Annals of the Deaf, 138,* 397–403.

Schirmer, B. R., Bailey, J., & Fitzgerald, S. M. (1999). Using a writing assessment rubric for writing development of children who are deaf. *Exceptional Children, 65,* 383–397.

Schirmer, B. R., & Bond, W. L. (1990). Enhancing the hearing impaired child's knowledge of story structure to improve comprehension of narrative text. *Reading Improvement, 27,* 242–254.

Schirmer, B. R., & Winter, C. R. (1993). Use of cognitive schema by children who are deaf for comprehending narrative text. *Reading Improvement, 30,* 26–34.

Schirmer, B. R., & Woolsey, M. L. (1997). Effect of teacher questions on the reading comprehension of deaf children. *Journal of Deaf Studies and Deaf Education, 2,* 47–56.

Schleper, D. R. (1995). Reading to deaf children: Learning from deaf adults. *Perspectives in Education and Deafness, 13*(4), 4–8.

Schmitt, M. C., & O'Brien, D. G. (1986). Story grammars: Some cautions about the translation of research into practice. *Reading Research and Instruction, 26,* 1–8.

Schroder, G. (1996). The elements of story writing: Using picture books to learn about the elements of chemistry. *Language Arts, 73,* 412–418.

Schroeder, B., & Strosnider, R. (1997). Box-and-whisker what? Deaf students learn—and write about—descriptive statistics. *Teaching Exceptional Children, 29,* 12–17.

Schrum, L., & Berenfeld, B. (1997). *Teaching and learning in the information age.* Boston: Allyn and Bacon.

Schuder, T., Clewell, S. F., & Jackson, N. (1989). Getting the gist of expository text. In K. D. Muth (Ed.), *Children's comprehension of text* (pp. 224–242). Newark, DE: International Reading Association.

Schwabe, A. M., Olswang, L. B., & Kriegsmann, E. (1986). Requests for information: Linguistic, cognitive, pragmatic, and environmental variables. *Language, Speech, and Hearing Services in Schools, 17,* 38–55.

Schwartz, R. M., & Raphael, T. E. (1985). Concept of definition: A key to improving students' vocabulary. *The Reading Teacher, 39,* 198–205.

Seidman, S. A. (1986). A survey of schoolteachers' utilization of media. *Educational Technology, 26*(10), 19–23.

Shah, D. C. (1986). Composing processes and writing instruction at the middle/junior high school level. *Theory into Practice, 25,* 109–116.

Shanahan, T. (1980). The impact of writing instruction on learning to read. *Reading World, 19,* 357–368.

Shanahan, T., & Barr, R. (1995). Reading Recovery: An independent evaluation of the effects of an early instructional intervention for at-risk learners. *Reading Research Quarterly, 30,* 958–996.

Shanahan, T., & Lomax, R. G. (1986). An analysis and comparison of theoretical models of the reading-writing relationship. *Journal of Educational Psychology, 78,* 116–123.

Shannon, P. (1982). Some subjective reasons for teacher's reliance on commercial reading materials. *The Reading Teacher, 35,* 884–889.

Shepard, A. (1994). From script to stage: Tips for Readers Theatre. *The Reading Teacher, 48,* 184–185.

Shuy, R. W. (1981). A holistic view of language. *Research in the Teaching of English, 15,* 101–111.

Shuy, R. W. (1987). Dialogue as the heart of learning. *Language Arts, 64,* 890–897.

Siedlecki, T., Votaw, M. C., Bonvillian, J. D., & Jordan, I. K. (1990). The effects of manual interference and reading level on deaf subjects' recall of word lists. *Applied Psycholinguistics, 11,* 185–199.

Simmons, J. (1990). Portfolios as large-scale assessment. *Language Arts, 67,* 262–268.

Simpson, A. (1995). Not the class novel: A different reading program. *Journal of Reading, 38,* 290–294.

Simpson, M. L., Stahl, N. A., & Hayes, C. G. (1989). PORPE: A research validation. *Journal of Reading, 33,* 22–28.

Sinatra, R., Stahl-Gemake, J., & Morgan, N. W. (1986). Using semantic mapping after reading to organize and write original discourse. *Journal of Reading, 30,* 4–13.

Sinatra, R. C., Stahl-Gemake, J., & Berg, D. N. (1984). Improving reading comprehension of disabled readers through semantic mapping. *The Reading Teacher, 38,* 22–29.

Singleton, D. (1995). A critical look at the critical period hypothesis in second language acquisition research. In D. Singleton & Z. Lengyel (Eds.), *The age factor in second language acquisition: A critical look at the critical period hypothesis* (pp. 1–29). Clevedon, England: Multilingual Matters.

Skarakis-Doyle, E., & Murphy, L. (1996). Discourse-based language intervention: An efficacy study. *Journal of Children's Communication Development, 17*(2), 1–22.

Slavin, R. E., Karweit, N. L., & Wasik, B. A. (Eds.). (1994). *Preventing early school failure: Research, policy, and practice.* Boston: Allyn and Bacon.

Slavin, R. E., Madden, N. A., Karweit, N. L., Livermon, B. J., & Dolan, L. (1990). Success for all: First year outcomes of a comprehensive plan for reforming urban education. *American Educational Research Journal, 27,* 255–278.

Smith, F. (1978). *Reading without nonsense.* New York: Teachers College, Columbia University.

Smith, F. (1983). Reading like a writer. *Language Arts, 60,* 558–567.

Smith, J. A., & Bowers, P. S. (1989). Approaches to using literature for teaching reading. *Reading Improvement, 26,* 345–348.

Smith, J. L., & Johnson, H. (1994). Models for implementing literature in content studies. *The Reading Teacher, 48,* 198–208.

Smith, P. L., & Tompkins, G. E. (1988). Structured notetaking: A new strategy for content area readers. *Journal of Reading, 32,* 46–53.

Snow, C. E. (1986). Conversations with children. In P. Fletcher & M. Garman (Eds.), *Language acquisition: Studies in first language development* (pp. 69–89). Cambridge, England: Cambridge University.

Snow, C. E., Burns, M. S., & Griffin, P. (Eds.). (1998). *Preventing reading difficulties in young children.* Washington, DC: National Academy Press.

Spiegel, D. L. (1992). Blending whole language and systematic direct instruction. *The Reading Teacher, 46,* 38–44.

Squire, J. R. (1984). Composing and comprehending: Two sides of the same basic process. In J. M. Jensen (Ed.), *Composing and comprehending* (pp. 23–31). Urbana, IL: National Conference on Research in English.

Staab, C. F. (1983). Language functions elicited by meaningful activities: A new dimension in language programs. *Language, Speech, and Hearing Services in Schools, 14,* 164–170.

Stahl, S. A. (1986). Three principles of effective vocabulary instruction. *Journal of Reading, 29,* 663–668.

Stahl, S. A., & Fairbanks, M. M. (1986). The effects of vocabulary instruction: A model-based meta-analysis. *Review of Educational Research, 56,* 72–110.

Stahl, S. A., & Kapinus, B. A. (1991). Possible sentences: Predicting word meanings to teach content area vocabulary. *The Reading Teacher, 45,* 36–43.

Stahl, S. A., & Vancil, S. J. (1986). Discussion is what makes semantic maps work in vocabulary instruction. *The Reading Teacher, 40,* 62–67.

Staton, J. (1985). Using dialogue journals for developing thinking, reading, and writing with hearing-impaired students. *The Volta Review, 87,* 127–154.

Staton, J. (1988). Dialogue journals. *Language Arts, 65,* 198–201.

Stauffer, R. G. (1969). *Teaching reading as a thinking process.* New York: Harper & Row.

Stein, N. L., & Glenn, C. G. (1979). An analysis of story comprehension in elementary school children. In R. O. Freedle (Ed.), *New directions in discourse processing* (pp. 53–120). Norwood, NJ: Ablex.

Stein, N. L., & Nezworski, T. (1978). The effects of organization and instructional set on story memory. *Discourse Processes, 1,* 177–193.

Stephens, M. I. (1988). Pragmatics. In M. A. Nippold (Ed.), *Later language development: Ages nine through nineteen* (pp. 247–262). San Diego, CA: Singular.

Stevens, K. C. (1980). The effect of background knowledge on the reading comprehension of ninth graders. *Journal of Reading Behavior, 12,* 151–154.

Stewart, D. A. (1987). Linguistic input for the American Sign Language/English bilingual. *A.C.E.H.I. Journal, 13*(2), 58–70.

Stoddard, B., & MacArthur, C. A. (1993). A peer editor strategy: Guiding learning-disabled students in response and revision. *Research in the Teaching of English, 27,* 76–103.

Stoefen-Fisher, J. M. (1987–88). Hearing impaired adolescents' comprehension of anaphoric relationships within conjoined sentences. *Journal of Special Education, 21,* 85–98.

Stokoe, W. (1971). *The study of sign language.* Silver Spring, MD: National Association of the Deaf.

Stone, P. (1988). *Blueprint for developing conversational competence: A planning/instruction model with detailed scenarios.* Washington, DC: Alexander Graham Bell Association for the Deaf.

Stotsky, S. (1983). Research on reading/writing relationships: A synthesis and suggested directions. *Language Arts, 60,* 627–642.

Strackbein, D., & Tillman, M. (1987). The joy of journals—with reservations. *Journal of Reading, 31,* 28–31.

Strassman, B. K. (1997). Metacognition and reading in children who are deaf: A review of the research. *Journal of Deaf Studies and Deaf Education, 2,* 140–149.

Strickland, D. S. (1982). Comprehending what's new in comprehension. *Reading Instruction Journal, 25,* 9–12.

Strickland, D. S., Dillon, R. M., Funkhouser, L., Glick, M., & Rogers, C. (1989). Classroom dialogue during literature response groups. *Language Arts, 66,* 192–200.

Strickland, D. S., & Morrow, L. M. (1988). Creating a print-rich environment. *The Reading Teacher, 42,* 156–157.

Strickland, D. S., & Morrow, L. M. (1989). Environments rich in print promote literacy behavior during play. *The Reading Teacher, 43,* 178–179.

Strickland, D. S., & Morrow, L. M. (1989b). *Emerging literacy: Young children learn to read and write.* Newark, DE: International Reading Association.

Strong, M. (1995). A review of bilingual/bicultural programs for deaf children in North America. *American Annals of the Deaf, 140,* 84–94.

Sulzby, E. (1982). Oral and written language mode adaptations in stories by kindergarten children. *Journal of Reading Behavior, 14,* 51–59.

Sulzby, E. (1989). Assessment of emergent writing and children's language while writing. In L. Morrow & J. Smith (Eds.), *Assessment for instruction in early literacy* (pp. 83–109). Englewood Cliffs, NJ: Prentice Hall.

Sulzby, E. (1992). Research directions: Transitions from emergent to conventional writing. *Language Arts, 69,* 290–297.

Summers, E. G., & McClelland, J. V. (1982). A field-based evaluation of sustained silent reading (SSR) in intermediate grades. *The Alberta Journal of Educational Research, 28,* 100–112.

Tager-Flusberg, H. (1997). Putting words together: Morphology and syntax in the preschool years. In J. B. Gleason (Ed.), *The development of language* (4th ed.) (pp. 154–209). Boston: Allyn and Bacon.

Tatham, S. M. (1978). Comprehension taxonomies: Their uses and abuses. *The Reading Teacher, 32,* 190–194.

Taylor, B. M., & Beach, R. W. (1984). The effects of text structure instruction on middle-grade students' comprehension and production of expository text. *Reading Research Quarterly, 19,* 134–146.

Taylor, B. M., Frye, B. J., & Maruyama, G. M. (1990). Time spent reading and reading growth. *American Educational Research Journal, 27,* 351–362.

Taylor, B. M., & Samuels, S. J. (1983). Children's use of text structure in the recall of expository material. *American Educational Research Journal, 20,* 517–528.

Taylor, N. E., & Connor, U. (1982). Silent vs. oral reading: The rational instructional use of both processes. *The Reading Teacher, 35,* 440–443.

Taylor, R. L. (1997). *Assessment of exceptional students* (4th ed.). Boston: Allyn and Bacon.

Teachers of English to Speakers of Other Languages. (1997). *ESL standards for pre-K–12 students.* Alexandria, VA: Author.

Teale, W. H. (1987). Emergent literacy: Reading and writing development in early childhood. In J. E. Readence & R. S. Baldwin (Eds.), *Research in literacy: Merging perspectives* (pp. 44–74). Rochester, NY: The National Reading Conference.

Teale, W. H., & Sulzby, E. (Eds.). (1986). *Emergent literacy: Writing and reading.* Norwood, NJ: Ablex.

Terrell, B. Y. (1985). Learning the rules of the game: Discourse skills in early childhood. In D. N. Ripich & F. M. Spinelli (Eds.), *School discourse problems* (pp. 13–27). San Diego, CA: College-Hill.

Thal, D., & Bates, E. (1988). Language and gesture in late talkers. *Journal of Speech and Hearing Research, 31,* 115–123.

Thompson, M., Biro, P., Vethivelu, S., Pious, C., & Hatfield, N. (1987). *Language assessment of hearing-impaired school age children.* Seattle: University of Washington.

Thorndyke, P. W. (1977). Cognitive structures in comprehension and memory of narrative discourse. *Cognitive Psychology, 9,* 77–110.

Thorndyke, P. W., & Hayes-Roth, B. (1979). The use of schemata in the acquisition and transfer of knowledge. *Cognitive Psychology, 11,* 82–106.

Thorum, A. R. (1981). *Language assessment instruments: Infancy through adulthood.* Springfield, IL: Charles C. Thomas.

Thurlow, M., Graden, J., Ysseldyke, J. E., & Algozzine, R. (1984). Student reading during reading class: The lost activity in reading instruction. *The Journal of Educational Research, 77,* 267–272.

Tierney, R. J., & Leys, M. (1986). What is the value of connecting reading and writing? In B. T. Peterson (Ed.), *Convergences: Transactions in readng and writing* (pp. 15–29). Urbana, IL: National Council of Teachers of English.

Tierney, R. J., & Pearson, P. D. (1983). Toward a composing model of reading. *Language Arts, 60,* 568–580.

Titus, J. C. (1996). The concept of fractional number among deaf and hard of hearing students. *American Annals of the Deaf, 140,* 255–263.

Tobin, K. (1986). Effects of teacher wait time on discourse characteristics in mathematics and language arts classes. *American Educational Research Journal, 23,* 191–200.

Tobin, K. (1987). The role of wait time in higher cognitive learning. *Review of Educational Research, 57,* 69–95.

Tomasello, M., & Mannle, S. (1985). Pragmatics of sibling speech to one-year-olds. *Child Development, 56,* 911–917.

Tomlinson-Keasey, C., Brawley, R., & Peterson, B. (1986). An analysis of an interactive videodisc system for teaching language skills to deaf students. *The Exceptional Child, 33,* 49–55.

Tompkins, G. E. (2000). *Teaching writing: Balancing process and product* (3rd ed.). Upper Saddle River, NJ: Merrill/Prentice Hall.

Townsend, M. A. R., & Clarihew, A. (1989). Facilitating children's comprehension through the use of advance organizers. *Journal of Reading Behavior, 21,* 15–35.

Trachtenburg, P., & Ferruggia, A. (1989). Big books from little voices: Reaching high risk beginning readers. *The Reading Teacher, 42,* 284–289.

Trelease, J. (1995). *The read-aloud handbook* (4th ed.). New York: Penguin.

Trout, M., & Foley, G. (1989). Working with families of handicapped infants and toddlers. *Topics in Language Disorders, 10*(1), 57–67.

Truax, R. (1985). Linking research to teaching to facilitate reading-writing-communication connections. *The Volta Review, 87,* 155–169.

Truax, R. (1992). Becoming literate: A sketch of a neverending cycle. *The Volta Review, 94,* 395–410.

Truax, R. R. (1987). Literacy learning in a secondary writing studio. *Teaching English to Deaf and Second-Language Students, 5*(3), 17–23.

Trueba, H. T. (1979). Bilingual-education models: Types and designs. In H. T. Trueba & C. Barnett-Mizrahi (Eds.), *Bilingual multicultural education and the professional: From theory to practice* (pp. 54–73). Rowley, MA: Newbury House.

Turnbull, A. P., Summers, J. A., & Brotherson, M. J. (1984). *Working with families with disabled members: A family systems approach.* Lawrence: University of Kansas.

Vacca, J. L., Vacca, R. T., & Gove, M. K. (2000). *Reading and learning to read* (4th ed.). New York: Longman.

Vacca, R. T., & Vacca, J. L. (1999). *Content area reading* (2nd ed.). New York: Longman.

Valli, C., & Lucas, C. (1995). *Linguistics of American Sign Language.* Washington, DC: Gallaudet University.

Vaughan, J. L., Castle, G., Gilbert, K., & Love, M. (1982). Varied approaches to preteaching vocabulary. In J. A. Niles & L. A. Harris (Eds.), *New inquiries in reading research and instruction* (pp. 94–98). Rochester, NY: The National Reading Conference.

Vernon, M. (1987). Controversy within sign language. *A.C.E.H.I. Journal, 12*(3), 155–164.

Vernon, M., & Andrews, J. F. (1990). *The psychology of deafness.* New York: Longman.

Vihman, M. M. (1982). The acquisition of morphology by a bilingual child: A whole-word approach. *Applied Psycholinguistics, 3,* 141–160.

Vihman, M. M. (1985). Language differentiation by the bilingual infant. *Journal of Child Language, 12,* 297–324.

Volterra, V. (1981). Gestures, signs, and words at two years: When does communication become language. *Sign Language Studies, 33,* 351–362.

Volterra, V., & Erting, C. J. (Eds.). (1990). *From gesture to language in hearing and deaf children.* Berlin, Germany: Springer-Verlag.

Vygotsky, L. S. (1962). *Thought and language.* Cambridge, MA: M.I.T. Press.

Wagner, B. J. (1985). Integrating the language arts. *Language Arts, 62,* 557–560.

Wagner, B. J. (1988). Does classroom drama effect the arts of language? *Language Arts, 65,* 46–55.

Wanska, S. K., & Bedrosian, J. L. (1985). Conversational structure and topic performance in mother-child interaction. *Journal of Speech and Hearing Research, 28,* 579–584.

Warren, A. R., & McCloskey, L. A. (1997). Language in social contexts. In J. B. Gleason (Ed.), *The development of language* (4th ed.) (pp. 210–258). Boston: Allyn and Bacon.

Warren, S. F., & Kaiser, A. P. (1986). Incidental language teaching: A critical review. *Journal of Speech and Hearing Disorders, 51,* 291–299.

Wasik, B. A., & Slavin, R. E. (1993). Preventing early reading failure with one-to-one tutoring: A review of five programs. *Reading Research Quarterly, 28,* 179–200.

Weaver, C. (1994). *Reading process and practice: From socio-psycholinguistics to whole language* (2nd ed.). Portsmouth, NH: Heinemann.

Weaver, P. A., & Dickinson, D. K. (1982). Scratching below the surface structure: Exploring the usefulness of story grammars. *Discourse Processes, 5,* 225–243.

Weiss, A. L. (1986). Classroom discourse and the hearing-impaired child. *Topics in Language Disorders, 6*(3), 60–70.

Wells, G. (1981). *Learning through interaction: The study of language development.* Cambridge, England: Cambridge University.

Wells, G. (1982). Story reading and the development of symbolic skills. *Australian Journal of Reading, 5,* 142–152.

Wells, G. (1986). *The meaning makers: Children learning language and using language to learn.* Portsmouth, NH: Heinemann.

Whaley, J. F. (1981). Readers' expectations for story structures. *Reading Research Quarterly, 17,* 90–114.

Whitesell, K., & Klein, H. L. (1995). Facilitating language and learning via scripts. *The Volta Review, 97*(5), 117–128.

Widomski, C. L. (1983). Building foundations for reading comprehension. *Reading World, 22,* 306–313.

Wiesendanger, K. D., & Bader, L. (1989). SSR: Its effects on students' reading habits after they complete the program. *Reading Horizons, 29,* 162–166.

Wilbur, R. B. (1987). *American Sign Language: Linguistic and applied dimensions* (2nd ed.). Austin, TX: Pro-Ed.

Wilbur, R. B., & Goodhart, W. C. (1985). Comprehension of indefinite pronouns and quantifers by hearing-impaired students. *Applied Psycholinguistics, 6,* 417–434.

Wilbur, R. B., Goodhart, W., & Montandon, E. (1983). Comprehension of nine syntactic structures by hearing-impaired students. *The Volta Review, 85,* 328–345.

Wilen, W. W. (1990). Forms and phases of discussion. In W. W. Wilen (Ed.), *Teaching and learning through discussion* (pp. 3–24). Springfield, IL: Charles C. Thomas.

Wilkinson, I., & Bain, J. (1984). Story comprehension and recall in poor readers: Everyone a schemer? *Australian Journal of Reading, 7,* 147–156.

Wilkinson, I. A. G., & Anderson, R. C. (1995). Sociocognitive processes in guided silent reading: A microanalysis of small-group lessons. *Reading Research Quarterly, 30,* 710–740.

Wilkinson, L. C., Wilkinson, A. C., Spinelli, F., & Chiang, C. P. (1984). Metalinguistic knowledge of pragmatic rules in school-age children. *Child Development, 55,* 2130–2140.

Williams, C. L. (1994). The language and literacy worlds of three profoundly deaf children. *Reading Research Quarterly, 29,* 125–155.

Williams, C. L., & McLean, M. M. (1997). Young deaf children's response to picture book reading in a preschool setting. *Research in the Teaching of English, 31,* 337–366.

Williams, J. P., Taylor, M. B., & deCani, J. S. (1984). Constructing macrostructure for expository text. *Journal of Educational Psychology, 76,* 1065–1075.

Williams, K. A. (1996). Reading assessment: Finding a balanced approach. *Balanced Reading Instruction, 3*(2), 1–14.

Winograd, K., & Higgins, K. M. (1995). Writing, reading, and talking mathematics: One interdisciplinary possibility. *The Reading Teacher, 48,* 310–318.

Winser, B. (1988). Readers getting control of reading. *Australian Journal of Reading, 11,* 257–268.

Winton, P. (1986). Effective strategies for involving families in intervention efforts. *Focus on Exceptional Children, 19*(2), 1–10, 12.

Wittrock, M. C. (1982). Three studies of generative reading comprehension. In J. A. Niles & L. A. Harris (Eds.), *New inquiries in reading research and instruction* (pp. 85–88). Rochester, NY: The National Reading Conference.

Wixson, K. K. (1986). Vocabulary instruction and children's comprehension of basal stories. *Reading Research Quarterly, 21,* 317–329.

Wolf, S. A. (1993). What's in a name? Labels and literacy in Readers Theatre. *The Reading Teacher, 46,* 540–545.

Wolf, S. A. (1994). Learning to act/acting to learn: Children as actors, critics, and characters in classroom theatre. *Research in the Teaching of English, 28,* 7–44.

Wolk, S., & Allen, T. E. (1984). A 5-year follow-up of reading comprehension achievement of hearing-impaired students in special education programs. *The Journal of Special Education, 18,* 161–176.

Wollman-Bonilla, J. E. (1994). Why don't they "just speak?" Attempting literature discussion with more and less able readers. *Research in the Teaching of English, 28,* 231–258.

Wong, B. Y. L. (1985). Self-questioning instructional research: A review. *Review of Educational Research, 55,* 227–268.

Wong, J. A. & Au, K. H. (1985). The concept-text-application approach: Helping elementary students comprehend expository text. *The Reading Teacher, 38,* 612–618.

Wood, D. J., Wood, H. A., Griffiths, A. J., Howarth, S. P., & Howarth, C. I. (1982). The structure of conversations with 6- to 10-year-old deaf children. *Journal of Child Psychology, Psychiatry, and Allied Disciplines, 23,* 295–308.

Wood, E., Winne, P. H., & Carney, P. A. (1995). Evaluating the effects of training high school students to use summarization when training includes analogically similar information. *Journal of Reading Behavior, 27,* 605–626.

Wood, H. A., & Wood, D. J. (1984). An experimental evaluation of the effects of five styles of teacher conversation on the language of hearing-impaired children. *Journal of Child Psychology, Psychiatry, and Allied Disciplines, 25,* 45–62.

Wood, K. D. (1988). Guiding students through informational text. *The Reading Teacher, 41,* 912–920.

Wood, M. (1985). Linking schema theory and metacognition research to the word identification strategies of beginning readers. *The New England Reading Association Journal, 20,* 18–24, 34.

Wood, M. (1989). Invented spelling revisited. *Reading Today, 6*(6), 22.

Yaden, D. (1988). Understanding stories through repeated read-alouds: How many does it take? *The Reading Teacher, 41,* 556–560.

Yawkey, T. D., & Hrncir, E. J. (1983). Pretend play tools for oral language growth in the preschool. *The Journal of Creative Behavior, 16,* 265–271.

Yoshinaga-Itano, C., & Downey, D. M. (1986). A hearing-impaired child's acquisition of schemata: Something's missing. *Topics in Language Disorders, 7,* 45–57.

Young, T. A., & Vardell, S. (1993). Weaving Readers Theatre and nonfiction into the curriculum. *The Reading Teacher, 46,* 396–406.

Ysseldyke, J. E., & Algozzine, B. (1983). Where to begin in diagnosing reading problems. *Topics in Learning and Learning Disabilities, 2*(4), 60–69.

Zakaluk, B. L., & Samuels, S. J. (1988). Toward a new approach to predicting text comprehensibility. In B. L. Zakaluk & S. J. Samuels (Eds.), *Readability: Its past, present, and future* (pp. 121–144). Newark, DE: International Reading Association.

Ziezula, F. R. (Ed.). (1982). *Assessment for hearing-impaired people: A guide for selecting psychological, educational, and vocational tests.* Washington, DC: Gallaudet College.

Zorfass, J. M. (1981). Metalinguistic awareness in young deaf children: A preliminary study. *Applied Psycholinguistics, 2,* 333–352.

INDEX